AF411335

Advanced Research in Pediatric Radiology and Nuclear Medicine

Advanced Research in Pediatric Radiology and Nuclear Medicine

Editor

Curtise K. C. Ng

MDPI • Basel • Beijing • Wuhan • Barcelona • Belgrade • Manchester • Tokyo • Cluj • Tianjin

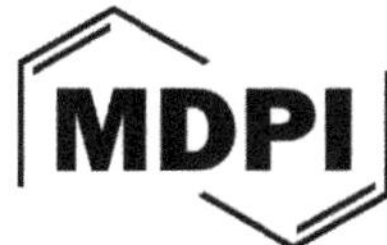

Editor
Curtise K. C. Ng
Curtin Medical School
Curtin University
Perth
Australia

Editorial Office
MDPI
St. Alban-Anlage 66
4052 Basel, Switzerland

This is a reprint of articles from the Special Issue published online in the open access journal *Children* (ISSN 2227-9067) (available at: www.mdpi.com/journal/children/special_issues/Pediatric_Radiology_Nuclear_Medicine).

For citation purposes, cite each article independently as indicated on the article page online and as indicated below:

LastName, A.A.; LastName, B.B.; LastName, C.C. Article Title. *Journal Name* **Year**, *Volume Number*, Page Range.

ISBN 978-3-0365-7959-7 (Hbk)
ISBN 978-3-0365-7958-0 (PDF)

Contents

About the Editor

Curtise K. C. Ng

Dr. Curtise K. C. Ng received his Bachelor of Science (Honours) Radiography degree in 2002 and Doctor of Philosophy degree in imaging informatics in 2007 from The Hong Kong Polytechnic University. In 2008, he decided to broaden his horizon and took up the Medical Imaging Lecturer position at Curtin University in Australia and has become a tenured Senior Lecturer since 2011. He has been awarded United Kingdom Higher Education Academy Senior Fellow status since 2021. Currently, he is a tenured Senior Lecturer of Curtin Medical School.

Dr. Ng is an active researcher in Radiology, Radiation Oncology, and Medical Radiation Science focussing on imaging informatics (including artificial intelligence) and education research. He was appointed as the Associate Editor of the *Journal of Medical Imaging and Radiation Sciences* (official journal of Canadian Association of Medical Radiation Technologists, Hong Kong Radiographers Association, Portuguese Association of Nuclear Medicine Technologists, Alliance in Nuclear Scintigraphy in Australia and Society of Medical Radiographers—Malta) between 2013 and 2019. Currently, he is the Guest Editor of a Special Issue of *Children* titled "Advanced Research in Pediatric Radiology and Nuclear Medicine (Volume II)" and is an Editorial Board Member of *BMC Medical Education* journal. He also serves as a reviewer for 30 journals such as *BMJ Open*, *International Journal of Medical Informatics*, *Knowledge-based Systems*, *Medicine*, *PLOS ONE* and *Scientific Reports*.

Preface to "Advanced Research in Pediatric Radiology and Nuclear Medicine"

Advancements in medical imaging modalities have resulted in increasing the importance and demand of pediatric radiology. This reprint showcases various examples of advanced research in pediatric radiology and nuclear medicine. These include the use of medical imaging modalities such as computed tomography, general radiography, magnetic resonance imaging, positron emission tomography, single-photon emission computed tomography, and ultrasound for diagnosis, as well as the performance of artificial intelligence (AI) in computer-aided detection and diagnosis in the pediatric population. The radiation dose issue of pediatric radiological examinations and emerging AI technology for dose reduction, as well as the use of three-dimensional printing based on medical images for pediatric surgical planning, healthcare professional education, and patient–clinician communication are also covered.

Curtise K. C. Ng
Editor

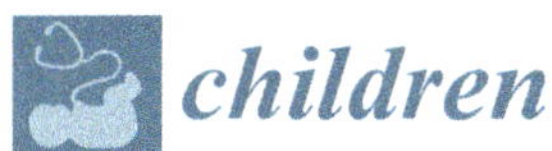

Review

Artificial Intelligence for Radiation Dose Optimization in Pediatric Radiology: A Systematic Review

Curtise K. C. Ng [1,2]

1   Curtin Medical School, Curtin University, GPO Box U1987, Perth, WA 6845, Australia;
curtise.ng@curtin.edu.au or curtise_ng@yahoo.com.hk; Tel.: +61-8-9266-7314; Fax: +61-8-9266-2377
2   Curtin Health Innovation Research Institute (CHIRI), Faculty of Health Sciences, Curtin University,
GPO Box U1987, Perth, WA 6845, Australia

Abstract: Radiation dose optimization is particularly important in pediatric radiology, as children are more susceptible to potential harmful effects of ionizing radiation. However, only one narrative review about artificial intelligence (AI) for dose optimization in pediatric computed tomography (CT) has been published yet. The purpose of this systematic review is to answer the question "What are the AI techniques and architectures introduced in pediatric radiology for dose optimization, their specific application areas, and performances?" Literature search with use of electronic databases was conducted on 3 June 2022. Sixteen articles that met selection criteria were included. The included studies showed deep convolutional neural network (CNN) was the most common AI technique and architecture used for dose optimization in pediatric radiology. All but three included studies evaluated AI performance in dose optimization of abdomen, chest, head, neck, and pelvis CT; CT angiography; and dual-energy CT through deep learning image reconstruction. Most studies demonstrated that AI could reduce radiation dose by 36–70% without losing diagnostic information. Despite the dominance of commercially available AI models based on deep CNN with promising outcomes, homegrown models could provide comparable performances. Future exploration of AI value for dose optimization in pediatric radiology is necessary due to small sample sizes and narrow scopes (only three modalities, CT, positron emission tomography/magnetic resonance imaging and mobile radiography, and not all examination types covered) of existing studies.

Keywords: as low as reasonably achievable; computed tomography; convolutional neural network; deep learning; dose reduction; generative adversarial network; image processing; machine learning; medical imaging; noise

Citation: Ng, C.K.C. Artificial Intelligence for Radiation Dose Optimization in Pediatric Radiology: A Systematic Review. *Children* **2022**, *9*, 1044. https://doi.org/10.3390/children9071044

Academic Editor: Ilias Tsiflikas

Received: 29 June 2022
Accepted: 11 July 2022
Published: 14 July 2022

Publisher's Note: MDPI stays neutral with regard to jurisdictional claims in published maps and institutional affiliations.

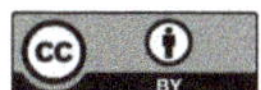

1. Introduction

Radiology is an indispensable part of modern healthcare. However, most of the medical imaging modalities, such as computed tomography (CT), positron emission tomography (PET), and general radiography, use ionizing radiation for image production [1–16]. Although the radiation dose involved in these imaging modalities is low (<100 mSv), and their real risk is unclear, some epidemiologic and biologic studies have demonstrated that these radiological examinations can cause cancers [17–23]. Hence, "as low as reasonably achievable" (ALARA) has become the fundamental principle of radiology practice [17,24,25]. International Commission on Radiological Protection (ICRP) has introduced the diagnostic reference levels (DRLs) initiative for radiological departments to identify examinations with radiation doses exceeding their corresponding DRLs and trigger the radiation dose-optimization process [26–32]. As the radiation used in radiological examinations is the source of signal, a reduction of the radiation amount results in a decrease of signal strength and an increase of image noise. Traditionally, the dose-optimization process involves the manipulation of a range of exposure/scan parameters and identification of parameters that deliver the lowest radiation dose but still producing images able to meet minimal diagnostic requirements [33–36]. Since the introduction of digital medical imaging, image processing has played an important role in the radiation dose optimization [37–39]. However, typical image processing techniques are unable to overcome the tradeoff between image noise and spatial resolution [9–12]. For the last few years, artificial intelligence (AI) has been introduced into radiology for radiation dose optimization. Studies have demonstrated its ability in pushing the limit, i.e., able to further reduce the radiation dose but without sacrificing image quality, such as noise and spatial resolution [1,6,9–12,15,16].

The dose optimization is particularly important for pediatric patients because they have longer life and more rapid cell proliferation, leading to two to three times more susceptibility to the potential harmful effects of ionizing radiation than the adult counterpart [17,33,36,40]. Nonetheless, dose optimization in pediatric radiology is challenging, as there is a greater variation of body size and composition within and across age groups [4,33]. Despite being an important and challenging topic area, apparently, only one narrative review article on this area has been published yet, and it is about deep learning (a subset of AI) image reconstruction (DLIR) for dose optimization in pediatric CT [17]. Hence, it is timely to conduct a systematic review about the use of AI for dose optimization in pediatric radiology. The purpose of this article is to systematically review published original studies to answer the question "What are the AI techniques and architectures introduced in pediatric radiology for dose optimization, their specific application areas, and performances?"

2. Materials and Methods

This systematic review on the AI for radiation dose optimization in pediatric radiology was conducted as per the PRISMA guidelines and patient/problem, intervention, comparison, and outcome (PICO) model [41,42]. This involved literature search, article selection, and data extraction and synthesis.

2.1. Literature Search

The literature search with use of electronic scholarly publication databases, including *Google Scholar, PubMed/Medline, ScienceDirect, Scopus*, and *Web of Science* was conducted on 3 June 2022 to identify articles about the AI for dose optimization in pediatric radiology published between 2017 and 2022. The search statement used was ("Artificial Intelligence" OR "Machine Learning" OR "Deep Learning") AND ("Dose Optimization" OR "Dose Reduction") AND ("Pediatric" OR "Children") AND ("Radiology" OR "Medical Imaging"). The keywords used in the search were based on the review focus. The year range was determined based on a narrative review about current and future applications of AI in radiology, which showed the use of AI for dose optimization in radiology not evident before 2017 [43].

2.2. Article Selection

A reviewer with more than 20 years of experience in conducting literature review was involved in the article selection process [44]. Only peer-reviewed original research articles that were written in English and focused on the use of AI for dose optimization in pediatric radiology were included. Grey literature, conference abstracts, editorials, review, perspective, opinion, commentary, and non-peer-reviewed (e.g., those published via the arXiv research-sharing platform, etc.) articles were excluded because of the following reasons: Well-established methodological guidelines were not available for proper selection of grey literature. Conference abstracts could not provide complete study information. Only secondary information was presented in editorials, review, perspective, opinion, and commentary articles. Non-peer-reviewed articles might provide unsubstantiated information [45,46].

Figure 1 illustrates details of the article selection process [41]. A three-stage screening process through assessing (1) article titles, (2) abstracts, and (3) full texts against the selection criteria was employed after duplicate article removal from results of the database search. Every non-duplicate article within the search results was retained until its exclusion could be decided. Lists of references of the included papers were reviewed for additional, relevant article identification [46].

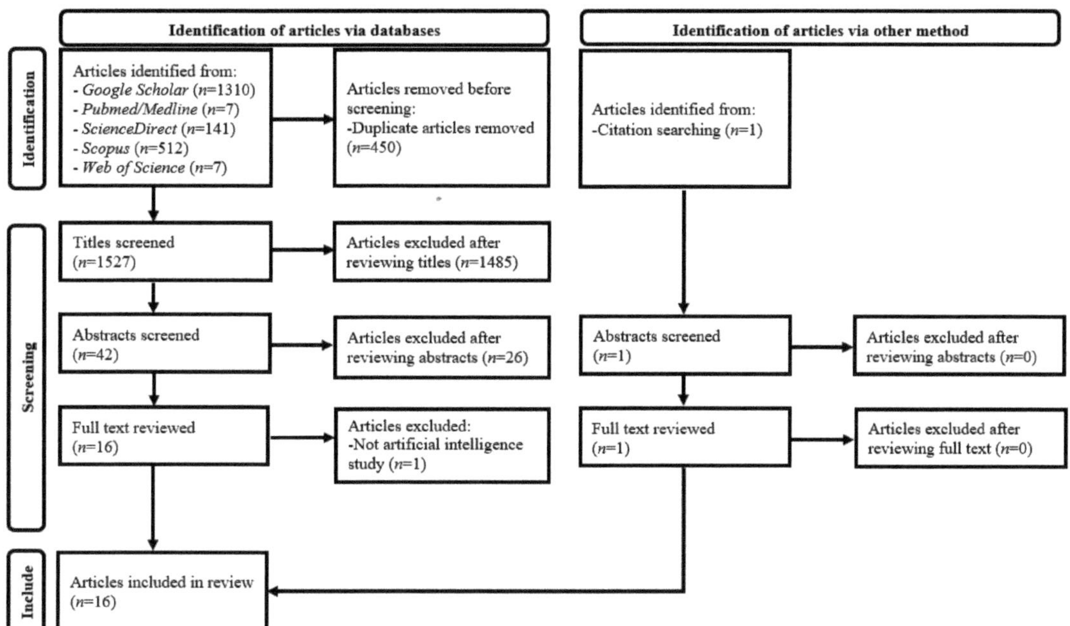

Figure 1. PRISMA flow diagram for systematic review of artificial intelligence for radiation dose optimization in pediatric radiology.

2.3. Data Extraction and Synthesis

A data extraction form (Table 1) was developed based on a recent systematic review on the use of AI in radiology [45]. The data, including names and countries of authors, publication years, clinical domains (radiology/nuclear medicine), AI techniques (such as machine learning and deep learning (DL)), model architectures (e.g., convolutional neural network (CNN), generative adversarial network (GAN), etc.), specific application areas (i.e., examination types and approaches that AI was used to achieve dose optimization), imaging modalities, details of AI model development (i.e., whether homegrown or commercially available model and arrangement of model training and testing), AI model evaluation approach (e.g., phantom study, clinical study, etc.), and key findings of AI model performance in dose optimization (including figures of dose reduction and diagnostic values and subjective and objective image assessment scores), were extracted from each included paper. To facilitate comparison of the AI model performance, percentage of dose reduction (if not reported) was synthesized based on the available absolute dose figures. When multiple image-quality-related figures were reported in a study, the most clinically relevant figures were presented. Diagnostic values were considered the most clinically relevant performance figures, while the objective image assessment scores were determined least relevant [47,48]. Quality assessment scores were determined for all included articles based on the quality assessment tool for studies with diverse designs (QATSDD) and expressed as percentages [49]. Less than 50%, 50–70%, and greater than 70% were considered low, moderate, and high study quality, respectively [46].

Table 1. Study characteristics of artificial intelligence for radiation dose optimization in pediatric radiology.

Author, Year, and Country	Clinical Domain	AI Technique and Architecture	Application Area for Dose Optimization	Imaging Modality	AI Model Development	AI Model Evaluation Approach	Key Findings of AI Model Performance
Brady et al. (2021), USA [1]	Radiology	DL-Convolutional neural network	DLIR of contrast-enhanced pediatric chest-abdomen-pelvis CT	CT	Commercially available model (AiCE, Canon Medical Systems, Tochigi, Japan) trained by image pairs of lower-dose CT with HIR and high-dose CT with MBIR and tested with datasets not involved in the training	Retrospective clinical study involving 19 children (mean age: 11 ± 5 y; range: 3–19 y)	With SBIR as reference, 52% dose reduction with noise texture and spatial resolution maintained, highest radiologists' confidence rating (scale 1–10) among 4 approaches (DLIR: 7 ± 1; SBIR & MBIR: 6.2 ± 1; FBP: 4.6 ± 1), and object detectability improved by 51%, 18%, and 11% when compared with FBP, SBIR, and MBIR, respectively.
Jeon et al. (2022), Republic of Korea [2]	Radiology	DL-Convolutional neural network	DLIR of non-contrast pediatric abdominal CT	CT	Commercially available model (AiCE, Canon Medical Systems) trained by image pairs of lower-dose CT with HIR and high-dose CT with MBIR and tested with datasets not involved in the training	Phantom study involving phantoms with diameters, 16 (pediatric) and 32 cm (adult)	For 80–120 kV, $CTDI_{vol}$ of DLIR images of pediatric phantom with CNR similar to corresponding FBP images was 5% of counterpart, representing 20-fold dose reduction potential.
Kim et al. (2017), Republic of Korea [3]	Radiology	DL-Gaussian mixture model	Post-processing of non-contrast pediatric abdominal CT images	CT	Homegrown model without training and testing details disclosed	Phantom study involving PMMA phantoms with diameters 12, 16, 20, 24, and 32 cm	Contrast-to-noise ratio dose increase by 1.7–4.9 times and 1.6–4.2 times for settings of 80–140 kV and fixed-tube current of 200 mA and 50–300 mA and fixed-tube potential of 120 kV, respectively.
Krueger et al. (2022), Germany [4]	Radiology	DL-Convolutional neural network	Post-processing of pediatric mobile chest and abdominal X-ray images acquired in intensive care units	Mobile radiography	Commercially available model (SimGrid, Samsung Electronics Co., Ltd., Suwon-si, Republic of Korea) trained by 30,000 images	Retrospective clinical study involving 210 images of 134 children (mean age: 4.2 y; range: 0–18 y)	Subjective image quality assessment demonstrated significant image quality improvement for patients with weight greater than 10 kg (odds ratio = 6.68, $p < 0.0001$), indicating its dose reduction potential.
Lee et al. (2021), Republic of Korea [5]	Radiology	DL-Convolutional neural network	Post-processing of pediatric abdominal DECT with lower CM concentration and noise-optimized virtual monoenergetic IR	CT	Commercially available model (ClariCT.AI, ClariPI, Seoul, Republic of Korea) trained by 410,000 image pairs of low- and standard-dose CT from 210 patients and tested with datasets not involved in the training	Retrospective clinical study involving 29 children (mean age: 10.1 y; range: 2–19 y)	19.6% $CTDI_{vol}$ and 14.3% CM concentration reductions in pediatric abdominal DECT with noise-optimized virtual monoenergetic IR when compared with those of standard CT.
Nagayama et al. (2022), Japan [6]	Radiology	DL-Convolutional neural network	DLIR of contrast-enhanced pediatric abdominal CT	CT	Commercially available model (AiCE Body Sharp, Canon Medical Systems) trained by image pairs of lower-dose CT with HIR and high-dose CT with MBIR and tested with datasets not involved in the training	Phantom and retrospective clinical study involving 20 cm diameter Catphan 700 phantom (The Phantom Laboratory, Greenwich, NY, USA) and 65 children (mean age: 25.0 ± 25.2 months; range: 0–81 months), respectively	In pediatric contrast-enhanced 80 kV abdominal CT, 53.7% SSDE reduction with better image quality (e.g., lower noise, noise texture, and edge sharpness improvements, etc.) when compared with standard-dose HIR.

Table 1. *Cont.*

Author, Year, and Country	Clinical Domain	AI Technique and Architecture	Application Area for Dose Optimization	Imaging Modality	AI Model Development	AI Model Evaluation Approach	Key Findings of AI Model Performance
Park et al. (2022), Republic of Korea [7]	Radiology	DL-Generative adversarial network	Post-processing of contrast-enhanced pediatric abdominal CT	CT	Homegrown model trained by 840 unpaired low- (42 patients; mean age: 7.2 ± 2.5 y) and standard-dose (42 patients; mean age: 6.2 ± 2.2 y) pediatric abdominal CT images and validated with 41 datasets (820 images; patient mean age: 7.4 ± 2.2 y) not involved in the training	Retrospective clinical study involving 660 images from 33 children	When compared with standard-dose CT, 36.6% $CTDI_{vol}$ reduction with image noise (7.1 ± 2.7) and CNR (portal vein: 21.2 ± 10.1; liver: 8.5 ± 4.3) similar to those of SAFIRE images (noise: 9.5 ± 4.0; CNR: 21.2 ± 9.8 (portal vein) and 8.5 ± 5.0 (liver)), and visual assessment (standard-dose and DL-processed image differentiation) yielded a sensitivity and specificity of 61.2% and 35.0%, indicating similar image quality.
Sun et al. (2021), People's Republic of China and USA [8]	Radiology	DL-Convolutional neural network	DLIR of pediatric neck, chest, and abdominal CT angiography	CT	Commercially available model (TrueFidelity, General Electric Healthcare, Chicago, IL, USA) trained by image pairs of low-dose CT projection (raw) data and higher-dose CT reconstructed by FBP from phantoms and patients	Retrospective clinical study involving 32 children with Takayasu's arteritis (mean age: 9.1 ± 4.5 y; range: 1–17 y)	High-strength DLIR had highest small artery detection and diagnostic confidence scores based on a 5-point scale (3.53 ± 0.51 and 4.09 ± 0.30) when compared with FBP (2.94 ± 0.25 and 2.91 ± 0.30), ASIR-V 50% (3.03 ± 0.18 and 3.03 ± 0.18), and ASIR-V 100% (2.84 ± 0.37 and 3.00 ± 0.00) groups, respectively, demonstrating its dose reduction potential.
Sun et al. (2021), People's Republic of China and USA [9]	Radiology	DL-Convolutional neural network	DLIR of pediatric chest CT angiography	CT	Commercially available model (TrueFidelity, General Electric Healthcare) trained by image pairs of low-dose CT projection (raw) data and higher-dose CT reconstructed by FBP from phantoms and patients	Retrospective clinical study involving 33 children (mean age: 5.9 ± 4.2 y; range: 4 months–13 y)	High-strength DLIR images had highest scores of subjective image assessment with a scale of 1–5 (noise: 4.05 ± 0.21 (little); vascular edge: 4.05 ± 0.58 (clear identification); vascular contrast: 4.14 ± 0.64 (good)) when compared with ASiR-V 100% (3.36 ± 0.58; 2.86 ± 0.56; 4.00 ± 0.62) and ASiR-V 50% (2.27 ± 0.55; 3.77 ± 0.61; 3.14 ± 0.64), respectively, demonstrating its potential for further dose reduction.
Sun et al. (2021), People's Republic of China and USA [10]	Radiology	DL-Convolutional neural network	DLIR of pediatric chest CT angiography	CT	Commercially available model (TrueFidelity, General Electric Healthcare) trained by image pairs of low-dose CT projection (raw) data and higher-dose CT reconstructed by FBP from phantoms and patients	Prospective case-control study involving 54 children (control group: $n = 27$; mean age: 9.5 ± 2.4 y; range: 5–13 y; and study group: $n = 27$; mean age: 9.3 ± 3.1 y; range: 5–14 y)	High-strength DLIR with 70 kV, NI of 22, and CM injection time of 4 s allowed 36% radiation dose and 53% CM dose reductions with scores of subjective image assessment against a 5-point scale similar to control group, ASiR-V 50% with 80 kV, NI of 19, and CM injection time of 8 s (artery contrast: 4.56 vs. 4.78; image quality: 3.67 vs 3.44; diagnostic confidence: 4.74 vs. 4.74; $p > 0.05$).

Table 1. *Cont.*

Author, Year, and Country	Clinical Domain	AI Technique and Architecture	Application Area for Dose Optimization	Imaging Modality	AI Model Development	AI Model Evaluation Approach	Key Findings of AI Model Performance
Sun et al. (2021), People's Republic of China and USA [11]	Radiology	DL-Convolutional neural network	DLIR of pediatric chest CT angiography	CT	Commercially available model (TrueFidelity, General Electric Healthcare) trained by image pairs of low-dose CT projection (raw) data and higher-dose CT reconstructed by FBP from phantoms and patients	Prospective case-control study involving 92 children (control group: $n = 46$; mean age: 5.9 ± 4.2 y; range: 4 months–13 y; and study group: $n = 46$; mean age: 5.9 ± 4.2 y; range: 4 months–13 y)	High-strength DLIR with 70 kV allowed 11% radiation dose and 20% CM dose reductions with higher scores of subjective image assessment against a 5-point scale (noise: 4 (little); vascular contrast: 4 (good); vascular edge: 4 (clear identification)) when compared with control group, ASiR-V 50% with 100 kV (noise: 2 (high); vascular contrast: 3 (fair); vascular edge: 3 (identifiable)).
Sun et al. (2021), People's Republic of China and USA [12]	Radiology	DL-Convolutional neural network	DLIR of non-contrast pediatric head CT	CT	Commercially available model (TrueFidelity, General Electric Healthcare) trained by image pairs of low-dose CT projection (raw) data and higher-dose CT reconstructed by FBP from phantoms and patients	Retrospective clinical study involving 50 children (median age: 2 y; range: 0.1–14 y)	High-strength DLIR images with 0.625 mm slice thickness had similar subjective image quality score and measured noise when compared with ASiR-V 50% 5 mm slice thickness images ($p > 0.05$) but able to reduce radiation dose by 85% and improve lesion detection (69 vs. 65 detected) due to spatial resolution increase.
Theruvath et al. (2021), USA [13]	Nuclear medicine	DL-2.5 dimensional encoder-decoder U-Net convolutional neural network	Post-processing of pediatric and adult whole-body PET images	PET/MRI	Commercially available model (SubtlePET 1.3, Subtle Medical, Menlo Park, CA, USA) trained by low- and high-count PET image pairs from whole-body PET/CT and PET/MRI studies of pediatric and adult patients and tested with adult brain and whole-body studies	Prospective clinical study involving 20 pediatric and adult lymphoma patients (mean age: 16.0 ± 6.0 y; range: 6–30 y)	Up to 50% ^{18}F-FDG dose reduction with 100% sensitivity and specificity for correct assessment of pediatric and adult lymphoma patients' treatment response.
Wang et al. (2021), USA and Germany [14]	Nuclear medicine	DL-Convolutional neural network	Post-processing of pediatric and adult ultra-low-dose whole-body PET/MRI images to synthesize standard-dose PET images	PET/MRI	Homegrown model development based on Lim et al.'s [50] open-source enhanced deep super-resolution network model through transfer learning with 17 standard-dose PET, simulated 6.25% ultra-low-dose PET and MRI training datasets, and 6 independent testing datasets acquired in USA	Prospective clinical study involving 34 pediatric and adult lymphoma patients in USA ($n = 23$; mean age: 17 ± 7 y, range: 6–30 y) and Germany ($n = 11$; mean age: 14 ± 5 y; range: 3–18 y)	Expert readers' agreements of tumor diagnosis between standard and AI-processed 6.25% ultra-low-dose PET images (kappa = 0.942 (USA datasets) and 0.912 (Germany datasets)) were significantly greater than the agreements between standard and 6.25% ultra-low-dose PET images (kappa = 0.650 (USA datasets) and 0.834 (Germany datasets)). Diagnostic accuracy of AI-processed 6.25% ultra-low-dose PET images was adequate, representing 93.75% dose reduction capability.

Table 1. *Cont.*

Author, Year, and Country	Clinical Domain	AI Technique and Architecture	Application Area for Dose Optimization	Imaging Modality	AI Model Development	AI Model Evaluation Approach	Key Findings of AI Model Performance
Yoon et al. (2021), Republic of Korea [15]	Radiology	DL-Convolutional neural network	DLIR of pediatric contrast enhanced abdominal and non-contrast and contrast enhanced chest CT	CT	Commercially available model (TrueFidelity, General Electric Healthcare) trained by image pairs of low-dose CT projection (raw) data and higher-dose CT reconstructed by FBP from phantoms and patients	Phantom and retrospective clinical study involving The Phantom Laboratory's 20 cm diameter Catphan 500 phantom and 51 pediatric patients (mean age: 11.5 $\pm$ 4.6 y; range: 1–18 y), respectively	When compared with ASiR-V 50%, medium- and high-strength DLIR images of contrast enhanced abdominal ($n = 23$) and non-contrast ($n = 16$) and contrast enhanced ($n = 12$) chest CT had statistically significantly higher subjective image quality score and lower noise ($p < 0.001$), illustrating its dose reduction potential.
Zhang et al. (2022), People's Republic of China [16]	Radiology	DL-Convolutional neural network	DLIR of non-contrast pediatric abdominal and chest CT	CT	Commercially available model (TrueFidelity, General Electric Healthcare) trained by image pairs of low-dose CT projection (raw) data and higher-dose CT reconstructed by FBP from phantoms and patients	Phantom and prospective clinical study involving a pediatric (equivalent to 5-year-old patient) whole body phantom (PBU−70, Kyoto Kagaku Co., Ltd., Kyoto, Japan) and 20 children (mean age: 5.4 $\pm$ 1.2 y; range: 4–6 y), respectively	When compared with ASiR-V 70%, high-strength DLIR achieved about 70% and 60% dose reductions for pediatric non-contrast abdominal ($n = 10$) and chest ($n = 10$) CT, respectively. However, high-strength DLIR did not statistically significantly improve subjective image assessment score of chest CT.

^{18}F-FDG, fluorine−18-fluorodeoxyglucose; AI, artificial intelligence; AiCE, Advanced Intelligent Clear-IQ Engine; ASiR-V, adaptive statistical iterative reconstruction-Veo; CM, contrast medium; CNR, contrast-to-noise ratio; CT, computed tomography; CTDI$_{vol}$, volume computed tomography dose index; DECT, dual-energy computed tomography; DL, deep learning; DLIR, deep learning image reconstruction; FBP, filtered back projection; HIR, hybrid iterative reconstruction; IR, image reconstruction; MBIR, model-based iterative reconstruction; MRI, magnetic resonance imaging; NI, noise index; No., number; PET, positron emission tomography; PMMA, polymethyl methacrylate; SAFIRE, sinogram affirmed iterative reconstruction; SBIR, statistical-based iterative reconstruction; SSDE, size-specific dose estimate; y, year.

3. Results

Sixteen articles met the selection criteria and were included in this review. Table 1 shows these study characteristics [1–16]. All but one article were published in the last two years, representing that the AI for dose optimization in pediatric radiology has only just become popular [1,2,4–16]. Nearly all (14) studies were determined high quality [1,4–16], and the lower quality ones were "pure" phantom studies [2,3]. All studies used the DL technique [1–16] and were conducted by 12 groups of researchers from USA (n = 8) [1,8–14], People's Republic of China (n = 6) [8–12,16], Republic of Korea (n = 5) [2,3,5,7,15], Germany (n = 2) [4,14], and Japan (n = 1) [6]. Only two studies were about nuclear medicine (whole-body PET/magnetic resonance imaging (MRI)) [13,14]. For the 14 radiology-related studies [1–12,15,16], all except one were related to CT, covering body parts such as the abdomen (n = 10) [1–8,15,16], chest (n = 8) [1,4,8–11,15,16], head (n = 1) [12], neck (n = 1) [8], and pelvis (n = 1) [1], and four focused on CT angiography [8–11] as well as one on dual-energy CT (DECT) [5]. Thirteen studies (81.3%) used commercially available AI models for dose optimization (TrueFidelity, General Electric Healthcare (GE): n = 7 [8–12,15,16]; AiCE, Canon Medical Systems: n = 3 [1,2,6]; ClariCT.AI, ClariPI: n = 1 [5]; SimGrid, Samsung Electronics Co., Ltd.: n = 1 [4]; SubtlePET 1.3, Subtle Medical: n = 1 [13]). Ten studies (62.5%) employed DLIR for CT dose optimization as a result of the dominance of GE TrueFidelity and Canon AiCE with the CNN architecture [1,2,6,8–12,15,16]. Hence, the CNN was the most popular (87.5%) AI architecture among the included studies [1,2,4–6,8–16].

Clinical evaluation of the AI model performance was conducted in all but two studies [1,4–16], and the use of phantom for an additional evaluation was also noted in three (21.4%) of the clinical studies [6,15,16]. Collectively, these clinical studies covered pediatric patients aged from 0 to 18 years [1,4–16]. All except one study recruited less than 100 patients for the model evaluation [1,5–16]. The only exception had 134 patients [4]. A retrospective approach was employed in about two-thirds (9 out of 14) of the clinical studies [1,4–9,12,15]. About 70% of (11) included studies reported absolute dose figures and/or dose reduction percentages. The performance of dose reduction of the AI models with acceptable image quality ranged from 11% to 95% [1,2,5–7,10–14,16]. More than half (6) of these studies reported that their AI models were able to achieve dose reductions between 36% and 70% [1,6,7,10,13,16] although three other studies showed dose reductions between 85% and 95% [2,12,14], and another two showed 11–20% dose reductions [5,11]. For the two most popular commercial AI models, GE TrueFidelity and Canon AiCE, great variations of their dose reduction performances, namely 11–85% and 52–95%, were noted, respectively [1,2,6,10–12,16].

4. Discussion

The findings of this systematic review on the AI for radiation dose optimization in pediatric radiology are consistent with several recent narrative reviews about the use of AI in radiology [17,43,51]. For the narrative review about the current and future applications of AI in radiology published in 2018 [43], only one study regarding low-dose CT denoising published in 2017 was cited [52]. However, recently, more studies about the use of AI for dose optimization have been published, resulting in a narrative review about the AI for dose optimization in pediatric CT available in 2021 [17]. This demonstrates that the use of AI for dose optimization in pediatric radiology has attracted the attention of the profession recently. That narrative review indicated the DLIR allowed 30–80% dose reduction in pediatric CT but was still able to produce images with diagnostic quality. This systematic review with inclusion of more studies about dose optimization in pediatric CT and covering other imaging modalities shows that the majority of the AI models were able to reduce the radiation dose by 36–70% [1,6,7,10,13,16]. Nonetheless, three studies included in this systematic review demonstrated that the use of AI could achieve further radiation dose reduction (up to 95%) [2,12,14]. Apparently, the large variation of dose reduction performances is due to the retrospective nature of many included studies [1,4–9,12,15], which did not allow further manipulation of examination/scan parameters to obtain ultra-low-dose images for evaluating whether the AI models could restore the quality of these ultra-low-dose images to close to the original [9]. Although there is a greater flexibility for phantom studies to manipulate the examination/scan parameters without any ethical and radiation dose concerns, enabling further exploration of the potential of these AI models, their evaluation outcomes tend to be less clinically relevant [47,48]. For example, Jeon et al. [2] reported that Canon AiCE was able to reduce the CT dose by 95% with the contrast-to-noise ratio values of the DLIR phantom images similar to those reconstructed by filtered back projection, but it is unclear whether these findings could be translated into clinical practice exactly. Nonetheless, Wang et al.'s [14] clinical prospective study showed that their homegrown AI denoising model developed through transfer learning with the use of 17 standard-dose PET simulated 6.25% ultra-low-dose PET, and MRI training datasets were able to reduce the radiation dose by 93.8% for the whole-body PET examinations with adequate diagnostic accuracy. This implies that it is feasible to use the AI denoising to achieve about 90% dose reduction in the clinical practice although all included studies had small sample sizes and/or number of training datasets [1,4–16], which is a common issue of AI studies in radiology due to limited availability of medical images [53]. Nevertheless, through the use of transfer learning (i.e., retraining an existing AI model using a smaller number of datasets with or without modification of its architecture) to develop an AI model for performing a similar task, such a model could provide a dose-optimization performance comparable to commercially available models (e.g., Canon AiCE, GE TrueFidelity, etc.) trained with more datasets [2,12,14,43].

It is within expectation that all but two studies used the AI models with the deep CNN architecture because the CNN architecture emerged in 1980s, and hence, it has been widely used in radiology, with satisfactory performances well-demonstrated [1,2,4–6,8–16,37]. However, one included study published in 2022 employed the more recent and advanced DL architecture: GAN, which was designed in 2014 [7,51]. According to a narrative review about the use of GAN in radiology published in 2021 [51], the CNN-based denoising models could cause CT images having a plastic-like appearance, which is similar to those produced by iterative reconstruction due to over-smoothing. In contrast, the GAN is a more complex architecture with a generator and a discriminator, which requires simultaneous training of these two, increasing the complexity of model development [37]. Nonetheless, the GAN-based denoising models are able to preserve texture details and hence produce images with quality matching standard images [51]. The GAN-based dose-optimization study included in this systematic review also demonstrated similar findings that their readers were unable to differentiate between the standard-dose and GAN-processed images although only 36.6% dose reduction was achieved in their study [7]. Another non-CNN-based dose-optimization study included in this review employed the Gaussian mixture model (GMM) architecture [3]. The use of GMM for medical image denoising was reported before the emergence of GAN [54]. However, it is not widely adopted in radiology, and its clinical performance in pediatric radiology dose optimization remains unclear [3,17,43,51].

This paper is the first systematic review on the AI for radiation dose optimization in pediatric radiology covering the imaging modalities of CT, PET/MRI, and mobile radiography and hence advancing the previous narrative review on the AI for dose optimization in pediatric CT published in 2021 [17]. Although it is well-known that radiation dose burden is a significant issue in pediatric CT [1–11,15,16], the dose involved in a PET scan is comparable to that of a CT examination [14]. Furthermore, general radiography is the most common radiological examination type for pediatric patients despite being a low-dose modality [36]. Nonetheless, as per the ALARA principle, the value of AI for dose optimization in other modalities that use ionizing radiation for pediatric examinations should be explored in the future [17,24,25]. Moreover, given the relatively narrow focus and small sample size of the included studies, future studies on this topic area for CT, PET, and general radiography need to have greater scale and wider scope [1,4–16]. Besides, further exploration of the use of GAN for dose optimization appears warranted [7,51].

This systematic review has two major limitations. Article selection, data extraction, and synthesis were performed by a single author, albeit one with more than 20 years of experience in conducting literature reviews. According to a recent methodological systematic review [44], this is an appropriate arrangement provided that the single reviewer is experienced. Additionally, through adherence to the PRISMA guidelines and the use of the data extraction form (Table 1) devised based on the recent systematic review on AI in radiology and QATSDD, the potential bias should be addressed to certain extent [41,45,46,49]. In addition, only articles written in English and published within last five years were included, potentially affecting comprehensiveness of this systematic review. Nevertheless, this review still has a wider coverage than the previous narrative review on the AI for dose optimization in pediatric CT [17].

5. Conclusions

This systematic review shows that the deep CNN was the most common AI technique and architecture used for radiation dose optimization in pediatric radiology. All but three included studies evaluated the AI performance in dose optimization of abdomen, chest, head, neck, and pelvis CT; CT angiography; and DECT through DLIR. The majority of studies demonstrated that the AI could reduce radiation dose by 36–70% without losing diagnostic information. Despite the dominance of commercially available AI models based on the deep CNN, the homegrown models, including the one with the more recent and advanced architecture, i.e., GAN, could provide comparable performances. Future exploration of the value of AI for dose optimization in pediatric radiology is necessary, as the sample sizes of the included studies appear small, and only three imaging modalities, namely CT, PET/MRI, and mobile radiography, rather than all examination types were covered.

Funding: This work received no external funding.

Institutional Review Board Statement: Not applicable.

Informed Consent Statement: Not applicable.

Data Availability Statement: Not applicable.

Conflicts of Interest: The author declares no conflict of interest.

References

1. Brady, S.L.; Trout, A.T.; Somasundaram, E.; Anton, C.G.; Li, Y.; Dillman, J.R. Improving image quality and reducing radiation dose for pediatric CT by using deep learning reconstruction. *Radiology* **2021**, *298*, 180–188. [CrossRef] [PubMed]
2. Jeon, P.H.; Kim, D.; Chung, M.A. Estimates of the image quality in accordance with radiation dose for pediatric imaging using deep learning CT: A phantom study. In Proceedings of the 2022 IEEE International Conference on Big Data and Smart Computing (BigComp), Daegu, Korea, 17–22 January 2022; pp. 352–356. [CrossRef]
3. Kim, S.H.; Seo, K.; Kang, S.H.; Bae, S.; Kwak, H.J.; Hong, J.W.; Hwang, Y.; Kang, S.M.; Choi, H.R.; Kim, G.Y.; et al. Study on feasibility for artificial intelligence (AI) noise reduction algorithm with various parameters in pediatric abdominal radio-magnetic computed tomography (CT). *J. Magn.* **2017**, *22*, 570–578. [CrossRef]
4. Krueger, P.C.; Ebeling, K.; Waginger, M.; Glutig, K.; Scheithauer, M.; Schlattmann, P.; Proquitté, H.; Mentzel, H.J. Evaluation of the post-processing algorithms SimGrid and S-Enhance for paediatric intensive care patients and neonates. *Pediatr. Radiol.* **2022**, *52*, 1029–1037. [CrossRef] [PubMed]
5. Lee, S.; Choi, Y.H.; Cho, Y.J.; Lee, S.B.; Cheon, J.E.; Kim, W.S.; Ahn, C.K.; Kim, J.H. Noise reduction approach in pediatric abdominal CT combining deep learning and dual-energy technique. *Eur. Radiol.* **2021**, *31*, 2218–2226. [CrossRef] [PubMed]
6. Nagayama, Y.; Goto, M.; Sakabe, D.; Emoto, T.; Shigematsu, S.; Oda, S.; Tanoue, S.; Kidoh, M.; Nakaura, T.; Funama, Y.; et al. Radiation dose reduction for 80-kVp pediatric CT using deep learning-based reconstruction: A clinical and phantom study. *AJR Am. J. Roentgenol.* **2022**, *23*, 1–10. [CrossRef] [PubMed]
7. Park, H.S.; Jeon, K.; Lee, J.; You, S.K. Denoising of pediatric low dose abdominal CT using deep learning based algorithm. *PLoS ONE* **2022**, *17*, e0260369. [CrossRef]
8. Sun, J.; Li, H.; Li, H.; Li, M.; Gao, Y.; Zhou, Z.; Peng, Y. Application of deep learning image reconstruction algorithm to improve image quality in CT angiography of children with Takayasu arteritis. *J. X-ray Sci. Technol.* **2022**, *30*, 177–184. [CrossRef]
9. Sun, J.; Li, H.; Li, J.; Yu, T.; Li, M.; Zhou, Z.; Peng, Y. Improving the image quality of pediatric chest CT angiography with low radiation dose and contrast volume using deep learning image reconstruction. *Quant. Imaging Med. Surg.* **2021**, *11*, 3051–3058. [CrossRef]

10. Sun, J.; Li, H.; Li, J.; Cao, Y.; Zhou, Z.; Li, M.; Peng, Y. Performance evaluation of using shorter contrast injection and 70 kVp with deep learning image reconstruction for reduced contrast medium dose and radiation dose in coronary CT angiography for children: A pilot study. *Quant. Imaging Med. Surg.* **2021**, *11*, 4162–4171. [CrossRef]

11. Sun, J.; Li, H.; Gao, J.; Li, J.; Li, M.; Zhou, Z.; Peng, Y. Performance evaluation of a deep learning image reconstruction (DLIR) algorithm in "double low" chest CTA in children: A feasibility study. *Radiol. Med.* **2021**, *126*, 1181–1188. [CrossRef]

12. Sun, J.; Li, H.; Wang, B.; Li, J.; Li, M.; Zhou, Z.; Peng, Y. Application of a deep learning image reconstruction (DLIR) algorithm in head CT imaging for children to improve image quality and lesion detection. *BMC Med. Imaging* **2021**, *21*, 108. [CrossRef]

13. Theruvath, A.J.; Siedek, F.; Yerneni, K.; Muehe, A.M.; Spunt, S.L.; Pribnow, A.; Moseley, M.; Lu, Y.; Zhao, Q.; Gulaka, P.; et al. Validation of deep learning-based augmentation for reduced 18F-FDG dose for PET/MRI in children and young adults with lymphoma. *Radiol. Artif. Intell.* **2021**, *3*, e200232. [CrossRef] [PubMed]

14. Wang, Y.J.; Baratto, L.; Hawk, K.E.; Theruvath, A.J.; Pribnow, A.; Thakor, A.S.; Gatidis, S.; Lu, R.; Gummidipundi, S.E.; Garcia-Diaz, J.; et al. Artificial intelligence enables whole-body positron emission tomography scans with minimal radiation exposure. *Eur. J. Nucl. Med. Mol. Imaging* **2021**, *48*, 2771–2781. [CrossRef] [PubMed]

15. Yoon, H.; Kim, J.; Lim, H.J.; Lee, M.J. Image quality assessment of pediatric chest and abdomen CT by deep learning reconstruction. *BMC Med. Imaging* **2021**, *21*, 146. [CrossRef] [PubMed]

16. Zhang, K.; Shi, X.; Xie, S.S.; Sun, J.H.; Liu, Z.H.; Zhang, S.; Song, J.Y.; Shen, W. Deep learning image reconstruction in pediatric abdominal and chest computed tomography: A comparison of image quality and radiation dose. *Quant. Imaging Med. Surg.* **2022**, *12*, 3238–3250. [CrossRef]

17. Nagayama, Y.; Sakabe, D.; Goto, M.; Emoto, T.; Oda, S.; Nakaura, T.; Kidoh, M.; Uetani, H.; Funama, Y.; Hirai, T. Deep learning-based reconstruction for lower-dose pediatric CT: Technical principles, image characteristics, and clinical implementations. *Radiographics* **2021**, *41*, 1936–1953. [CrossRef]

18. Pearce, M.S.; Salotti, J.A.; Little, M.P.; McHugh, K.; Lee, C.; Kim, K.P.; Howe, N.L.; Ronckers, C.M.; Rajaraman, P.; Sir Craft, A.W.; et al. Radiation exposure from CT scans in childhood and subsequent risk of leukaemia and brain tumours: A retrospective cohort study. *Lancet* **2012**, *380*, 499–505. [CrossRef]

19. de Gonzalez, A.B.; Salotti, J.A.; McHugh, K.; Little, M.P.; Harbron, R.W.; Lee, C.; Ntowe, E.; Braganza, M.Z.; Parker, L.; Rajaraman, P.; et al. Relationship between paediatric CT scans and subsequent risk of leukaemia and brain tumours: Assessment of the impact of underlying conditions. *Br. J. Cancer* **2016**, *114*, 388–394. [CrossRef]

20. Lee, K.H.; Lee, S.; Park, J.H.; Lee, S.S.; Kim, H.Y.; Lee, W.J.; Cha, E.S.; Kim, K.P.; Lee, W.; Lee, J.Y.; et al. Risk of hematologic malignant neoplasms from abdominopelvic computed tomographic radiation in patients who underwent appendectomy. *JAMA Surg.* **2021**, *156*, 343–351. [CrossRef]

21. Mathews, J.D.; Forsythe, A.V.; Brady, Z.; Butler, M.W.; Goergen, S.K.; Byrnes, G.B.; Giles, G.G.; Wallace, A.B.; Anderson, P.R.; Guiver, T.A.; et al. Cancer risk in 680,000 people exposed to computed tomography scans in childhood or adolescence: Data linkage study of 11 million Australians. *BMJ* **2013**, *346*, f2360. [CrossRef]

22. Halm, B.M.; Franke, A.A.; Lai, J.F.; Turner, H.C.; Brenner, D.J.; Zohrabian, V.M.; DiMauro, R. γ-H2AX foci are increased in lymphocytes in vivo in young children 1 h after very low-dose X-irradiation: A pilot study. *Pediatr. Radiol.* **2014**, *44*, 1310–1317. [CrossRef] [PubMed]

23. Vandevoorde, C.; Franck, C.; Bacher, K.; Breysem, L.; Smet, M.H.; Ernst, C.; De Backer, A.; Van De Moortele, K.; Smeets, P.; Thierens, H. γ-H2AX foci as in vivo effect biomarker in children emphasize the importance to minimize X-ray doses in paediatric CT imaging. *Eur. Radiol.* **2015**, *25*, 800–811. [CrossRef] [PubMed]

24. Ng, C.K.C.; Sun, Z. Development of an online automatic computed radiography dose data mining program: A preliminary study. *Comput. Methods Programs Biomed.* **2010**, *97*, 48–52. [CrossRef]

25. MacKay, M.; Hancy, C.; Crowe, A.; D'Rozario, R.; Ng, C.K.C. Attitudes of medical imaging technologists on use of gonad shielding in general radiography. *Radiographer* **2012**, *59*, 35–39. [CrossRef]

26. Ng, C.K.C.; Sun, Z. Development of an online automatic diagnostic reference levels management system for digital radiography: A pilot experience. *Comput. Methods Programs Biomed.* **2011**, *103*, 145–150. [CrossRef] [PubMed]

27. Ng, C.K.C.; Sun, Z.; Parry, H.; Burrage, J. Local diagnostic reference levels for x-ray examinations in an Australian tertiary hospital. *J. Med. Imaging Health Inform.* **2014**, *4*, 297–302. [CrossRef]

28. Sun, Z.; Ng, C.K.C.; Wong, Y.H.; Yeong, C.H. 3D-printed coronary plaques to simulate high calcification in the coronary arteries for investigation of blooming artifacts. *Biomolecules* **2021**, *11*, 1307. [CrossRef]

29. Sun, Z.; Ng, C.K.C.; Sá Dos Reis, C. Synchrotron radiation computed tomography versus conventional computed tomography for assessment of four types of stent grafts used for endovascular treatment of thoracic and abdominal aortic aneurysms. *Quant. Imaging Med. Surg.* **2018**, *8*, 609–620. [CrossRef]

30. Sun, Z.; Ng, C.K.C.; Squelch, A. Synchrotron radiation computed tomography assessment of calcified plaques and coronary stenosis with different slice thicknesses and beam energies on 3D printed coronary models. *Quant. Imaging Med. Surg.* **2019**, *9*, 6–22. [CrossRef]

31. Sun, Z.; Ng, C.K.C. Use of synchrotron radiation to accurately assess cross-sectional area reduction of the aortic branch ostia caused by suprarenal stent wires. *J. Endovasc. Ther.* **2017**, *24*, 870–879. [CrossRef]

32. Sun, Z.; Ng, C.K.C. Synchrotron radiation imaging of aortic stent grafting: An in vitro phantom study. *J. Med. Imaging Health Inform.* **2017**, *7*, 890–896. [CrossRef]

33. Al Mahrooqi, K.M.S.; Ng, C.K.C.; Sun, Z. Pediatric computed tomography dose optimization strategies: A literature review. *J. Med. Imaging Radiat. Sci.* **2015**, *46*, 241–249. [CrossRef] [PubMed]

34. Sun, Z.; Ng, C. Dual-source CT angiography in aortic stent grafting: An in vitro aorta phantom study of image noise and radiation dose. *Acad. Radiol.* **2010**, *17*, 884–893. [CrossRef] [PubMed]

35. Almutairi, A.M.; Sun, Z.; Ng, C.; Al-Safran, Z.A.; Al-Mulla, A.A.; Al-Jamaan, A.I. Optimal scanning protocols of 64-slice CT angiography in coronary artery stents: An in vitro phantom study. *Eur. J. Radiol.* **2010**, *74*, 156–160. [CrossRef]

36. Feghali, J.A.; Chambers, G.; Delépierre, J.; Chapeliere, S.; Mannes, I.; Adamsbaum, C. New image quality and dose reduction technique for pediatric digital radiography. *Diagn. Interv. Imaging* **2021**, *102*, 463–470. [CrossRef]

37. Sun, Z.; Ng, C.K.C. Artificial intelligence (enhanced super-resolution generative adversarial network) for calcium deblooming in coronary computed tomography angiography: A feasibility study. *Diagnostics* **2022**, *12*, 991. [CrossRef]

38. Sun, Z.; Ng, C.K.C. High calcium scores in coronary CT angiography: Effects of image post-processing on visualization and measurement of coronary lumen diameter. *J. Med. Imaging Health Inform.* **2015**, *5*, 110–116. [CrossRef]

39. Sun, Z.; Ng, C.K.C.; Xu, L.; Fan, Z.; Lei, J. Coronary CT angiography in heavily calcified coronary arteries: Improvement of coronary lumen visualization and coronary stenosis assessment with image postprocessing methods. *Medicine* **2015**, *94*, e2148. [CrossRef]

40. Christie, S.; Ng, C.K.C.; Sá Dos Reis, C. Australasian radiographers' choices of immobilisation strategies for paediatric radiological examinations. *Radiography* **2020**, *26*, 27–34. [CrossRef]

41. PRISMA: Transparent Reporting of Systematic Reviews and Meta-Analyses. Available online: https://www.prisma-statement.org (accessed on 24 June 2022).

42. Eriksen, M.B.; Frandsen, T.F. The impact of patient, intervention, comparison, outcome (PICO) as a search strategy tool on literature search quality: A systematic review. *J. Med. Libr. Assoc.* **2018**, *106*, 420–431. [CrossRef]

43. Choy, G.; Khalilzadeh, O.; Michalski, M.; Do, S.; Samir, A.E.; Pianykh, O.S.; Geis, J.R.; Pandharipande, P.V.; Brink, J.A.; Dreyer, K.J. Current applications and future impact of machine learning in radiology. *Radiology* **2018**, *288*, 318–328. [CrossRef] [PubMed]

44. Waffenschmidt, S.; Knelangen, M.; Sieben, W.; Bühn, S.; Pieper, D. Single screening versus conventional double screening for study selection in systematic reviews: A methodological systematic review. *BMC Med. Res. Methodol.* **2019**, *19*, 132. [CrossRef] [PubMed]

45. Jeong, J.J.; Tariq, A.; Adejumo, T.; Trivedi, H.; Gichoya, J.W.; Banerjee, I. Systematic review of generative adversarial networks (GANs) for medical image classification and segmentation. *J. Digit. Imaging* **2022**, *35*, 137–152. [CrossRef] [PubMed]

46. Ng, C.K.C. A review of the impact of the COVID-19 pandemic on pre-registration medical radiation science education. *Radiography* **2022**, *28*, 222–231. [CrossRef] [PubMed]

47. Petri, S.A.; Ng, C.K.C. Comparison of the performance of computed radiography and direct radiography in glass soft tissue foreign body visualisation. *S. Afr. Radiogr.* **2018**, *56*, 18–25.

48. Kleinfelder, T.R.; Ng, C.K.C. Effects of image postprocessing in digital radiography to detect wooden, soft tissue foreign bodies. *Radiol. Technol.* **2022**, *93*, 544–554. Available online: https://pubmed.ncbi.nlm.nih.gov/35790309/ (accessed on 28 June 2022)

49. Sirriyeh, R.; Lawton, R.; Gardner, P.; Armitage, G. Reviewing studies with diverse designs: The development and evaluation of a new tool. *J. Eval. Clin. Pract.* **2012**, *18*, 746–752. [CrossRef]

50. Lim, B.; Son, S.; Kim, H.; Nah, S.; Lee, K.M. Enhanced deep residual networks for single image super-resolution. In Proceedings of the 2017 IEEE Conference on Computer Vision and Pattern Recognition Workshops (CVPRW), Honolulu, HI, USA, 21–26 July 2017; pp. 1132–1140. [CrossRef]

51. Wolterink, J.M.; Mukhopadhyay, A.; Leiner, T.; Vogl, T.J.; Bucher, A.M.; Išgum, I. Generative adversarial networks: A primer for radiologists. *Radiographics* **2021**, *41*, 840–857. [CrossRef]

52. Wolterink, J.M.; Leiner, T.; Viergever, M.A.; Isgum, I. Generative adversarial networks for noise reduction in low-dose CT. *IEEE Trans. Med. Imaging* **2017**, *36*, 2536–2545. [CrossRef]

53. Kimy, H.E.; Cosa-Linan, A.; Santhanam, N.; Jannesari, M.; Maros, M.E.; Ganslandt, T. Transfer learning for medical image classification: A literature review. *BMC Med. Imaging* **2022**, *22*, 69. [CrossRef]

54. Garg, G.; Prasad, G.; Coyle, D. Gaussian mixture model-based noise reduction in resting state fMRI data. *J. Neurosci. Methods* **2013**, *215*, 71–77. [CrossRef] [PubMed]

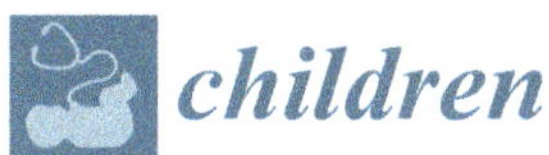

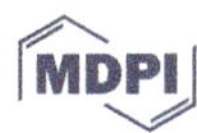

Review

Diagnostic Performance of Artificial Intelligence-Based Computer-Aided Detection and Diagnosis in Pediatric Radiology: A Systematic Review

Curtise K. C. Ng [1,2]

1 Curtin Medical School, Curtin University, GPO Box U1987, Perth, WA 6845, Australia; curtise.ng@curtin.edu.au or curtise_ng@yahoo.com.hk; Tel.: +61-8-9266-7314; Fax: +61-8-9266-2377
2 Curtin Health Innovation Research Institute (CHIRI), Faculty of Health Sciences, Curtin University, GPO Box U1987, Perth, WA 6845, Australia

Abstract: Artificial intelligence (AI)-based computer-aided detection and diagnosis (CAD) is an important research area in radiology. However, only two narrative reviews about general uses of AI in pediatric radiology and AI-based CAD in pediatric chest imaging have been published yet. The purpose of this systematic review is to investigate the AI-based CAD applications in pediatric radiology, their diagnostic performances and methods for their performance evaluation. A literature search with the use of electronic databases was conducted on 11 January 2023. Twenty-three articles that met the selection criteria were included. This review shows that the AI-based CAD could be applied in pediatric brain, respiratory, musculoskeletal, urologic and cardiac imaging, and especially for pneumonia detection. Most of the studies (93.3%, 14/15; 77.8%, 14/18; 73.3%, 11/15; 80.0%, 8/10; 66.6%, 2/3; 84.2%, 16/19; 80.0%, 8/10) reported model performances of at least 0.83 (area under receiver operating characteristic curve), 0.84 (sensitivity), 0.80 (specificity), 0.89 (positive predictive value), 0.63 (negative predictive value), 0.87 (accuracy), and 0.82 (F1 score), respectively. However, a range of methodological weaknesses (especially a lack of model external validation) are found in the included studies. In the future, more AI-based CAD studies in pediatric radiology with robust methodology should be conducted for convincing clinical centers to adopt CAD and realizing its benefits in a wider context.

Keywords: children; confusion matrix; convolutional neural network; deep learning; diagnostic accuracy; disease identification; image interpretation; machine learning; medical imaging; pneumonia

Citation: Ng, C.K.C. Diagnostic Performance of Artificial Intelligence-Based Computer-Aided Detection and Diagnosis in Pediatric Radiology: A Systematic Review. *Children* **2023**, *10*, 525. https://doi.org/10.3390/children10030525

Academic Editor: Paul R. Carney

Received: 31 January 2023
Revised: 13 February 2023
Accepted: 7 March 2023
Published: 8 March 2023

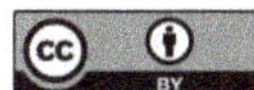

1. Introduction

Artificial intelligence (AI) is an active research area in radiology [1–4]. However, the investigation of use of AI for computer-aided detection and diagnosis (CAD) in radiology started in 1955. Any CAD systems are AI applications and can be subdivided into two types: computer-aided detection (CADe) and computer-aided diagnosis (CADx) [5–7]. The former focuses on the automatic detection of anomalies (e.g., tumor, etc.) on medical images, while the latter is capable of automatically characterizing anomaly types such as benign and malignant [7]. Since the 1980s, more researchers have become interested in the CAD system development due to availabilities of digital medical imaging and powerful computers. The first CAD system approved by The United States of America Food and Drug Administration was commercially available in 1998 for breast cancer detection [6].

Early AI-based CAD systems in radiology were entirely rule based, and their algorithms could not improve automatically. In contrast, machine learning (ML)-based and deep learning (DL)-based CAD systems can automatically improve their performances through training, and hence, they have become dominant. DL is a subset of ML, and its models have more layers than those of ML. The DL algorithms are capable of modeling high-level abstractions in medical images without predetermined inputs [5,8,9].

A recent systematic review has shown that the DL-based CAD systems in radiology have been developed for a range of areas including breast, cardiovascular, gastrointestinal, hepatological, neurological, respiratory, rheumatic, thyroid and urologic diseases, and trauma. The performances of these CAD systems matched expert readers' capabilities (pooled sensitivity and specificity: 87.0% vs. 86.4% and 92.5% vs. 90.5%), respectively [10]. Apparently, the current AI-based CAD systems might help to address radiologist shortage problems [9–11]. Nevertheless, various systematic reviews have criticized that the diagnostic performance figures reported in many AI-based CAD studies were not trustworthy because of their methodological weaknesses [10,12,13].

Pediatric radiology is a subset of radiology [14–17]. The aforementioned systematic review findings may not be applicable to the pediatric radiology [10,12,13,16,17]. For example, the AI-based CAD systems for breast and prostate cancer detections seem not relevant to children [10,12,13,17]. Although the AI-based CAD is an important topic area in radiology [10,12,13], apparently, only two narrative reviews about various uses of AI in pediatric radiology (e.g., examination booking, image acquisition and post-processing, CAD, etc.) [17] and AI-based CAD in pediatric chest imaging have been published to date [16]. Hence, it is timely to conduct a systematic review about the diagnostic performance of AI-based CAD in pediatric radiology. The purpose of this article is to systematically review the original studies to answer the question: "What are the AI-based CAD applications in pediatric radiology, their diagnostic performances and methods for their performance evaluation?"

2. Materials and Methods

This systematic review of the diagnostic performance of the AI-based CAD in pediatric radiology was conducted as per the preferred reporting items for systematic reviews and meta-analyses (PRISMA) guidelines and patient/population, intervention, comparison, and outcome model. This involved a literature search, article selection, and data extraction and synthesis [10,12–14,18].

2.1. Literature Search

The literature search with the use of electronic scholarly publication databases, including EBSCOhost/Cumulative Index of Nursing and Allied Health Literature Ultimate, Ovid/Embase, PubMed/Medline, ScienceDirect, Scopus, SpringerLink, Web of Science, and Wiley Online Library was conducted on 11 January 2023 to identify articles investigating the diagnostic performance of the AI-based CAD in the pediatric radiology with no publication year restriction [12,19,20]. The search statement used was ("Artificial Intelligence" OR "Machine Learning" OR "Deep Learning") AND ("Computer-Aided Diagnosis" OR "Computer-Aided Detection") AND ("Pediatric" OR "Children") AND ("Radiology" OR "Medical Imaging"). The keywords used in the search were based on the review focus and systematic reviews on the diagnostic performance of the AI-based CAD in radiology [19–23].

2.2. Article Selection

A reviewer with more than 20 years of experience in conducting literature reviews was involved in the article selection process [14,24]. Only peer-reviewed original research articles that were written in English and focused on the AI-based CAD in pediatric radiology with the diagnostic accuracy measures were included. Gray literature, conference proceedings, editorials, review, perspective, opinion, commentary, and non-peer-reviewed (e.g., those published via the arXiv research-sharing platform, etc.) articles were excluded because this systematic review focused on the diagnostic performance of the AI-based CAD in the pediatric radiology and appraisal of the associated methodology reported in the refereed original articles. Papers mainly about image segmentation or clinical prediction instead of disease identification or classification were also excluded [12].

Figure 1 illustrates the details of the article selection process. A three-stage screening process through assessing (1) article titles, (2) abstracts, and (3) full texts against the selection criteria was employed after duplicate article removal from the results of the database search. Every non-duplicate article within the search results was retained until its exclusion could be decided [14,25,26].

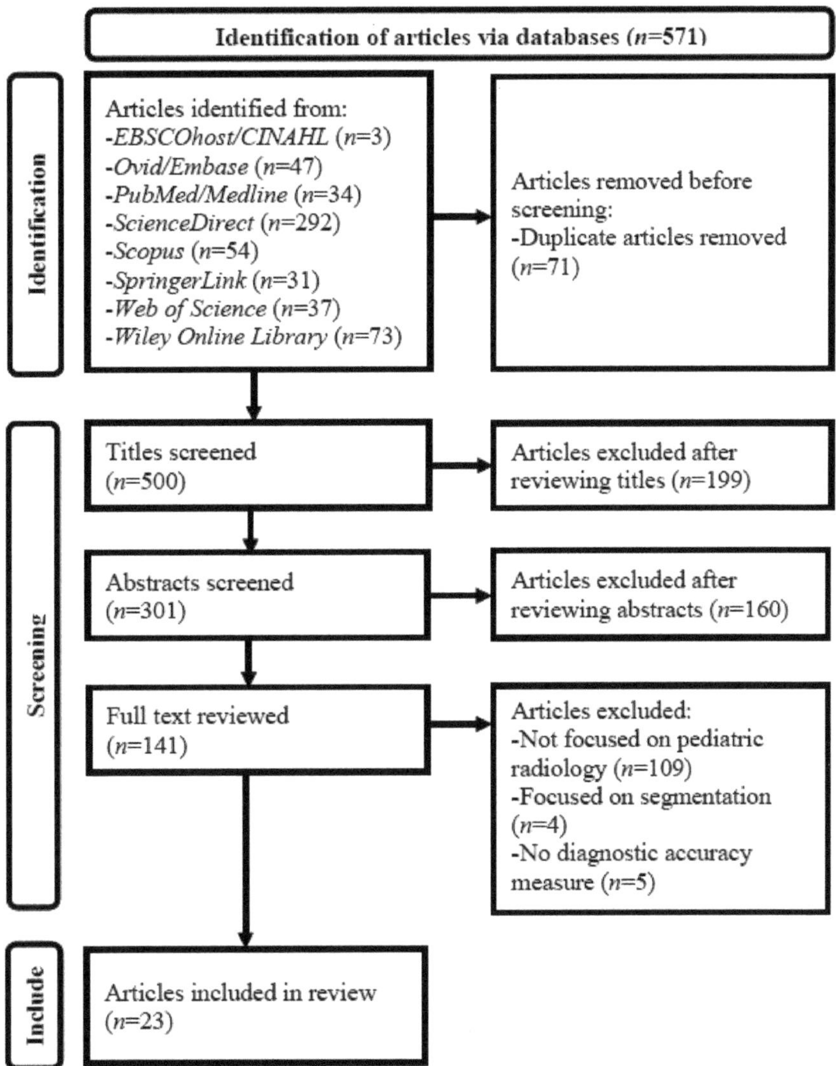

Figure 1. Preferred reporting items for systematic reviews and meta-analyses flow diagram for systematic review of diagnostic performance of artificial intelligence-based computer-aided detection and diagnosis in pediatric radiology. CINAHL, Cumulative Index of Nursing and Allied Health Literature.

2.3. Data Extraction and Synthesis

Two data extraction forms (Tables 1 and 2) were developed based on a recent systematic review on the diagnostic performance of AI-based CAD in radiology [12]. The data, including author name and country, publication year, imaging modality, diagnosis, diagnostic performance of AI-based CAD system (area under receiver operating characteristic curve (AUC), sensitivity, specificity, positive predictive value (PPV), negative predictive value (NPV), accuracy and F1 score), AI type (such as ML and DL) and model (e.g., support vector machine, convolutional neural network (CNN), etc.) for developing the CAD system, study design (either prospective or retrospective), source (such as public dataset by Guangzhou Women and Children's Medical Center, China) and size (e.g., 5858 images, etc.) of dataset for testing the CAD system, patient/population (such as 1–5-year-old children), any sample size calculation, model internal validation type (e.g., 10-fold cross-validation, etc.), any model external validation (i.e., any model testing with use of dataset not involved in internal validation and acquired from different setting), reference standard for ground truth establishment (such as histology and expert consensus), any model performance comparison with clinician and model commercial availability were extracted from each included paper. When diagnostic performance findings were reported for multiple AI-based CAD models in a study, only the values of the best performing model were presented [27]. Meta-analysis was not conducted because this systematic review covered a range of imaging modalities and pathologies, and hence, high study heterogeneity was expected, affecting its usefulness [12,13,28]. The Revised Quality Assessment of Diagnostic Accuracy Studies (QUADAS-2) tool was used to assess the quality of all included studies [9,12,13,19,23,27,29].

3. Results

Twenty-three articles met the selection criteria and were included in this review [30–52]. Table 1 shows their AI-based CAD application areas in the pediatric radiology and the diagnostic performances. These studies covered brain ($n = 9$) [30–38], respiratory ($n = 9$) [42–50], musculoskeletal ($n = 2$) [40,41], urologic ($n = 2$) [51,52] and cardiac imaging ($n = 1$) [39]. The commonest AI-based CAD application area (30.4%, 7/23) was pediatric pneumonia [43,45–50]. No study reported all seven diagnostic accuracy measures [30–52]. Most commonly, the papers (30.4%, 7/23) reported four metrics [30,32,35,42,44,45,52]. Accuracy ($n = 19$) and sensitivity ($n = 18$) were the two most frequently used evaluation metrics [30–39,41–52]. One study only used one measure, AUC [40]. Most of the articles (93.3%, 14/15; 77.8%, 14/18; 73.3%, 11/15; 80.0%, 8/10; 66.6%, 2/3; 84.2%, 16/19; 80.0%, 8/10) reported AI-based CAD model performances of at least 0.83 (AUC), 0.84 (sensitivity), 0.80 (specificity), 0.89 (PPV), 0.63 (NPV), 0.87 (accuracy), and 0.82 (F1 score), respectively. The ranges of the reported performance values were 0.698–0.999 (AUC), 0.420–0.987 (sensitivity), 0.585–1.000 (specificity), 0.600–1.000 (PPV), 0.260–0.971 (NPV), 0.643–0.986 (accuracy), and 0.626–0.983 (F1 score) [30–52]. For the seven studies about AI-based CAD for pneumonia, their model performances were at least 0.850 (AUC), 0.760 (sensitivity), 0.800 (specificity), 0.891 (PPV), 0.905 (accuracy) and 0.903 (F1 score).

Table 1. Artificial intelligence-based computer-aided detection and diagnosis application areas in pediatric radiology and their diagnostic performances.

Author, Year and Country	Modality	Diagnosis	Diagnostic Performance						
			AUC	Sensitivity	Specificity	PPV	NPV	Accuracy	F1 Score
			Brain Imaging						
Dou et al. (2022)—China [30]	MRI	Bipolar disorder	0.830	0.909	0.769	NR	NR	0.854	NR
Kuttala et al. (2022)—Australia, India & United Arab Emirates [31]	MRI	ADHD and ASD	0.850 (ADHA); 0.910 (ASD)	NR	NR	NR	NR	0.854 (ADHA); 0.978 (ASD)	NR
Li et al. (2020)—China [32]	MRI	Posterior fossa tumors	0.865	0.929	0.800	NR	NR	0.878	NR
Peruzzo et al. (2016)—Italy [33]	MRI	Malformations of corpus callosum	0.953	0.923	0.904	0.906	NR	0.914	NR
Prince et al. (2020)—USA [34]	CT & MRI	ACP	0.978	NR	NR	NR	NR	0.979	NR
Tan et al. (2013)—USA [35]	MRI	Congenital sensori-neural hearing loss	0.900	0.890	0.860	NR	NR	0.870	NR
Xiao et al. (2019)—China [36]	MRI	ASD	NR	0.980	0.936	0.959	0.971	0.963	NR
Zahia et al. (2020)—Spain [37]	MRI	Dyslexia	NR	0.750	0.714	0.600	NR	0.727	0.670
Zhou et al. (2021)—China [38]	MRI	ADHD	0.698	0.609	0.676	NR	NR	0.643	0.626
			Cardiac Imaging						
Lee et al. (2022)—South Korea [39]	US	Kawasaki disease	NR	0.841	0.585	0.811	0.633	0.759	0.826
			Musculoskeletal Imaging						
Petibon et al. (2021)—Canada, Israel and USA [40]	SPECT	Low back pain	0.830	NR	NR	NR	NR	NR	NR
Sezer and Sezer (2020)—France and Turkey [41]	US	DDH	NR	0.962	0.980	NR	NR	0.977	NR
			Respiratory Imaging						
Behzadi—Khormouji et al. (2020)—Iran and USA [42]	X-ray	Pulmonary consolidation	0.995	0.987	0.864	NR	NR	0.945	NR

Table 1. *Cont.*

Author, Year and Country	Modality	Diagnosis	Diagnostic Performance						
			AUC	Sensitivity	Specificity	PPV	NPV	Accuracy	F1 Score
Bodapati and Rohith (2022)—India [43]	X-ray	Pneumonia	0.939	NR	NR	NR	NR	0.948	0.959
Helm et al. (2009)—Canada, UK and USA [44]	CT	Pulmonary nodules	NR	0.420	1.000	1.000	0.260	NR	NR
Jiang and Chen (2022)-China [45]	X-ray	Pneumonia	NR	0.894	NR	0.918	NR	0.912	0.903
Liang and Zheng (2020)-China [46]	X-ray	Pneumonia	0.953	0.967	NR	0.891	NR	0.905	0.927
Mahomed et al. (2020)-Netherlands and South Africa [47]	X-ray	Primary-endpoint pneumonia	0.850	0.760	0.800	NR	NR	NR	NR
Shouman et al. (2022)-Egypt and Saudi Arabia [48]	X-ray	Bacterial and viral pneumonia	0.999	0.987	0.987	0.979	NR	0.986	0.983
Silva et al. (2022)-Brazil [49]	X-ray	Pneumonia	NR	0.945	NR	0.957	NR	NR	0.951
Vrbančič and Podgorelec (2022)-Slovenia [50]	X-ray	Pneumonia	0.952	0.976	0.927	0.973	NR	0.963	0.974
Urologic Imaging									
Guan et al. (2022)-China [51]	US	Hydronephrosis	NR	NR	NR	NR	NR	0.891	0.895
Zheng et al. (2019)-China and USA [52]	US	CAKUT	0.920	0.86	0.880	NR	NR	0.870	NR

ACP, adamantinomatous craniopharyngioma; ADHD, attention deficit hyperactivity disorder; ASD, autism spectrum disorder; AUC, area under receiver operating characteristic curve; CAKUT, congenital abnormalities of kidney and urinary tract; CT, computed tomography; DDH, developmental dysplasia of hip; MRI, magnetic resonance imaging; NPV, negative predictive value; NR, not reported; PPV, positive predictive value; SPECT, single-photon emission computed tomography; UK, United Kingdom; US, ultrasound; USA, United States of America.

Table 2 presents the included study characteristics. Overall, 18 out of 23 (78.3%) studies were published in the last three years [30–32,34,37–43,45–51]. Most of them (72.7%, 16/22) developed the DL-based CAD systems [31,34,36,37,39–43,45,46,48–52]. Of these 16 DL-based systems, 75% (*n* = 12) used the CNN model [34,37,39–43,46,48–51]. Magnetic resonance imaging (MRI) (*n* = 9) [30–38] and X-ray (*n* = 8) [42,43,45–50] were most frequently used by the AI-based CAD models for the brain and respiratory disease diagnoses, respectively. The majority of studies (69.6%, 16/23) collected the datasets retrospectively [31,33,34,36,38–40,42–46,48–50,52]. Of these 16 retrospective studies, about one-third (*n* = 11) relied on the public datasets [31,34,36,38,42,43,45,46,48–50]; most of them (*n* = 7) used the chest X-ray dataset consisting of 1741 normal and 4346 pneumonia images of 6087 1–5-year-old children collected from the Guangzhou Women and Children's Medical Center, China [42,43,45,46,48–50]. No study calculated the sample size for the data collection [30–52]. Most of the studies (60.9%, 14/23) collected less than 233 cases [30–41,44,52], and about one-third (*n* = 7) collected data of less than 87 patients for testing their systems [30,32,34,35,37,40,44]. Hence, for the model internal validation, more than half of the studies (*n* = 13) used the cross-validation to address the small test set issue [30,33–40,47,50–52]. However, all but one did not conduct the external validation [30–43,45–52]. The only exception conducted external validation for a commercial AI-based CAD system evaluation [44]. Less than one-fifth of the included studies (*n* = 4) used the consensus diagnosis as the reference standard (ground truth) for the model training and performance evaluation [33,42,44,47], and one-quarter (*n* = 6) did not report the reference standard [31,43,45,46,48,49]. Only about one-fifth (*n* = 5) compared their model performances with those of clinicians [33,34,40,44,47], and most of these (60%, 3/5) were the studies using the consensus diagnosis as the reference standard [33,44,47].

Figure 2 shows the quality assessment summary of all (23) studies based on the QUADAS-2 tool. Only around one-third of the studies had a low risk of bias [34–38,41,44,52] and concern regarding applicability for the patient selection category [30,34–38,41,44,52]. The low risk of bias of the reference standard was only noted in about half of them [32–38,40,42,47,50,52].

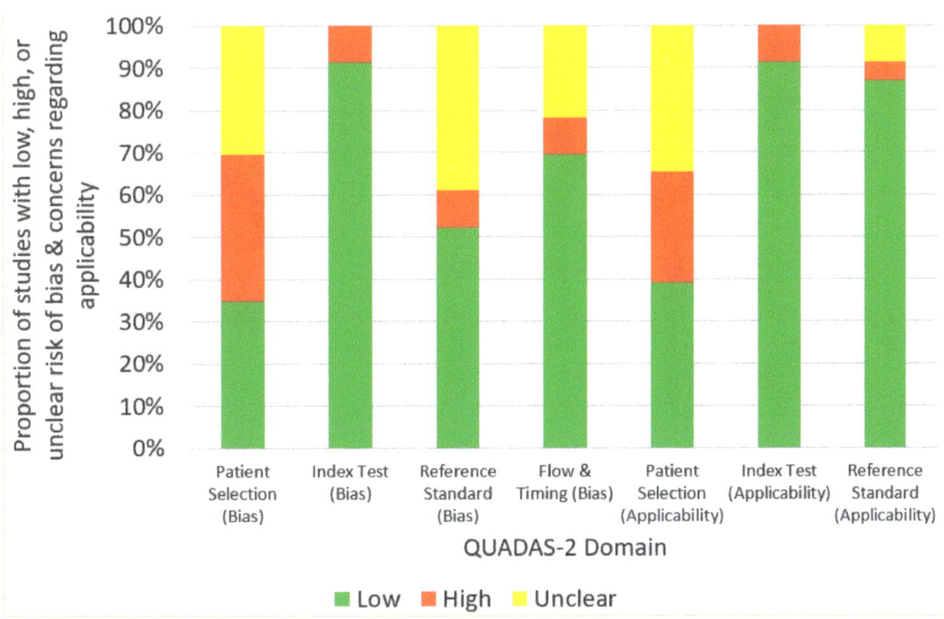

Figure 2. Quality assessment summary of all (23) included studies based on Revised Quality Assessment of Diagnostic Accuracy Studies tool.

Table 2. Study characteristics of artificial intelligence-based computer-aided detection and diagnosis in pediatric radiology.

Author, Year and Country	Modality	Diagnosis	AI Type and Model	Study Design	Dataset Source	Test Set Size	Patient/ Population	Sample Size Calculation	Internal Validation Type	External Validation	Reference Standard	AI vs. Clinician	Commercial Availability
						Brain Imaging							
Dou et al. (2022)—China [30]	MRI	Bipolar disorder	ML-LR	Prospective	Private dataset by Second Xiangya Hospital, China	52 scans	12–18-year-old children	No	2-fold cross-validation	No	Clinical diagnosis	No	No
Kuttala et al. (2022)— Australia, India and United Arab Emirates [31]	MRI	ADHD and ASD	DL-GAN and softmax	Retrospective	Public datasets (ADHD-200 and Autism Brain Imaging Data Exchange II)	217 scans	Children (median ages for baseline and follow-up scans: 12 and 15 years, respectively)	No	NR	No	NR	No	No
Li et al. (2020)—China [32]	MRI	Posterior fossa tumors	ML-SVM	Prospective	Private dataset by Affiliated Hospital of Zhengzhou University, China	45 scans	0–14-year-old children	No	Repeated hold-out with 70:30 random split	No	Histology	No	No
Peruzzo et al. (2016)—Italy [33]	MRI	Malformations of corpus callosum	ML-SVM	Retrospective	Private dataset by Scientific Institute "Eugenio Medea", Italy	104 scans	2–12-year-old children	No	Leave-one-out cross validation	No	Expert consensus	Yes	No
Prince et al. (2020)—USA [34]	CT and MRI	ACP	DL-CNN	Retrospective	Public dataset (ATPC Consortium) and private datasets by Children's Hospital Colorado and St. Jude Children's Research Hospital, USA	86 CT-MRI scans	Children	No	60:40 random split and 5-fold cross validation	No	Histology	Yes	No
Tan et al. (2013)—USA [35]	MRI	Congenital sensori-neural hearing loss	ML-SVM	Prospective	Private dataset by Cincinnati Children's Hospital Medical Center, USA	39 scans	8–24-month-old children	No	Leave-one-out cross-validation	No	Follow-up	No	No
Xiao et al. (2019)—China [36]	MRI	ASD	DL-SAE and softmax	Retrospective	Public dataset (Autism Brain Imaging Data Exchange II)	198 scans	5–12-year-old children	No	11-, 33-, 66-, 99- and 198-fold cross-validation	No	Clinical diagnosis	No	No

Table 2. *Cont.*

Author, Year and Country	Modality	Diagnosis	AI Type and Model	Study Design	Dataset Source	Test Set Size	Patient/ Population	Sample Size Calculation	Internal Validation Type	External Valida-tion	Reference Standard	AI vs. Clinician	Commercial Availability
Zahia et al. (2020)—Spain [37]	MRI	Dyslexia	DL-CNN	Prospective	Private dataset by University Hospital of Cruces, Spain	55 scans	9–12-year-old children	No	4-fold cross validation	No	Clinical diagnosis	No	No
Zhou et al. (2021)—China [38]	MRI	ADHD	ML-SVM	Retrospective	Public dataset (Adolescent Brain Cognitive Development Data Repository)	232 scans	9–10-year-old children	No	10-fold cross-validation	No	Clinical diagnosis	No	No
Cardiac Imaging													
Lee et al. (2022)—South Korea [39]	US	Kawasaki disease	DL-CNN	Retrospective	Private dataset by Yonsei University Gangnam Severance Hospital, South Korea	203 scans	Children	No	10-fold cross-validation	No	Single expert reader	No	No
Musculoskeletal Imaging													
Petibon et al. (2021)—Canada, Israel and USA [40]	SPECT	Low back pain	DL-CNN	Retrospective	Private dataset by Boston Children's Hospital, USA	65 scans	10–17 years old children	No	3-fold cross-validation	No	Other-ground truth established by artificial lesion insertion	Yes	No
Sezer and Sezer (2020)—France and Turkey [41]	US	DDH	DL-CNN	Prospective	Private dataset	203 scans	0–6-month-old children	No	70:30 random split	No	Single expert reader	No	No

Table 2. *Cont.*

Author, Year and Country	Modality	Diagnosis	AI Type and Model	Study Design	Dataset Source	Test Set Size	Patient/ Population	Sample Size Calculation	Internal Validation Type	External Valida-tion	Reference Standard	AI vs. Clinician	Commercial Availability
					Respiratory Imaging								
Behzadi—Khormouji et al. (2020)—Iran and USA [42]	X-ray	Pulmonary consolida-tion	DL-CNN	Retrospective	Public dataset by Guangzhou Women and Children's Medical Center, China	582 images	1–5-year-old children	No	90:10 random split	No	Expert consensus	No	No
Bodapati and Rohith (2022)—India [43]	X-ray	Pneumonia	DL-CNN and CapsNet	Retrospective	Public dataset by Guangzhou Women and Children's Medical Center, China	640 images	1–5-year-old children	No	NR	No	NR	No	No
Helm et al. (2009)—Canada, UK and USA [44]	CT	Pulmonary nodules	NR	Retrospective	Private dataset by a tertiary pediatric hospital	29 scans	3 years and 11 months to 18-year-old children	No	NR	Yes	Expert and reader consensus	Yes	Yes
Jiang and Chen (2022)—China [45]	X-ray	Pneumonia	DL-ViT	Retrospective	Public dataset by Guangzhou Women and Children's Medical Center, China	624 images	1–5-year-old children	No	NR	No	NR	No	No
Liang and Zheng (2020)—China [46]	X-ray	Pneumonia	DL-CNN	Retrospective	Public dataset by Guangzhou Women and Children's Medical Center, China	624 images	1–5-year-old children	No	90:10 random split	No	NR	No	No
Mahomed et al. (2020)—Netherlands and South Africa [47]	X-ray	Primary-endpoint pneumo-nia	ML-SVM	Prospective	Private dataset by Chris Hani Baragwanath Academic Hospital, South Africa	858 digitized images	1–59-month-old children	No	10-fold cross-validation	No	Reader consensus	Yes	No

23

Table 2. *Cont.*

Author, Year and Country	Modality	Diagnosis	AI Type and Model	Study Design	Dataset Source	Test Set Size	Patient/ Population	Sample Size Calculation	Internal Validation Type	External Validation	Reference Standard	AI vs. Clinician	Commercial Availability
Shouman et al. (2022)—Egypt and Saudi Arabia [48]	X-ray	Bacterial and viral pneumonia	DL-CNN and LSTM	Retrospective	Public dataset by Guangzhou Women and Children's Medical Center, China	586 images	1–5-year-old children	No	90:10 random split	No	NR	No	No
Silva et al. (2022)—Brazil [49]	X-ray	Pneumonia	DL-CNN	Retrospective	Public dataset by Guangzhou Women and Children's Medical Center, China	1172 images	1–5-year-old children	No	NR	No	NR	No	No
Vrbančič and Podgorelec (2022)—Slovenia [50]	X-ray	Pneumonia	DL-CNN and SGD	Retrospective	Public dataset by Guangzhou Women and Children's Medical Center, China	5858 images	1–5-year-old children	No	10-fold cross-validation	No	Expert readers	No	No
Urologic Imaging													
Guan et al. (2022)—China [51]	US	Hydronephrosis	DL-CNN	Prospective	Private dataset by Beijing Children's Hospital, China	3257 images	Children	No	10-fold cross-validation	No	Readers and experts without consensus	No	No
Zheng et al. (2019)—China and USA [52]	US	CAKUT	DL-SVM	Retrospective	Private dataset by Children's Hospital of Philadelphia, USA	100 scans	Children with mean age of 111 days (SD: 262)	No	10-fold cross-validation	No	Clinical diagnosis	No	No

ACP, adamantinomatous craniopharyngioma; ADHD, attention deficit hyperactivity disorder; AI, artificial intelligence; ASD, autism spectrum disorder; ATPC, Advancing Treatment for Pediatric Craniopharyngioma; CAKUT, congenital abnormalities of kidney and urinary tract; CapsNet, capsule network; CNN, convolutional neural network; CT, computed tomography; DDH, developmental dysplasia of hip; DL, deep learning; GAN, generative adversarial network; LR, logistic regression; LSTM, long short-term memory; ML, machine learning; MRI, magnetic resonance imaging; NR, not reported; SAE, stacked auto-encoder; SD, standard deviation; SGD, stochastic gradient descent; SPECT, single-photon emission computed tomography; SVM, support vector machine; UK, United Kingdom; US, ultrasound; USA, United States of America; ViT, vision transformer.

4. Discussion

This article is the first systematic review on the diagnostic performance of the AI-based CAD in the pediatric radiology covering the brain [30–38], respiratory [42–50], musculoskeletal [40,41], urologic [51,52] and cardiac imaging [39]. Hence, it advances the previous two narrative reviews about various uses of AI in the pediatric radiology [17] and the AI-based CAD in the pediatric chest imaging [16] published in 2021 and 2022, respectively. Most of the included studies reported AI-based CAD model performances of at least 0.83 (AUC), 0.84 (sensitivity), 0.80 (specificity), 0.89 (PPV), 0.63 (NPV), 0.87 (accuracy), and 0.82 (F1 score) [30–52]. However, the diagnostic performances of these CAD systems appeared a bit lower than those reported in the systematic review of the AI-based CAD in the radiology (pooled sensitivity and specificity: 0.87 and 0.93, respectively) [10]. In addition, the pediatric pneumonia was the only disease that was investigated by more than two studies [43,45–50]. Although these studies reported that their CAD performances for the pneumonia diagnosis were at least 0.850 (AUC), 0.760 (sensitivity), 0.800 (specificity), 0.891 (PPV), 0.905 (accuracy) and 0.903 (F1 score), which would be sufficient to support less experienced pediatric radiologists in image interpretation, all but one were the retrospective studies and relied on the chest X-ray dataset consisting of 1741 normal and 4346 pneumonia images of 6087 1–5-year-old children collected from the Guangzhou Women and Children's Medical Center, China [13,43–50]. It is noted that the use of the public dataset could facilitate AI-based CAD model performance comparison with other similar studies [43]. On the other hand, this approach would affect the model generalization ability (i.e., unable to maintain the performance when applying to different settings), causing the model to be unfit for real clinical situations [10,46]. Although techniques such as the cross-validation can be used to improve the AI-based CAD model generalization ability [37], only one of these studies used the cross-validation approach [50], while half of them did not report the internal validation type [43,45,49]. In addition, some ground truths given in the public datasets might be inaccurate, indicating potential reference standard issues [10,42]. These studies did not calculate the required sample size; perform the external validation; and compare their model performances with radiologists, but they are essential for the demonstration of the trustworthiness of study findings [43,45,46,48–50]. As per Table 2, the aforementioned methodological issues were also common for other included studies. These issues are found in many studies about the AI-based CAD in the radiology as well [10,12,13].

Table 2 reveals that the DL and its model, CNN, were commonly used for the development of the AI-based CAD systems in the pediatric radiology similar to the situation in the radiology [13]. According to the recent narrative review about the AI-based CAD in the pediatric chest imaging published in 2022, 144 Conformité Européenne-marked AI-based CAD systems for brain (35%), respiratory, (27%), musculoskeletal (11%), breast (11%), other (7%), abdominal (6%) and cardiac (4%) imaging were commercially available in the radiology [16]. The proportions of these systems are comparable to the findings of this systematic review that the brain, respiratory and musculoskeletal imaging were the three most popular application areas of the AI-based CAD in the pediatric radiology and the cardiac imaging was the least (Table 1). However, except for Helm et al.'s retrospective study about the detection of pediatric pulmonary nodules in 29 3–18-year-old patients with the use of the AI-based CAD system developed for adults [44], no commercial system was involved in the included studies (Table 2) [30–43,45–52]. Helm et al.'s study [44] was the only one that performed the external validation of the CAD system with the reference standard established by the consensus of six radiologists, and one of the few compared the CAD performance with the clinicians. However, that study only used four evaluation measures: sensitivity (0.42), specificity (1.00), PPV (1.00) and NPV (0.26), and the other metrics commonly used in more clinically focused studies, AUC and accuracy, were not reported [10,12,44,53]. This highlights that even for a more clinically focused AI-based CAD study in the pediatric radiology with the better design, the common methodological weaknesses such as the retrospective data collection with limited information of patient characteristics reported and cases included, and no sample size calculation, were still prevalent (Table 2) [44,54,55]. Hence, these explain the findings in Figure 2 that the concern regarding applicability was found in the patient selection, and the risk of bias was noted in both patient selection and reference standard categories, although similar results were also reported in the systematic reviews of the AI-based CAD in the radiology [10,12].

Apparently, the AI-based CAD in the pediatric radiology is less developed when compared to its adult counterpart. For example, not many studies were published before 2020 [33,35,36,44,52,56–76], and the studies mainly focused on the MRI and X-ray and particular patient cohorts [30–52] (Table 2). Although Schalekamp et al.'s [16] narrative review published in 2022 suggested the use of the AI-based CAD designed for the adult population in children, Helm et al.'s [44] study demonstrated that this approach yielded low sensitivity (0.42) and NPV (0.26) in detecting pediatric pulmonary nodules because of the smaller nodule sizes in children. Hence, AI-based CAD systems specifically designed/finetuned for the pediatric radiology by researchers and/or commercial companies seem necessary in the future. In addition, for further research, more robust study designs that can address the aforementioned methodological issues (especially the lack of the external validation) are essential for providing trustworthy findings to convince clinical centers to adopt the AI-based CAD in the pediatric radiology. In this way, the potential benefits of the CAD could be realized in a wider context [5,10,12,13].

This systematic review has two major limitations. The article selection, data extraction, and synthesis were performed by a single author, albeit one with more than 20 years of experience in conducting the literature reviews [14]. According to a recent methodological systematic review, this is an appropriate arrangement provided that the single reviewer is experienced [14,24,77–79]. Additionally, through adherence to the PRISMA guidelines and the use of the data extraction forms (Tables 1 and 2) devised based on the recent systematic review on the diagnostic performance of the AI-based CAD in the radiology and the QUADAS-2 tool, the potential bias should be addressed to a certain extent [12,14,26,29]. In addition, only articles in English identified via databases were included, potentially affecting the comprehensiveness of this systematic review [9,21,26,27,80]. Nevertheless, this review still has a wider coverage about the AI-based CAD in the pediatric radiology than the previous two narrative reviews [16,17].

5. Conclusions

This systematic review shows that the AI-based CAD for the pediatric radiology could be applied in the brain, respiratory, musculoskeletal, urologic and cardiac imaging. Most of the studies (93.3%, 14/15; 77.8%, 14/18; 73.3%, 11/15; 80.0%, 8/10; 66.6%, 2/3; 84.2%, 16/19; 80.0%, 8/10) reported AI-based CAD model performances of at least 0.83 (AUC), 0.84 (sensitivity), 0.80 (specificity), 0.89 (PPV), 0.63 (NPV), 0.87 (accuracy), and 0.82 (F1 score), respectively. The pediatric pneumonia was the most common pathology covered in the included studies. They reported that their CAD performances for pneumonia diagnosis were at least 0.850 (AUC), 0.760 (sensitivity), 0.800 (specificity), 0.891 (PPV), 0.905 (accuracy) and 0.903 (F1 score). Although these diagnostic performances appear sufficient to support the less experienced pediatric radiologists in the image interpretation, a range of methodological weaknesses such as the retrospective data collection, no sample size calculation, overreliance on public dataset, small test set size, limited patient cohort coverage, use of diagnostic accuracy measures and cross-validation, lack of model external validation and model performance comparison with clinicians, and risk of bias of reference standard are found in the included studies. Hence, their AI-based CAD systems might be unfit for the real clinical situations due to a lack of generalization ability. In the future, more AI-based CAD systems specifically designed/fine-tuned for a wider range of imaging modalities and pathologies in the pediatric radiology should be developed. In addition, more robust study designs should be used in further research to address the aforementioned methodological issues for providing the trustworthy findings to convince the clinical centers to adopt the AI-based CAD in the pediatric radiology. In this way, the potential benefits of the CAD could be realized in a wider context.

Funding: This work received no external funding.

Institutional Review Board Statement: Not applicable.

Informed Consent Statement: Not applicable.

Data Availability Statement: Not applicable.

Conflicts of Interest: The author declares no conflict of interest.

References

1. Lu, Y.; Zheng, N.; Ye, M.; Zhu, Y.; Zhang, G.; Nazemi, E.; He, J. Proposing intelligent approach to predicting air kerma within radiation beams of medical x-ray imaging systems. *Diagnostics* **2023**, *13*, 190. [CrossRef] [PubMed]
2. Sun, Z.; Ng, C.K.C. Artificial intelligence (enhanced super-resolution generative adversarial network) for calcium deblooming in coronary computed tomography angiography: A feasibility study. *Diagnostics* **2022**, *12*, 991. [CrossRef]
3. Sun, Z.; Ng, C.K.C. Finetuned super-resolution generative adversarial network (artificial intelligence) model for calcium deblooming in coronary computed tomography angiography. *J. Pers. Med.* **2022**, *12*, 1354. [CrossRef]
4. Ng, C.K.C.; Leung, V.W.S.; Hung, R.H.M. Clinical evaluation of deep learning and atlas-based auto-contouring for head and neck radiation therapy. *Appl. Sci.* **2022**, *12*, 11681. [CrossRef]
5. Choy, G.; Khalilzadeh, O.; Michalski, M.; Do, S.; Samir, A.E.; Pianykh, O.S.; Geis, J.R.; Pandharipande, P.V.; Brink, J.A.; Dreyer, K.J. Current applications and future impact of machine learning in radiology. *Radiology* **2018**, *288*, 318–328. [CrossRef] [PubMed]
6. Chan, H.P.; Hadjiiski, L.M.; Samala, R.K. Computer-aided diagnosis in the era of deep learning. *Med. Phys.* **2020**, *47*, e218–e227. [CrossRef]
7. Suzuki, K. A review of computer-aided diagnosis in thoracic and colonic imaging. *Quant. Imaging Med. Surg.* **2012**, *2*, 163–176. [CrossRef] [PubMed]
8. Wardlaw, J.M.; Mair, G.; von Kummer, R.; Williams, M.C.; Li, W.; Storkey, A.J.; Trucco, E.; Liebeskind, D.S.; Farrall, A.; Bath, P.M.; et al. Accuracy of automated computer-aided diagnosis for stroke imaging: A critical evaluation of current evidence. *Stroke* **2022**, *53*, 2393–2403. [CrossRef]
9. Harris, M.; Qi, A.; Jeagal, L.; Torabi, N.; Menzies, D.; Korobitsyn, A.; Pai, M.; Nathavitharana, R.R.; Ahmad Khan, F. A systematic review of the diagnostic accuracy of artificial intelligence-based computer programs to analyze chest x-rays for pulmonary tuberculosis. *PLoS ONE* **2019**, *14*, e0221339. [CrossRef]
10. Liu, X.; Faes, L.; Kale, A.U.; Wagner, S.K.; Fu, D.J.; Bruynseels, A.; Mahendiran, T.; Moraes, G.; Shamdas, M.; Kern, C.; et al. A comparison of deep learning performance against health-care professionals in detecting diseases from medical imaging: A systematic review and meta-analysis. *Lancet Digit. Heal.* **2019**, *1*, e271–e297. [CrossRef]
11. Masud, R.; Al-Rei, M.; Lokker, C. Computer-aided detection for breast cancer screening in clinical settings: Scoping review. *JMIR Med. Inform.* **2019**, *7*, e12660. [CrossRef]
12. Aggarwal, R.; Sounderajah, V.; Martin, G.; Ting, D.S.W.; Karthikesalingam, A.; King, D.; Ashrafian, H.; Darzi, A. Diagnostic accuracy of deep learning in medical imaging: A systematic review and meta-analysis. *NPJ Digit. Med.* **2021**, *4*, 65. [CrossRef]
13. Vasey, B.; Ursprung, S.; Beddoe, B.; Taylor, E.H.; Marlow, N.; Bilbro, N.; Watkinson, P.; McCulloch, P. Association of clinician diagnostic performance with machine learning-based decision support systems: A systematic review. *JAMA Netw. Open* **2021**, *4*, e211276. [CrossRef]
14. Ng, C.K.C. Artificial intelligence for radiation dose optimization in pediatric radiology: A systematic review. *Children* **2022**, *9*, 1044. [CrossRef] [PubMed]
15. Al Mahrooqi, K.M.S.; Ng, C.K.C.; Sun, Z. Pediatric computed tomography dose optimization strategies: A literature review. *J. Med. Imaging Radiat. Sci.* **2015**, *46*, 241–249. [CrossRef]
16. Schalekamp, S.; Klein, W.M.; van Leeuwen, K.G. Current and emerging artificial intelligence applications in chest imaging: A pediatric perspective. *Pediatr. Radiol.* **2022**, *52*, 2120–2130. [CrossRef] [PubMed]
17. Davendralingam, N.; Sebire, N.J.; Arthurs, O.J.; Shelmerdine, S.C. Artificial intelligence in paediatric radiology: Future opportunities. *Br. J. Radiol.* **2021**, *94*, 20200975. [CrossRef] [PubMed]
18. Kim, K.W.; Lee, J.; Choi, S.H.; Huh, J.; Park, S.H. Systematic review and meta-analysis of studies evaluating diagnostic test accuracy: A practical review for clinical researchers-Part I. general guidance and tips. *Korean J. Radiol.* **2015**, *16*, 1175–1187. [CrossRef] [PubMed]
19. Zhao, W.J.; Fu, L.R.; Huang, Z.M.; Zhu, J.Q.; Ma, B.Y. Effectiveness evaluation of computer-aided diagnosis system for the diagnosis of thyroid nodules on ultrasound: A systematic review and meta-analysis. *Medicine* **2019**, *98*, e16379. [CrossRef]
20. Devnath, L.; Summons, P.; Luo, S.; Wang, D.; Shaukat, K.; Hameed, I.A.; Aljuaid, H. Computer-aided diagnosis of coal workers' pneumoconiosis in chest x-ray radiographs using machine learning: A systematic literature review. *Int. J. Environ. Res. Public Health* **2022**, *19*, 6439. [CrossRef]
21. Groen, A.M.; Kraan, R.; Amirkhan, S.F.; Daams, J.G.; Maas, M. A systematic review on the use of explainability in deep learning systems for computer aided diagnosis in radiology: Limited use of explainable AI? *Eur. J. Radiol.* **2022**, *157*, 110592. [CrossRef] [PubMed]

22. Henriksen, E.L.; Carlsen, J.F.; Vejborg, I.M.; Nielsen, M.B.; Lauridsen, C.A. The efficacy of using computer-aided detection (CAD) for detection of breast cancer in mammography screening: A systematic review. *Acta Radiol.* **2019**, *60*, 13–18. [CrossRef] [PubMed]
23. Gundry, M.; Knapp, K.; Meertens, R.; Meakin, J.R. Computer-aided detection in musculoskeletal projection radiography: A systematic review. *Radiography* **2018**, *24*, 165–174. [CrossRef]
24. Waffenschmidt, S.; Knelangen, M.; Sieben, W.; Bühn, S.; Pieper, D. Single screening versus conventional double screening for study selection in systematic reviews: A methodological systematic review. *BMC Med. Res. Methodol.* **2019**, *19*, 132. [CrossRef]
25. Ng, C.K.C. A review of the impact of the COVID-19 pandemic on pre-registration medical radiation science education. *Radiography* **2022**, *28*, 222–231. [CrossRef]
26. PRISMA: Transparent Reporting of Systematic Reviews and Meta-Analyses. Available online: https://www.prisma-statement.org (accessed on 25 January 2023).
27. Xu, L.; Gao, J.; Wang, Q.; Yin, J.; Yu, P.; Bai, B.; Pei, R.; Chen, D.; Yang, G.; Wang, S.; et al. Computer-aided diagnosis systems in diagnosing malignant thyroid nodules on ultrasonography: A systematic review and meta-analysis. *Eur. Thyroid J.* **2020**, *9*, 186–193. [CrossRef]
28. Imrey, P.B. Limitations of meta-analyses of studies with high heterogeneity. *JAMA Netw. Open* **2020**, *3*, e1919325. [CrossRef]
29. Whiting, P.F.; Rutjes, A.W.; Westwood, M.E.; Mallett, S.; Deeks, J.J.; Reitsma, J.B.; Leeflang, M.M.; Sterne, J.A.; Bossuyt, P.M.; QUADAS-2 Group. QUADAS-2: A revised tool for the quality assessment of diagnostic accuracy studies. *Ann. Intern. Med.* **2011**, *155*, 529–536. [CrossRef]
30. Dou, R.; Gao, W.; Meng, Q.; Zhang, X.; Cao, W.; Kuang, L.; Niu, J.; Guo, Y.; Cui, D.; Jiao, Q.; et al. Machine learning algorithm performance evaluation in structural magnetic resonance imaging-based classification of pediatric bipolar disorders type I patients. *Front. Comput. Neurosci.* **2022**, *16*, 915477. [CrossRef]
31. Kuttala, D.; Mahapatra, D.; Subramanian, R.; Oruganti, V.R.M. Dense attentive GAN-based one-class model for detection of autism and ADHD. *J. King Saud Univ. Comput. Inf. Sci.* **2022**, *34*, 10444–10458. [CrossRef]
32. Li, M.; Wang, H.; Shang, Z.; Yang, Z.; Zhang, Y.; Wan, H. Ependymoma and pilocytic astrocytoma: Differentiation using radiomics approach based on machine learning. *J. Clin. Neurosci.* **2020**, *78*, 175–180. [CrossRef]
33. Peruzzo, D.; Arrigoni, F.; Triulzi, F.; Righini, A.; Parazzini, C.; Castellani, U. A framework for the automatic detection and characterization of brain malformations: Validation on the corpus callosum. *Med. Image Anal.* **2016**, *32*, 233–242. [CrossRef]
34. Prince, E.W.; Whelan, R.; Mirsky, D.M.; Stence, N.; Staulcup, S.; Klimo, P.; Anderson, R.C.E.; Niazi, T.N.; Grant, G.; Souweidane, M.; et al. Robust deep learning classification of adamantinomatous craniopharyngioma from limited preoperative radiographic images. *Sci. Rep.* **2020**, *10*, 16885. [CrossRef]
35. Tan, L.; Chen, Y.; Maloney, T.C.; Caré, M.M.; Holland, S.K.; Lu, L.J. Combined analysis of sMRI and fMRI imaging data provides accurate disease markers for hearing impairment. *Neuroimage Clin.* **2013**, *3*, 416–428. [CrossRef]
36. Xiao, Z.; Wu, J.; Wang, C.; Jia, N.; Yang, X. Computer-aided diagnosis of school-aged children with ASD using full frequency bands and enhanced SAE: A multi-institution study. *Exp. Ther. Med.* **2019**, *17*, 4055–4063. [CrossRef]
37. Zahia, S.; Garcia-Zapirain, B.; Saralegui, I.; Fernandez-Ruanova, B. Dyslexia detection using 3D convolutional neural networks and functional magnetic resonance imaging. *Comput. Methods Programs Biomed.* **2020**, *197*, 105726. [CrossRef]
38. Zhou, X.; Lin, Q.; Gui, Y.; Wang, Z.; Liu, M.; Lu, H. Multimodal MR images-based diagnosis of early adolescent attention-deficit/hyperactivity disorder using multiple kernel learning. *Front. Neurosci.* **2021**, *15*, 710133. [CrossRef]
39. Lee, H.; Eun, Y.; Hwang, J.Y.; Eun, L.Y. Explainable deep learning algorithm for distinguishing incomplete Kawasaki disease by coronary artery lesions on echocardiographic imaging. *Comput. Methods Programs Biomed.* **2022**, *223*, 106970. [CrossRef]
40. Petibon, Y.; Fahey, F.; Cao, X.; Levin, Z.; Sexton-Stallone, B.; Falone, A.; Zukotynski, K.; Kwatra, N.; Lim, R.; Bar-Sever, Z.; et al. Detecting lumbar lesions in 99m Tc-MDP SPECT by deep learning: Comparison with physicians. *Med. Phys.* **2021**, *48*, 4249–4261. [CrossRef]
41. Sezer, A.; Sezer, H.B. Deep convolutional neural network-based automatic classification of neonatal hip ultrasound images: A novel data augmentation approach with speckle noise reduction. *Ultrasound Med. Biol.* **2020**, *46*, 735–749. [CrossRef]
42. Behzadi-Khormouji, H.; Rostami, H.; Salehi, S.; Derakhshande-Rishehri, T.; Masoumi, M.; Salemi, S.; Keshavarz, A.; Gholamrezanezhad, A.; Assadi, M.; Batouli, A. Deep learning, reusable and problem-based architectures for detection of consolidation on chest x-ray images. *Comput. Methods Programs Biomed.* **2020**, *185*, 105162. [CrossRef]
43. Bodapati, J.D.; Rohith, V.N. ChxCapsNet: Deep capsule network with transfer learning for evaluating pneumonia in paediatric chest radiographs. *Measurement* **2022**, *188*, 110491. [CrossRef]
44. Helm, E.J.; Silva, C.T.; Roberts, H.C.; Manson, D.; Seed, M.T.; Amaral, J.G.; Babyn, P.S. Computer-aided detection for the identification of pulmonary nodules in pediatric oncology patients: Initial experience. *Pediatr. Radiol.* **2009**, *39*, 685–693. [CrossRef]
45. Jiang, Z.; Chen, L. Multisemantic level patch merger vision transformer for diagnosis of pneumonia. *Comput. Math. Method Med.* **2022**, *2022*, 7852958. [CrossRef]
46. Liang, G.; Zheng, L. A transfer learning method with deep residual network for pediatric pneumonia diagnosis. *Comput. Methods Programs Biomed.* **2020**, *187*, 104964. [CrossRef]
47. Mahomed, N.; van Ginneken, B.; Philipsen, R.H.H.M.; Melendez, J.; Moore, D.P.; Moodley, H.; Sewchuran, T.; Mathew, D.; Madhi, S.A. Computer-aided diagnosis for World Health Organization-defined chest radiograph primary-endpoint pneumonia in children. *Pediatr. Radiol.* **2020**, *50*, 482–491. [CrossRef]

48. Shouman, M.A.; El-Fiky, A.; Hamada, S.; El-Sayed, A.; Karar, M.E. Computer-assisted lung diseases detection from pediatric chest radiography using long short-term memory networks. *Comput. Electr. Eng.* **2022**, *103*, 108402. [CrossRef]

49. Silva, L.; Araújo, L.; Ferreira, V.; Neto, R.; Santos, A. Convolutional neural networks applied in the detection of pneumonia by x-ray images. *Int. J. Innov. Comput. Appl.* **2022**, *13*, 187–197. [CrossRef]

50. Vrbančič, G.; Podgorelec, V. Efficient ensemble for image-based identification of pneumonia utilizing deep CNN and SGD with warm restarts. *Expert Syst. Appl.* **2022**, *187*, 115834. [CrossRef]

51. Guan, Y.; Peng, H.; Li, J.; Wang, Q. A mutual promotion encoder-decoder method for ultrasonic hydronephrosis diagnosis. *Methods* **2022**, *203*, 78–89. [CrossRef]

52. Zheng, Q.; Furth, S.L.; Tasian, G.E.; Fan, Y. Computer-aided diagnosis of congenital abnormalities of the kidney and urinary tract in children based on ultrasound imaging data by integrating texture image features and deep transfer learning image features. *J. Pediatr. Urol.* **2019**, *15*, 75.e1–75.e7. [CrossRef]

53. Kleinfelder, T.R.; Ng, C.K.C. Effects of image postprocessing in digital radiography to detect wooden, soft tissue foreign bodies. *Radiol. Technol.* **2022**, *93*, 544–554. Available online: https://pubmed.ncbi.nlm.nih.gov/35790309/ (accessed on 30 January 2023).

54. Sun, Z.; Ng, C.K.C.; Wong, Y.H.; Yeong, C.H. 3D-printed coronary plaques to simulate high calcification in the coronary arteries for investigation of blooming artifacts. *Biomolecules* **2021**, *11*, 1307. [CrossRef] [PubMed]

55. Ng, C.K.C.; Sun, Z. Development of an online automatic computed radiography dose data mining program: A preliminary study. *Comput. Methods Programs Biomed.* **2010**, *97*, 48–52. [CrossRef]

56. Christe, A.; Peters, A.A.; Drakopoulos, D.; Heverhagen, J.T.; Geiser, T.; Stathopoulou, T.; Christodoulidis, S.; Anthimopoulos, M.; Mougiakakou, S.G.; Ebner, L. Computer-aided diagnosis of pulmonary fibrosis using deep learning and CT images. *Investig. Radiol.* **2019**, *54*, 627–632. [CrossRef]

57. Tanaka, H.; Chiu, S.W.; Watanabe, T.; Kaoku, S.; Yamaguchi, T. Computer-aided diagnosis system for breast ultrasound images using deep learning. *Phys. Med. Biol.* **2019**, *64*, 235013. [CrossRef] [PubMed]

58. Kim, H.L.; Ha, E.J.; Han, M. Real-world performance of computer-aided diagnosis system for thyroid nodules using ultrasonography. *Ultrasound Med. Biol.* **2019**, *45*, 2672–2678. [CrossRef] [PubMed]

59. Jeongy, E.Y.; Kim, H.L.; Ha, E.J.; Park, S.Y.; Cho, Y.J.; Han, M. Computer-aided diagnosis system for thyroid nodules on ultrasonography: Diagnostic performance and reproducibility based on the experience level of operators. *Eur. Radiol.* **2019**, *29*, 1978–1985. [CrossRef]

60. Park, H.J.; Kim, S.M.; La Yun, B.; Jang, M.; Kim, B.; Jang, J.Y.; Lee, J.Y.; Lee, S.H. A computer-aided diagnosis system using artificial intelligence for the diagnosis and characterization of breast masses on ultrasound: Added value for the inexperienced breast radiologist. *Medicine* **2019**, *98*, e14146. [CrossRef]

61. Zhang, S.; Sun, F.; Wang, N.; Zhang, C.; Yu, Q.; Zhang, M.; Babyn, P.; Zhong, H. Computer-aided diagnosis (CAD) of pulmonary nodule of thoracic CT image using transfer learning. *J. Digit. Imaging* **2019**, *32*, 995–1007. [CrossRef]

62. Wei, R.; Lin, K.; Yan, W.; Guo, Y.; Wang, Y.; Li, J.; Zhu, J. Computer-aided diagnosis of pancreas serous cystic neoplasms: A radiomics method on preoperative MDCT images. *Technol. Cancer Res. Treat.* **2019**, *18*, 1533033818824339. [CrossRef]

63. Chen, C.H.; Lee, Y.W.; Huang, Y.S.; Lan, W.R.; Chang, R.F.; Tu, C.Y.; Chen, C.Y.; Liao, W.C. Computer-aided diagnosis of endobronchial ultrasound images using convolutional neural network. *Comput. Methods Programs Biomed.* **2019**, *177*, 175–182. [CrossRef] [PubMed]

64. Gong, J.; Liu, J.; Hao, W.; Nie, S.; Wang, S.; Peng, W. Computer-aided diagnosis of ground-glass opacity pulmonary nodules using radiomic features analysis. *Phys. Med. Biol.* **2019**, *64*, 135015. [CrossRef]

65. Li, L.; Liu, Z.; Huang, H.; Lin, M.; Luo, D. Evaluating the performance of a deep learning-based computer-aided diagnosis (DL-CAD) system for detecting and characterizing lung nodules: Comparison with the performance of double reading by radiologists. *Thorac. Cancer.* **2019**, *10*, 183–192. [CrossRef]

66. Bajaj, V.; Pawar, M.; Meena, V.K.; Kumar, M.; Sengur, A.; Guo, Y. Computer-aided diagnosis of breast cancer using bi-dimensional empirical mode decomposition. *Neural Comput. Appl.* **2019**, *31*, 3307–3315. [CrossRef]

67. Nayak, A.; Baidya Kayal, E.; Arya, M.; Culli, J.; Krishan, S.; Agarwal, S.; Mehndiratta, A. Computer-aided diagnosis of cirrhosis and hepatocellular carcinoma using multi-phase abdomen CT. *Int. J. Comput. Assist. Radiol. Surg.* **2019**, *14*, 1341–1352. [CrossRef] [PubMed]

68. Greer, M.D.; Lay, N.; Shih, J.H.; Barrett, T.; Bittencourt, L.K.; Borofsky, S.; Kabakus, I.; Law, Y.M.; Marko, J.; Shebel, H.; et al. Computer-aided diagnosis prior to conventional interpretation of prostate mpMRI: An international multi-reader study. *Eur. Radiol.* **2018**, *28*, 4407–4417. [CrossRef] [PubMed]

69. Ishioka, J.; Matsuoka, Y.; Uehara, S.; Yasuda, Y.; Kijima, T.; Yoshida, S.; Yokoyama, M.; Saito, K.; Kihara, K.; Numao, N.; et al. Computer-aided diagnosis of prostate cancer on magnetic resonance imaging using a convolutional neural network algorithm. *BJU Int.* **2018**, *122*, 411–417. [CrossRef]

70. Song, Y.; Zhang, Y.D.; Yan, X.; Liu, H.; Zhou, M.; Hu, B.; Yang, G. Computer-aided diagnosis of prostate cancer using a deep convolutional neural network from multiparametric MRI. *J. Magn. Reason. Imaging.* **2018**, *48*, 1570–1577. [CrossRef]

71. Yoo, Y.J.; Ha, E.J.; Cho, Y.J.; Kim, H.L.; Han, M.; Kang, S.Y. Computer-aided diagnosis of thyroid nodules via ultrasonography: Initial clinical experience. *Korean J. Radiol.* **2018**, *19*, 665–672. [CrossRef]

72. Al-Antari, M.A.; Al-Masni, M.A.; Choi, M.T.; Han, S.M.; Kim, T.S. A fully integrated computer-aided diagnosis system for digital x-ray mammograms via deep learning detection, segmentation, and classification. *Int. J. Med. Inform.* **2018**, *117*, 44–54. [CrossRef] [PubMed]

73. Choi, Y.J.; Baek, J.H.; Park, H.S.; Shim, W.H.; Kim, T.Y.; Shong, Y.K.; Lee, J.H. A computer-aided diagnosis system using artificial intelligence for the diagnosis and characterization of thyroid nodules on ultrasound: Initial clinical assessment. *Thyroid* **2017**, *27*, 546–552. [CrossRef] [PubMed]

74. Li, S.; Jiang, H.; Wang, Z.; Zhang, G.; Yao, Y.D. An effective computer aided diagnosis model for pancreas cancer on PET/CT images. *Comput. Methods Programs Biomed.* **2018**, *165*, 205–214. [CrossRef]

75. Chang, C.C.; Chen, H.H.; Chang, Y.C.; Yang, M.Y.; Lo, C.M.; Ko, W.C.; Lee, Y.F.; Liu, K.L.; Chang, R.F. Computer-aided diagnosis of liver tumors on computed tomography images. *Comput. Methods Programs Biomed.* **2017**, *145*, 45–51. [CrossRef]

76. Cho, E.; Kim, E.K.; Song, M.K.; Yoon, J.H. Application of computer-aided diagnosis on breast ultrasonography: Evaluation of diagnostic performances and agreement of radiologists according to different levels of experience. *J. Ultrasound Med.* **2018**, *37*, 209–216. [CrossRef]

77. Sun, Z.; Ng, C.K.C.; Sá Dos Reis, C. Synchrotron radiation computed tomography versus conventional computed tomography for assessment of four types of stent grafts used for endovascular treatment of thoracic and abdominal aortic aneurysms. *Quant. Imaging Med. Surg.* **2018**, *8*, 609–620. [CrossRef]

78. Almutairi, A.M.; Sun, Z.; Ng, C.; Al-Safran, Z.A.; Al-Mulla, A.A.; Al-Jamaan, A.I. Optimal scanning protocols of 64-slice CT angiography in coronary artery stents: An in vitro phantom study. *Eur. J. Radiol.* **2010**, *74*, 156–160. [CrossRef] [PubMed]

79. Sun, Z.; Ng, C.K.C. Use of synchrotron radiation to accurately assess cross-sectional area reduction of the aortic branch ostia caused by suprarenal stent wires. *J. Endovasc. Ther.* **2017**, *24*, 870–879. [CrossRef]

80. Zebari, D.A.; Ibrahim, D.A.; Zeebaree, D.Q.; Haron, H.; Salih, M.S.; Damaševičius, R.; Mohammed, M.A. Systematic review of computing approaches for breast cancer detection based computer aided diagnosis using mammogram images. *Appl. Artif. Intell.* **2021**, *35*, 2157–2203. [CrossRef]

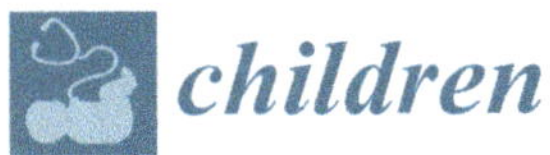

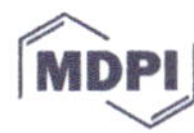

Review

Efficacy of Artificial Intelligence in the Categorisation of Paediatric Pneumonia on Chest Radiographs: A Systematic Review

Erica Louise Field [1], Winnie Tam [2,*], Niamh Moore [1] and Mark McEntee [1]

1   Discipline of Medical Imaging and Radiation Therapy, University College Cork, College Road, T12 K8AF Cork, Ireland
2   Department of Midwifery and Radiography, University of London, Northampton Square, London EC1V 0HB, UK
*   Correspondence: winnie.tam@city.ac.uk

Abstract: This study aimed to systematically review the literature to synthesise and summarise the evidence surrounding the efficacy of artificial intelligence (AI) in classifying paediatric pneumonia on chest radiographs (CXRs). Following the initial search of studies that matched the pre-set criteria, their data were extracted using a data extraction tool, and the included studies were assessed via critical appraisal tools and risk of bias. Results were accumulated, and outcome measures analysed included sensitivity, specificity, accuracy, and area under the curve (AUC). Five studies met the inclusion criteria. The highest sensitivity was by an ensemble AI algorithm (96.3%). DenseNet201 obtained the highest level of specificity and accuracy (94%, 95%). The most outstanding AUC value was achieved by the VGG16 algorithm (96.2%). Some of the AI models achieved close to 100% diagnostic accuracy. To assess the efficacy of AI in a clinical setting, these AI models should be compared to that of radiologists. The included and evaluated AI algorithms showed promising results. These algorithms can potentially ease and speed up diagnosis once the studies are replicated and their performances are assessed in clinical settings, potentially saving millions of lives.

Keywords: artificial intelligence (AI); deep learning (DL); paediatric pneumonia; chest radiograph; computer-aided detection (CAD)

Citation: Field, E.L.; Tam, W.; Moore, N.; McEntee, M. Efficacy of Artificial Intelligence in the Categorisation of Paediatric Pneumonia on Chest Radiographs: A Systematic Review. *Children* **2023**, *10*, 576. https://doi.org/10.3390/children10030576

Academic Editor: Francesca Santamaria

Received: 8 February 2023
Revised: 4 March 2023
Accepted: 15 March 2023
Published: 17 March 2023

1. Introduction

Pneumonia is one of the leading causes of global mortality and morbidity [1] and the leading cause of death among children under five years of age [2]. The chest X-ray (CXR) is the primary diagnostic tool in both the detection and diagnosis of paediatric pneumonia [1] due to the unspecific and subjective signs and symptoms of the infection [3], while sputum cultures are often extremely difficult to ascertain [4]. A lack of expert radiologists, particularly in resource-constrained countries, where paediatric pneumonia is endemic with shockingly high mortality rates [5], might have significantly contributed to the high mortality rates.

Pneumonia, as a whole, often manifests on a chest radiograph as areas of increased opacity [6]. Bacterial and viral pneumonia, the two most common aetiologies, have different appearances on CXRs and have different treatment regimes [7]. Bacterial pneumonia often manifests as a lobar and focal consolidation, whereas viral pneumonia can present as an interstitial pattern. Although the different appearances on CXRs, interpretation of the aetiologies on CXR varies amongst physicians [3] as the opacification presented is often variable and irregular [8].

There are roughly two billion CXRs performed in the United States annually [9], with approximately two million of these being on paediatric patients [10]. The accumulation of imaging data and the increasing complexity of medical history pose new challenges in modern medicine but also open up new opportunities in implementing artificial intelligence (AI) for effective detection and diagnosis [3].

AI is defined, by the father of AI, Marvin Minsky, as "the science of making machines do things that would require intelligence if done by men" [11]. Machine learning (ML) and deep learning (DL) are both under the umbrella of AI. In ML, the system identifies patterns by learning from data and makes decisions with minimal programming and human interventions [12,13]. On the other hand, DL involves multiple processing layers, with individual layers extracting a large number of features from unstructured data before progressing to the next layer [14]. Higher levels typically represent more abstract concepts [15] and can give a more comprehensive depiction or decision after passing through the entire network [14].

Computer-aided detection (CAD) was first introduced between 1963–1973 [16–21], and utilised in facets of radiology, predominantly the identification of lung, colorectal, breast, and prostate cancer, over the past 20 years [22–33]. CAD is trained in a regimental fashion and can only be improved by inputting more data, while AI has the autonomous learning element in which explicit programming and human instructions are not necessary for its improvement [34].

AI interpretation of medical images can also potentially be utilised in low- to middle-income countries, where the availability of radiologists is limited. Currently, interpretations rely on teleradiology [35], though it is not flawless. Cross-border teleradiology, in particular, is challenging due to liability in case of malpractice, healthcare professional registration restrictions, data protection, quality of the reporting, healthcare system, and cultural differences [36]. This is where AI can potentially come in to make the diagnostic and treatment pathway of patients smoother, especially in these developing nations [35].

Recent studies exhibited that AI algorithms outperformed radiologists in the detection of skin cancer [37], diabetic retinopathy [38], and haemorrhage identification [39], probably owing to the recent AI model advancement [40] and widening availability of electronic health record, providing more training materials. The winner of the Turning Prize said in 2016, "We should stop training radiologists now. It's just completely obvious that within five years, DL is going to do better than radiologists" [41].

These successes have sparked interest in the automated diagnosis of paediatric pneumonia in CXRs, reflected by the increased number of studies regarding the diagnostic accuracy of AI for paediatric pneumonia over the last number of years. When being asked about AI's role in diagnosing pneumonia, Andrew Ng, the co-founder and head of Google Brain, went further—"radiologists should be worried about their jobs" [42]. A recent study by Kermany et al. [43] showed that a customised AI model demonstrated a good level of classification of paediatric pneumonia on CXR. By systematically reviewing the current literature regarding AI and paediatric pneumonia, the current gap in literature may be filled and potentially result in a dramatic improvement of accuracy and efficiency in differentiating bacterial and viral pneumonia in paediatric CXRs in a clinical setting [44].

2. Materials and Methods

2.1. Literature Search Strategy

A comprehensive search of the literature was conducted in accordance with the Preferred Reporting Items for Systematic Reviews and Meta-Analyses (PRISMA) guidelines [45] in February 2021. A number of pre-determined keywords were pooled for this systematic search, and subsequent medical subject headings (MeSH terms) were generated. The MeSH terms used for this systematic search include: ('artificial intelligence' OR 'deep learning' OR 'CNN' OR 'convolutional neural network' OR 'deep residual network'), ('paediatric pneumonia' OR 'pediatric pneumonia' OR 'child* pneumonia'), 'classification', ('chest xray' OR 'chest x ray' OR 'chest x-ray' OR 'CXR' OR 'chest radiograph'). The pre-determined MeSH terms were then linked using Boolean operators specific to each database (PubMed, Science Direct, Embase, ProQuest, and Scopus) to retrieve all relevant articles evaluating the diagnostic efficacy of AI models in the classification of paediatric pneumonia in CXRs. These databases were chosen as opposed to others due to their scientific reliability and coverage. Google Scholar and the reference lists of relevant studies were also screened to ensure as much grey literature was captured as possible. In addition to these criteria, only peer-reviewed articles published in English were included in this review.

2.2. Study Selection and Eligibility Criteria

The initial selection involved screening the paper title and abstract. After gathering all of the potential papers, a full-text assessment was undertaken. Studies were included if they met the following inclusion criteria: only original cross-sectional studies, cohort or case-control studies, randomised control trials (RCTs), or diagnostic accuracy studies in the format of either journal articles, dissertations, conference proceedings, or grey literature, disseminated between 2015–2021, were included. In addition, the paper must analyse/evaluate the AI performances on the classification of pneumonia aetiology (bacterial or viral) using CXR test datasets of children under the age of 16 years in acute healthcare settings. These studies should also evaluate the AI performance using at least three of the following parameters: accuracy, sensitivity, specificity, and area under the curve (AUC). Studies which did not meet one of the inclusion criteria, or inaccessible full-text articles, were excluded.

2.3. Data Extraction

Data extraction was performed on included studies using the amended version of the Cochrane 'Data collection form for Intervention Reviews for RCTs and Non-RCTS—Template' [46]. A general overview of the data extracted is as follows: general information (report title, study ID, date form completed, etc.), study eligibility, characteristics of study (the aim of the study, design, etc.), participants (description of images from dataset, setting, age, etc.), AI model (AI type, mode, detail, etc.), outcomes (sensitivity, specificity, accuracy, AUC), and other information (key conclusions, future work, etc.). Each data extraction form was reviewed by two independent reviewers, and any discrepancies were resolved by consensus. The original data extraction form applied to each included study can be obtained from the author on request.

2.4. Quality Assessment and Risk of Bias

A quality assessment of each included study was examined using the Critical Appraisal Skills Programme (CASP) Diagnostic Study Checklist, which focuses on the result validity, measuring parameters and transparency, and generalisability [47]. A risk of bias (ROB) assessment was also completed for each included study. The tool utilised for the ROB was adjusted from Hung et al.'s QUADAS-2 tool, whose systematic review investigated the use and performance of AI applications in the maxillofacial and dental radiology [48]. This adapted ROB consists of four key domains: patient selection, index test, reference standard, and study flow and timing with regard to both applicability and general ROB. Each domain was assessed using a three-point scale, low (green), high (red), or unclear (yellow), to reflect the level of bias concerns accordingly. All CASP and ROB checklists were reviewed by two independent reviewers, and any discrepancies were resolved by consensus.

3. Results

3.1. Study Selection

A total of 114 papers were identified following the initial systematic search from the six databases previously mentioned, combined with subsequent manual searches of reference lists based on the relevance of their title to the research question. After the removal of duplicates, 82 papers were considered for abstract screening, and 24 out of 82 were considered suitable and underwent full-text assessment. Of these 24 papers, 19 did not meet the required inclusion criteria due to a broad spectrum of reasons, such as the study did not classify pneumonia subtypes, the study did not include the desired (number of) outcome measures, and the dataset used was inapplicable. Five papers were included at last. The PRISMA flowchart exhibiting the study eligibility and selection process is presented in Figure 1. The two independent reviewers agreed with the initial search and study selection/eligibility process, with no discrepancies found.

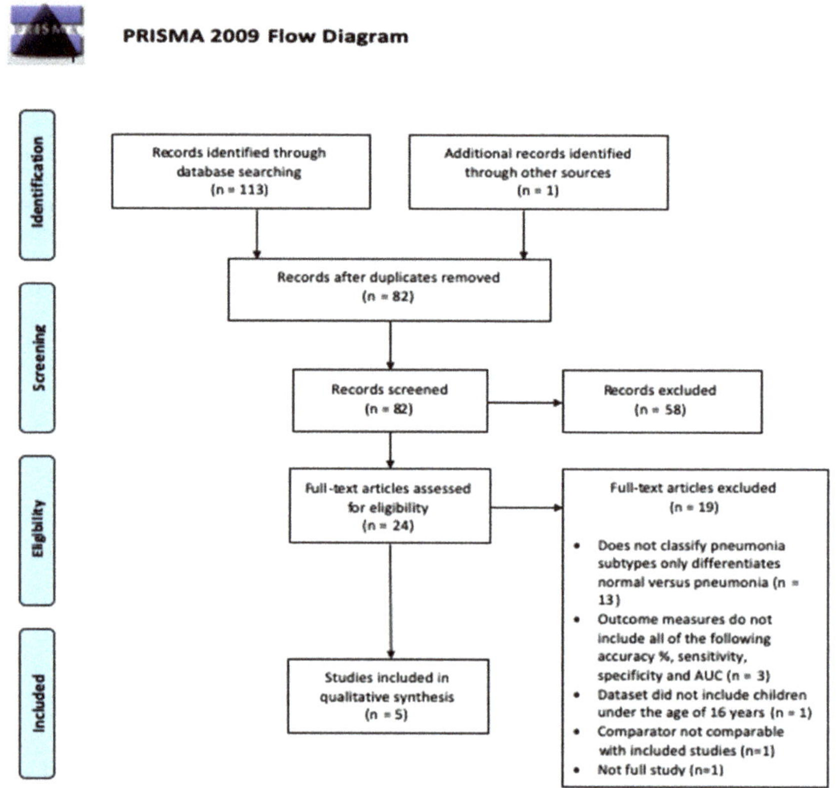

Figure 1. A PRISMA flow chart illustrating the filtering and gathering of eligible studies.

3.2. Study Quality Assessment

The quality assessment of each included study can be seen in Figure 2. All five papers were considered as having a "low" risk of concern in the workflow, and both reference standard domains. Gu et al.'s study [44] was regarded as a "high" risk in the subject selection domain because the authors omitted CXRs without the condition of interest. In the index test domain, Rajaraman et al.'s [5] and Karthikeyan's studies [49] were graded as "unclear", while Ferreira et al.'s study [50] was considered a "high" risk, in the same domain due to the fact that the performance of the AI model was not evaluated by an independent testing dataset that was excluded in the development of the AI model. Since the QUADAS-2 tool allows a study to contain one element ascertaining a high risk of bias without being eliminated [48], none of the selected studies were eliminated at this stage.

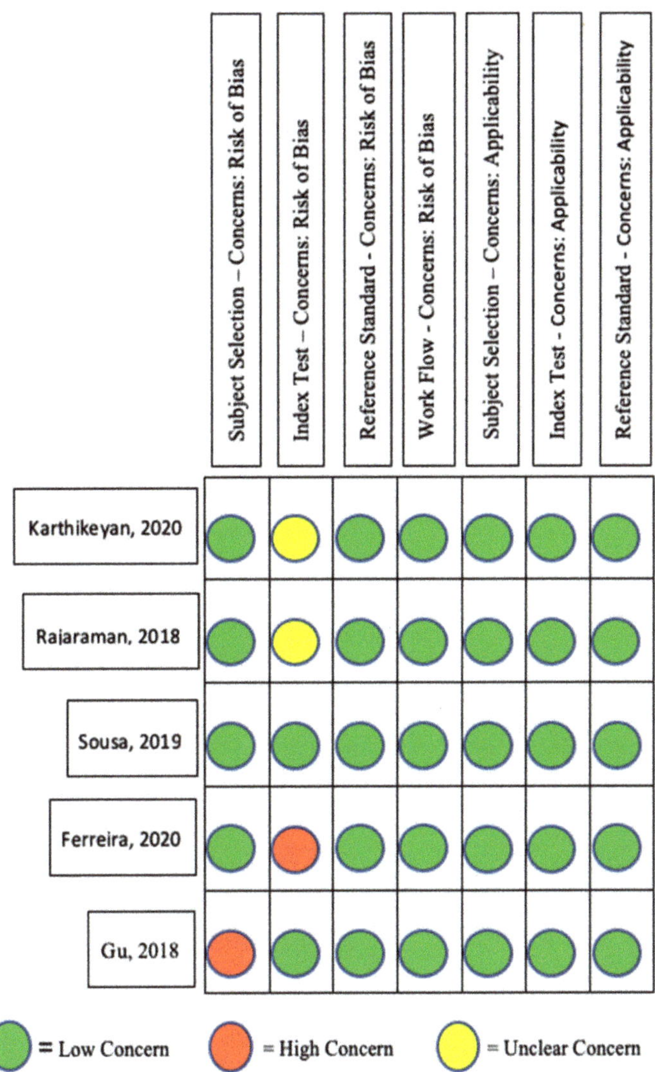

Figure 2. A risk of bias table of the five included studies from the adapted version of the QUADAS-2 ROB tool with a three-point scale indicating low, high and unclear concern [5,44,49–51].

3.3. Study Characteristics

Table 1 presents the characteristics of the included papers. All included papers utilised the same public dataset obtained from Guangzhou Women and Children's Medical Centre; however, each paper varied regarding the number of images used for training, testing and validation sets. All studies, apart from Gu et al.'s study [44], included 'normal' radiographs, as well as bacterial and viral pneumonia, labelled radiographs in their dataset. There were some similarities and overlaps with regard to pre-processing methods employed, though none of the studies utilised precisely the same pre-processing strategy.

Table 1. Characteristics of the AI algorithm employed, pre-processing methods utilised, as well as detailed descriptions of each dataset used in each of the included studies. Abbreviations: N/A (not applicable), ROI (region of interest), CLAHE (contrast limited adaptive histogram equalisation), CNN (convolutional neural network).

Author, Year	Algorithm Employed	Type of AI	Age of Participants (Years)	No. of Images (by Aetiology)					No. of Images Used in				Pre-Processing Methods
				Normal	Pneumonia			Total	Training	Validation	Testing		
					Bacterial	Viral	Total						
Gu et al., 2018 [44]	• AlexNet, • 3 Handcrafted Features (Gray level co-concurrence matrix-based feature extraction, Haar wavelet transform feature extraction, Histogram of oriented gradient-based feature extraction)	DL	5.5 ± 4.2	0	2665	1848	4513	4513	3211	802	500	• All input ROIs images were resized to 256 × 256 matrices. • An AlexNet-based fully convolutional networks model was applied for the segmentation of lung regions.
Ferreira et al., 2020 [50]	• VGG16, • Inception V3 architecture	DL	1–5	1349	2538	1345	3883	5232	5232	0	624	• CLAHE method • Chest cavity cropped from radiograph images • Combination of the above
Sousa et al., 2019 [51]	• CNN, • Inception V3 Architecture	DL	1–5	1349	2538	1345	3883	5232	624	0	624	• All of the images were re-dimensioned to a 300 × 300 pixels resolution and saved in a one-dimensional format
Rajaraman et al., 2018 [5]	• Sequential CNN, • Residual CNN, • Inception CNN, • Customised VGG16	DL	1–5	1349	2538	1345	3883	5232	5232	0	624	• Both baseline and cropped images are resampled to 1024 × 1024 pixel • Cropped using an algorithm based on anatomical atlases to detect the lung ROI automatically
Karthikeyan 2020 [49]	• AlexNet, • ResNet18, • DenseNet201, • SqueezeNet	DL	1–5	1341	2561	1345	3906	5247	4500	0	398	• The images were resized to 227 × 227 pixels

15. Bengio, Y. Deep Learning of Representations: Looking Forward. In *Statistical Language and Speech Processing [Internet]*; Lecture Notes in Computer Science; Dediu, A.H., Martín-Vide, C., Mitkov, R., Truthe, B., Eds.; Springer: Berlin/Heidelberg, Germany, 2013; Volume 7978, pp. 1–37. Available online: http://link.springer.com/10.1007/978-3-642-39593-2_1 (accessed on 28 September 2022).
16. Lodwick, G.S.; Haun, C.L.; Smith, W.E.; Keller, R.F.; Robertson, E.D. Computer Diagnosis of Primary Bone Tumors: A Preliminary Report. *Radiology* **1963**, *80*, 273–275. [CrossRef]
17. Meyers, P.H.; Nice, C.M.; Becker, H.C.; Nettleton, W.J.; Sweeney, J.W.; Meckstroth, G.R. Automated Computer Analysis of Radiographic Images. *Radiology* **1964**, *83*, 1029–1034. [CrossRef]
18. Winsberg, F.; Elkin, M.; Macy, J.; Bordaz, V.; Weymouth, W. Detection of Radiographic Abnormalities in Mammograms by Means of Optical Scanning and Computer Analysis. *Radiology* **1967**, *89*, 211–215. [CrossRef]
19. Kruger, R.P.; Townes, J.R.; Hall, D.L.; Dwyer, S.J.; Lodwick, G.S. Automated Radiographic Diagnosis via Feature Extraction and Classification of Cardiac Size and Shape Descriptors. *IEEE Trans. Biomed. Eng.* **1972**, *19*, 174–186. [CrossRef]
20. Kruger, R.P.; Thompson, W.B.; Turner, A.F. Computer Diagnosis of Pneumoconiosis. *IEEE Trans. Syst. Man. Cybern.* **1974**, *4*, 40–49. [CrossRef]
21. Yamamoto, Y.; Nishiyama, Y.; Sota, T.; Miyai, M.; Uchibe, T.; Yada, N.; Nishiyama, Y.; Kitagaki, H. Improvement in the Quantification of Striatal Tracer Uptake in Single-photon Emission Computed Tomography With 123I-ioflupane Using a Cadmium-zinc-telluride Semiconductor Camera. *Shimane J. Med. Sci.* **2017**, *34*, 35–40.
22. Hadjiiski, L.; Sahiner, B.; Chan, H.-P. Advances in computer-aided diagnosis for breast cancer. *Curr. Opin. Obstet. Gynecol.* **2006**, *18*, 64–70. [CrossRef]
23. Hambrock, T.; Vos, P.C.; Hulsbergen–van de Kaa, C.A.; Barentsz, J.O.; Huisman, H.J. Prostate Cancer: Computer-aided Diagnosis with Multiparametric 3-T MR Imaging—Effect on Observer Performance. *Radiology* **2013**, *266*, 521–530. [CrossRef]
24. Dromain, C.; Boyer, B.; Ferré, R.; Canale, S.; Delaloge, S.; Balleyguier, C. Computed-aided diagnosis (CAD) in the detection of breast cancer. *Eur. J. Radiol.* **2013**, *82*, 417–423. [CrossRef]
25. Firmino, M.; Morais, A.H.; Mendoça, R.M.; Dantas, M.R.; Hekis, H.R.; Valentim, R. Computer-aided detection system for lung cancer in computed tomography scans: Review and future prospects. *Biomed. Eng. Online* **2014**, *13*, 41. [CrossRef]
26. Mosquera-Lopez, C.; Agaian, S.; Velez-Hoyos, A.; Thompson, I. Computer-aided prostate cancer diagnosis from digitized histopathology: A review on texture-based systems. *IEEE Rev. Biomed. Eng.* **2014**, *8*, 98–113. [CrossRef] [PubMed]
27. El Abbadi, N.K.; AL, J.; Taee, E. Breast Cancer Diagnosis by CAD. *Int. J. Comput. Appl.* **2014**, *100*, 25–29.
28. Brown, M.S.; Lo, P.; Goldin, J.; Barnoy, E.; Kim, G.H.J.; McNItt-Gray, M.; Aberle, D.R. Toward clinically usable CAD for lung cancer screening with computed tomography. *Eur. Radiol.* **2014**, *24*, 2719–2728. [CrossRef] [PubMed]
29. Mittal, A.; Kaur, M. Computer-aided-diagnosis in colorectal cancer: A survey of state of the art techniques. In Proceedings of the 2016 International Conference on Inventive Computation Technologies (ICICT), Coimbatore, India, 26–27 August 2016.
30. Shariaty, F.; Mousavi, M. Application of CAD systems for the automatic detection of lung nodules. *Inform. Med. Unlocked* **2019**, *15*, 100173. [CrossRef]
31. Chan, H.P.; Samala, R.K.; Hadjiiski, L.M. CAD and AI for breast cancer—Recent development and challenges. *Br. J. Radiol.* **2020**, *93*, 20190580. [CrossRef]
32. Oliveira, S.P.; Neto, P.C.; Fraga, J.; Montezuma, D.; Monteiro, A.; Monteiro, J.; Ribeiro, L.; Gonçalves, S.; Pinto, I.M.; Cardoso, J.S. CAD systems for colorectal cancer from WSI are still not ready for clinical acceptance. *Sci. Rep.* **2021**, *11*, 14358. [CrossRef]
33. Porto-Álvarez, J.; Barnes, G.T.; Villanueva, A.; García-Figueiras, R.; Baleato-González, S.; Zapico, E.H.; Souto-Bayarri, M. Digital Medical X-ray Imaging, CAD in Lung Cancer and Radiomics in Colorectal Cancer: Past, Present and Future. *Appl. Sci.* **2023**, *13*, 2218. [CrossRef]
34. European Society of Radiology (ESR). What the radiologist should know about artificial intelligence—An ESR white paper. *Insights Imaging* **2019**, *10*, 44. [CrossRef]
35. Frija, G.; Blažić, I.; Frush, D.P.; Hierath, M.; Kawooya, M.; Donoso-Bach, L.; Brkljačić, B. How to improve access to medical imaging in low- and middle-income countries ? *Eclinicalmedicine* **2021**, *38*, 101034. [CrossRef]
36. Legido-Quigley, H.; Doering, N.; McKee, M. Challenges facing teleradiology services across borders in the European union: A qualitative study. *Health Policy Technol.* **2014**, *3*, 160–166. [CrossRef]
37. Esteva, A.; Kuprel, B.; Novoa, R.A.; Ko, J.; Swetter, S.M.; Blau, H.M.; Thrun, S. Dermatologist-level classification of skin cancer with deep neural networks. *Nature* **2017**, *542*, 115–118. [CrossRef]
38. Son, J.; Shin, J.Y.; Kim, H.D.; Jung, K.-H.; Park, K.H.; Park, S.J. Development and Validation of Deep Learning Models for Screening Multiple Abnormal Findings in Retinal Fundus Images. *Ophthalmology* **2020**, *127*, 85–94. [CrossRef]
39. Grewal, M.; Srivastava, M.M.; Kumar, P.; Varadarajan, S. RADnet: Radiologist level accuracy using deep learning for hemorrhage detection in CT scans. In Proceedings of the 2018 IEEE 15th International Symposium on Biomedical Imaging (ISBI 2018), Washington, DC, USA, 4–7 April 2018; pp. 281–284. Available online: https://ieeexplore.ieee.org/document/8363574/ (accessed on 28 September 2022).
40. Stephen, O.; Sain, M.; Maduh, U.J.; Jeong, D.-U. An Efficient Deep Learning Approach to Pneumonia Classification in Healthcare. *J. Healthc. Eng.* **2019**, *2019*, 1–7. [CrossRef]
41. Siddhartha, M.A.I. Versus M.D.—What happens when diagnosis is automated? *The New Yorker*, 27 March 2017; Annals of Medicine.
42. The Economist. Images Aren't Everything. Economists, 9 June 2018; Leaders Section. Available online: https://www.economist.com/leaders/2018/06/07/ai-radiology-and-the-future-of-work (accessed on 28 September 2022).

43. Kermany, D.S.; Goldbaum, M.; Cai, W.; Valentim, C.C.S.; Liang, H.; Baxter, S.L.; McKeown, A.; Yang, G.; Wu, X.; Yan, F.; et al. Identifying Medical Diagnoses and Treatable Diseases by Image-Based Deep Learning. *Cell* **2018**, *172*, 1122–1131.e9. [CrossRef]

44. Gu, X.; Pan, L.; Liang, H.; Yang, R. Classification of Bacterial and Viral Childhood Pneumonia Using Deep Learning in Chest Radiography. In Proceedings of the 3rd International Conference on Multimedia and Image Processing—ICMIP 2018 [Internet], Guiyang, China, 16–18 March 2018; ACM Press: New York, NY, USA, 2018. Available online: http://dl.acm.org/citation.cfm?doid=3195588.3195597 (accessed on 28 September 2022).

45. Page, M.J.; McKenzie, J.E.; Bossuyt, P.M.; Boutron, I.; Hoffmann, T.C.; Mulrow, C.D.; Shamseer, L.; Tetzlaff, J.M.; Akl, E.A.; Brennan, S.E.; et al. The PRISMA 2020 statement: An updated guideline for reporting systematic reviews. *BMJ* **2021**, *372*, n71. [CrossRef]

46. Chandler, J.; Cumpston, M.; Li, T.; Page, M.J.; Welch, V.A. (Eds.) *Cochrane Handbook for Systematic Reviews of Interventions [Internet], Version 6.3*; Cochrane, 2022; Available online: www.training.cochrane.org/handbook (accessed on 28 September 2022).

47. Critical Appraisal Skills Programme. CASP Diagnostic Study Checklist [Internet]. 2022. Available online: https://casp-uk.net/images/checklist/documents/CASP-Diagnostic-Study-Checklist/CASP-Diagnostic-Checklist-2018_fillable_form.pdf (accessed on 28 September 2022).

48. Hung, K.; Montalvao, C.; Tanaka, R.; Kawai, T.; Bornstein, M.M. The use and performance of artificial intelligence applications in dental and maxillofacial radiology: A systematic review. *Dentomaxillofac. Radiol.* **2020**, *49*, 20190107. [CrossRef]

49. Karthikeyan, M.P. An Efficient Deep Learning Approach to Pneumonia Classification in Healthcare. *Int. J. Adv. Res. Sci. Technol. IJARST* **2019**, *2019*, 4180949. Available online: https://ijarsct.co.in/Paper158.pdf (accessed on 28 September 2022).

50. Ferreira, J.R.; Armando Cardona Cardenas, D.; Moreno, R.A.; de Fatima de Sa Rebelo, M.; Krieger, J.E.; Antonio Gutierrez, M. Multi-View Ensemble Convolutional Neural Network to Improve Classification of Pneumonia in Low Contrast Chest X-ray Images. In Proceedings of the 2020 42nd Annual International Conference of the IEEE Engineering in Medicine & Biology Society (EMBC) [Internet], Montreal, QC, Canada, 11 July 2020; pp. 1238–1241. Available online: https://ieeexplore.ieee.org/document/9176517/ (accessed on 28 September 2022).

51. Sousa, G.G.B.; Fernandes, V.R.M.; de Paiva, A.C. Optimized Deep Learning Architecture for the Diagnosis of Pneumonia Through Chest X-rays. In *Image Analysis and Recognition*; Lecture Notes in Computer Science; Karray, F., Campilho, A., Yu, A., Eds.; Springer International Publishing: Berlin/Heidelberg, Germany, 2019; Volume 11663, pp. 353–361. Available online: http://link.springer.com/10.1007/978-3-030-27272-2_31 (accessed on 28 September 2022).

52. Hoo, Z.H.; Candlish, J.; Teare, D. What is an ROC curve? *Emerg. Med. J.* **2017**, *34*, 357. [CrossRef]

53. O'Grady, K.A.F.; Torzillo, P.J.; Frawley, K.; Chang, A.B. The radiological diagnosis of pneumonia in children. *Pneumonia* **2014**, *5*, 38–51. [CrossRef]

54. McAllister, D.A.; Liu, L.; Shi, T.; Chu, Y.; Reed, C.; Burrows, J.; Adeloye, D.; Rudan, I.; Black, R.E.; Campbell, H.; et al. Global, regional, and national estimates of pneumonia morbidity and mortality in children younger than 5 years between 2000 and 2015: A systematic analysis. *Lancet Glob. Health* **2018**, *7*, e47–e57. [CrossRef]

55. GBD 2015. Estimates of the global, regional, and national morbidity, mortality, and aetiologies of lower respiratory tract infections in 195 countries: A systematic analysis for the Global Burden of Disease Study 2015. *Lancet Infect. Dis.* **2017**, *17*, 1133–1161. [CrossRef]

56. Longjiang, E.; Zhao, B.; Liu, H.; Zheng, C.; Song, X.; Cai, Y.; Liang, H. Image-based deep learning in diagnosing the etiology of pneumonia on pediatric chest X-rays. *Pediatr. Pulmonol.* **2021**, *56*, 1036–1044.

57. Shelmerdine, S.C.; Martin, H.; Shirodkar, K.; Shamshuddin, S.; Weir-McCall, J.R. Can artificial intelligence pass the Fellowship of the Royal College of Radiologists examination? Multi-reader diagnostic accuracy study. *BMJ* **2022**, *379*, e072826. [CrossRef] [PubMed]

58. Ng, M.Y.; Ramamurthy, N. A career in radiology. *BMJ* **2012**, *345*, e8142. [CrossRef]

59. Gertych, A.; Zhang, A.; Sayre, J.; Pospiech-Kurkowska, S.; Huang, H. Bone age assessment of children using a digital hand atlas. *Comput. Med. Imaging Graph.* **2007**, *31*, 322–331. [CrossRef]

60. Rajpurkar, P.; Irvin, J.; Bagul, A.; Ding, D.; Duan, T.; Mehta, H.; Yang, B.; Zhu, K.; Laird, D.; Ball, L.R.; et al. Mura: Large dataset for abnormality detection in musculoskeletal radiographs. *arXiv* **2017**, arXiv:171206957.

61. Wang, X.; Peng, Y.; Lu, L.; Lu, Z.; Bagheri, M.; Summers, R.M. ChestX-Ray8: Hospital-Scale Chest X-Ray Database and Benchmarks on Weakly-Supervised Classification and Localization of Common Thorax Diseases. In Proceedings of the 2017 IEEE Conference on Computer Vision and Pattern Recognition (CVPR) [Internet], Honolulu, HI, USA, 21–26 July 2017; pp. 3462–3471. Available online: http://ieeexplore.ieee.org/document/8099852/ (accessed on 28 September 2022).

62. Irvin, J.; Rajpurkar, P.; Ko, M.; Yu, Y.; Ciurea-Ilcus, S.; Chute, C.; Marklund, H.; Haghgoo, B.; Ball, R.; Shpanskaya, K.; et al. Chexpert: A large chest radiograph dataset with uncertainty labels and expert comparison. In Proceedings of the AAAI Conference on Artificial Intelligence, Honolulu, HA, USA, 27 January–1 February 2019; Volume 33, pp. 590–597.

63. Johnson, A.E.; Pollard, T.J.; Berkowitz, S.J.; Greenbaum, N.R.; Lungren, M.P.; Deng, C.Y.; Mark, R.G.; Horng, S. MIMIC-CXR, a de-identified publicly available database of chest radiographs with free-text reports. *Sci. Data* **2019**, *6*, 317. [CrossRef]

64. Halabi, S.S.; Prevedello, L.; Kalpathy-Cramer, J.; Mamonov, A.B.; Bilbily, A.; Cicero, M.; Pan, I.; Pereira, L.A.; Sousa, R.; Abdala, N.; et al. The RSNA pediatric bone age machine learning challenge. *Radiology* **2019**, *290*, 498–503. [CrossRef]

65. Bustos, A.; Pertusa, A.; Salinas, J.M.; de la Iglesia-Vayá, M. PadChest: A large chest X-ray image dataset with multi-label annotated reports. *Med. Image Anal.* **2020**, *66*, 101797. [CrossRef]

66. Selby, I. Automated Quality Control of Chest X-ray [Internet]. Oral Presentation Presented at: European Congress of Radiology 3 March 2023; Vienna. Available online: https://connect.myesr.org/?esrc_course=using-ai-for-quality-control-in-radiography (accessed on 28 September 2022).

67. Ying, X. An Overview of Overfitting and its Solutions. *J. Phys. Conf. Ser.* **2019**, *1168*, 022022. [CrossRef]
68. Whiteson, S.; Tanner, B.; Taylor, M.E.; Stone, P. Protecting against evaluation overfitting in empirical reinforcement learning. In Proceedings of the 2011 IEEE Symposium on Adaptive Dynamic Programming and Reinforcement Learning (ADPRL), Paris, France, 12–14 April 2011; pp. 120–127. Available online: http://ieeexplore.ieee.org/document/5967363/ (accessed on 28 September 2022).
69. Dieterich, T. Overfitting and undercomputing in machine learning. *ACM Comput. Surv. CSUR* **1995**, *27*, 326–327. [CrossRef]
70. Mutasa, S.; Sun, S.; Ha, R. Understanding artificial intelligence based radiology studies: What is overfitting? *Clin. Imaging* **2020**, *65*, 96–99. [CrossRef]
71. Anderson, D.; Burnham, K. *Model Selection and Multi-Model Inference*, 2nd ed.; Springer: New York, NY, USA, 2004; Volume 63, p. 10.
72. England, J.R.; Cheng, P.M. Artificial intelligence for medical image analysis: A guide for authors and reviewers. *Am. J. Roentgenol.* **2019**, *212*, 513–519. [CrossRef]
73. Sun, Y.; Wang, X.; Tang, X. Deep Learning Face Representation from Predicting 10,000 Classes. In Proceedings of the 2014 IEEE Conference on Computer Vision and Pattern Recognition, Columbus, OH, USA, 23–28 June 2014; pp. 1891–1898.
74. Gonçalves, I.; Silva, S.; Melo, J.B.; Carreiras, J.M.B. Random Sampling Technique for Overfitting Control in Genetic Programming. In *Genetic Programming*; Moraglio, A., Silva, S., Krawiec, K., Machado, P., Cotta, C., Eds.; Springer: Berlin/Heidelberg, Germany, 2012; pp. 218–229.
75. Parmar, C.; Barry, J.D.; Hosny, A.; Quackenbush, J.; Aerts, H.J.W.L. Data Analysis Strategies in Medical Imaging. *Clin. Cancer Res.* **2018**, *24*, 3492–3499. [CrossRef]
76. Chartrand, G.; Cheng, P.M.; Vorontsov, E.; Drozdzal, M.; Turcotte, S.; Pal, C.J.; Kadoury, S.; Tang, A. Deep Learning: A Primer for Radiologists. *RadioGraphics* **2017**, *37*, 2113–2131. [CrossRef]
77. Yamashita, R.; Nishio, M.; Do, R.K.G.; Togashi, K. Convolutional neural networks: An overview and application in radiology. *Insights Into Imaging* **2018**, *9*, 611–629. [CrossRef]
78. Kim, D.; MacKinnon, T. Artificial intelligence in fracture detection: Transfer learning from deep convolutional neural networks. *Clin. Radiol.* **2018**, *73*, 439–445. [CrossRef]
79. Ha, R.; Mutasa, S.; Karcich, J.; Gupta, N.; Pascual Van Sant, E.; Nemer, J.; Sun, M.; Chang, P.; Liu, M.Z.; Jambawalikar, S. Predicting Breast Cancer Molecular Subtype with MRI Dataset Utilizing Convolutional Neural Network Algorithm. *J. Digit. Imaging* **2019**, *32*, 276–282. [CrossRef]
80. Fry, H. *Hello World: How to Be Human in the Age of the Machine [Internet]*; Transworld, 2018; Available online: https://books.google.co.uk/books?id=72FCDwAAQBAJ (accessed on 28 September 2022).

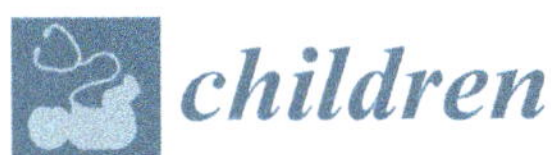

Systematic Review

Radiographic Features of COVID-19 in Children—A Systematic Review

Niamh Bergin, Niamh Moore, Shauna Doyle, Andrew England * and Mark F. McEntee

Discipline of Medical Imaging & Radiation Therapy, University College Cork, T12 AK54 Cork, Ireland
* Correspondence: aengland@ucc.ie; Tel.: +44-(07743)-318459

Abstract: INTRODUCTION: The SARS-CoV-19 (COVID-19) pandemic has become a global problem but has affected the paediatric population less so than in adults. The clinical picture in paediatrics can be different to adults but nonetheless both groups have been subject to frequent imaging. The overall aim of this study was to comprehensively summarise the findings of the available literature describing the chest radiograph (CXR) findings of paediatric patients with confirmed COVID-19. The COVID-19 landscape is rapidly changing, new information is being constantly brought to light, it is therefore important to appraise clinicians and the wider scientific community on the radiographic features of COVID-19 in children. METHODS: Four databases, which included, PubMed; Medline; CINAHL; ScienceDirect were searched from the 30 November 2020 to the 5 March 2021. The review was conducted using the "Preferred Reporting Items for Systematic Reviews and Meta-Analysis, PRISMA" guidelines. Studies were included for (1) publications with full text available, (2) patients with confirmed COVID-19 diagnoses, (3) CXR imaging features of COVID-19 were reported, (4) the age of patients was 0–18 years, (5) studies were limited to human subjects and (6) a language restriction of English was placed on the search. Quality assessment of included articles used the National of Health Quality Assessment Tool for Case Series Studies. RESULTS: Eight studies met our criteria for inclusion in the review. All eight studies documented the number of CXRs obtained, along with the number of abnormal CXRs. Seven out of the eight studies noted greater than 50% of the CXRs taken were abnormal. Opacification was the number one feature that was recorded in all eight studies, followed by pleural effusion which was seen in six studies. Consolidation and peri-bronchial thickening features were both evident in four studies. Opacification was sub-divided into common types of opacities i.e., consolidation, ground glass opacities, interstitial, alveolar and hazy. Consolidation was reported in half of the studies followed by ground glass opacities and interstitial opacities which was seen in three out of the eight studies. CONCLUSION: This systematic review provides insight into the common COVID-19 features that are seen on CXRs in paediatric patients. Opacification was the most common feature reported, with consolidation, ground glass and interstitial opacities the top three opacifications seen. Peri-bronchial thickening is reported. in the paediatric population but this differs from the adult population and was not reported as a common radiographic finding typically seen in adults. ADVANCES IN KNOWLEDGE: This systematic review highlights the CXR appearances of paediatric patients with confirmed SARS-CoV-19, to gain insight into the disease pathophysiology and provide a comprehensive summary of the features for clinicians aiding optimal management.

Keywords: child; paediatric; infant; adolescent; chest X-ray; CXR; chest radiography; COVID-19; SARS-CoV-2; coronavirus

Citation: Bergin, N.; Moore, N.; Doyle, S.; England, A.; McEntee, M.F. Radiographic Features of COVID-19 in Children—A Systematic Review. *Children* **2022**, *9*, 1620. https://doi.org/10.3390/children9111620

Academic Editor: Ilias Tsiflikas

Received: 28 September 2022
Accepted: 20 October 2022
Published: 25 October 2022

1. Introduction

In Wuhan China, in December 2019, a group of patients presented with fever, cough, and pneumonia of an unknown source. Initial investigations found that this illness was the result of a novel coronavirus (SARS-CoV-2). The SARS-CoV-2 'coronavirus' more commonly known as 'COVID-19', rapidly spread across the globe and led to COVID-19 being declared as a worldwide pandemic in March 2020. On the 20 May 2021, according to World Health Organisation (WHO), there had been 164,409,804 confirmed cases and 3,409,220 deaths [1].

Many published studies stated that the individuals most frequently affected during the Pandemic were adults over 60 years of age, there has also been many COVID-19 cases seen in paediatrics, including infants, children and young adults. In 2021, the WHO, stated that children and young adults would face many challenges based on their phase of life and from both the COVID-19 disease and the measures created to contain the disease [1]. Children and young people typically comprise only 1–2% of cases of COVID-19 worldwide [2]. COVID-19 has appeared to have a minimal effect on children, with reports of only a low number of symptomatic and severe cases compared to adults [3,4]. In the majority children will be symptomatic for only a few of days and symptoms will resolve naturally. Although children tend to have milder symptoms, like all humans they can be agents for transmission and are therefore important to identify promptly.

The early detection and treatment of individuals affected by COVID-19 is critical. Lung imaging plays an important role and to date the most frequently used imaging modalities are chest radiography (CXR) and computed tomography (CT) [5]. CT has become extremely valuable in the screening, diagnosis and aftercare of patients with COVID-19 and provides medical practitioners with important diagnostic information. Radiological studies are less frequently requested in children due to the overall lower rates of infection [6] and the generally milder nature of the disease. COVID-19 features on imaging appear to be changeable with age and there are possible distinct features in infants, children and adolescents. Appearances of COVID-19 on lung imaging in adults have been previously documented in the literature, but by comparison documentation of the lung disease patterns of COVID-19 in a paediatric population remains less clear [7]. Paediatric clinicians also face additional challenges when attempting to differentiate early stages of COVID-19 infection from other types of viral lower respiratory tract infections. In addition, a small number of COVID-19 positive children will go on to develop Paediatric Inflammatory Multisystem Syndrome (PIMS). PIMS can present with a range of symptoms and evaluation in severe cases may include imaging.

Although, imaging is commonly used in the management of adults with COVID-19, radiology is likely not to be routinely required in paediatric cases, especially if the child is asymptomatic [4]. A child is more sensitive to radiation exposure; therefore, routine use of CT is not recommended, which makes a distinct difference in their radiological work-up in contrast to adults [8]. Also, the American College of Radiology [9] does not recommend medical imaging examinations as a formal method of COVID-19 diagnosis, and confirmation of COVID-19 by PCR testing is key even if the radiological appearances are highly suggestive of COVID-19 [6].

Referral for imaging is part of the management plan for clinicians [5]. It is vitally important that clinicians of all specialties recognise the appearances of COVID-19 on radiographic images, especially when the clinicians are suspecting something other than COVID-19.

The overall aim of this study was to undertake a comprehensive evaluation of the findings of published literature which have described the CXR features in children with confirmed COVID-19. To achieve the aim, the research team undertook a systematic review of the published literature across different databases to identify (1) the number of children with normal chest radiography, (2) the incidence of different radiographic (CXR) abnormalities reported in PCR-confirmed paediatric SARS-CoV-2 cases. Considering the low number of children which will require imaging it is important to provide up to date information regarding the appearances of COVID-19 on chest radiography. This in turn will help improve knowledge of COVID-19 and improve diagnosis and management.

2. Materials and Methods

2.1. Search Strategy

An extensive electronic search was conducted in the following databases PubMed, MEDLINE, ScienceDirect and CINAHL. All procedures in the review were executed in accordance with the "Preferred Reporting Items for Systematic reviews and Meta-Analyses, PRISMA," [10] guidelines (Figure 1). A methodological search of literature was undertaken from the 30 November 2020 to the 5 March 2021. An initial search of the literature was performed on 17 February 2021 and a second 'repeat' search was run on 5 March 2021. As this continues to be an ever-evolving field there is a rapid number of studies being published every day. The above systematic search was reviewed by a second researcher to ensure transparency throughout the searching process.

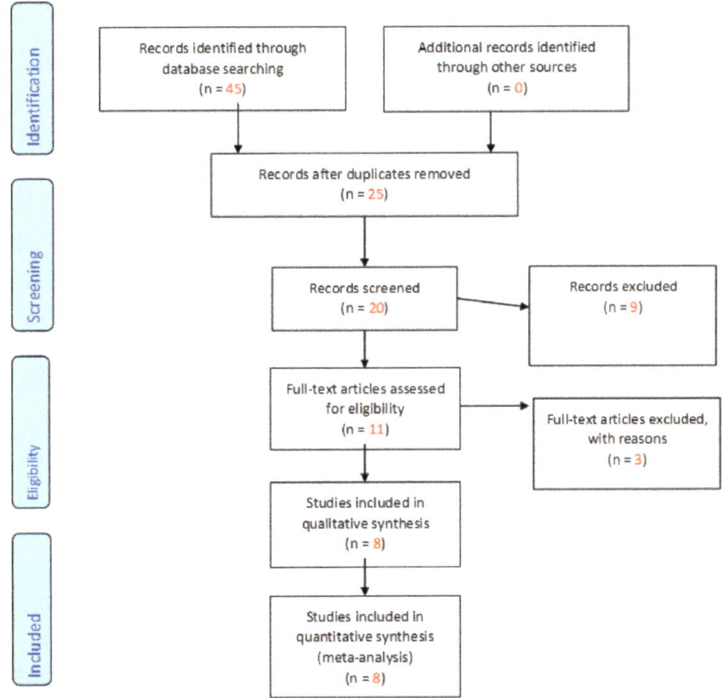

Figure 1. Diagram of retrieval of studies, using "Preferred Reporting Items for Systematic reviews and Meta-Analyses, PRISMA".

2.2. Inclusion and Exclusion Criteria

Studies were selected for potential inclusion based on full text analysis of the title, abstract and keywords. Criteria for inclusion included all studies which described or investigated chest radiography findings of COVID-19 confirmed infections in children. Studies were eligible for inclusion if (1) publications were available in full text, (2) contained patients who had confirmed COVID-19 diagnoses, (3) CXR imaging features of COVID-19 were included in the publication, (4) the age of patients was between 0–18 years, (5) studies were limited only to humans and (6) articles had to have been published in English.

Studies were excluded if they were (1) letters, theses, books, editorials or posters, (2) studies on the adult population, (3) any studies reporting on a mixed paediatric/adult cohort and specifically where imaging results for the paediatric cohort could not be extracted, (4) lack of clinical data presented, (5) no PCR-confirmation of COVID-19 infection and (6) duplicate studies.

2.3. Risk of Bias

Quality assessment of the included literature was determined using the National Institutes of Health (NIH) Quality Assessment Tool for Case Series Studies [11], from this general quality ratings were categorized as poor, fair, or good (Table 1). Two reviewers independently graded the quality of the selected articles. Any disagreements between reviewers were resolved through discussion, and if necessary, a third reviewer was introduced to make the final decision.

Table 1. Summary of the quality ratings, according to the National Institute of Health (NIH) Quality Assessment Tool for Case Studies, of the included studies.

Article:	Bayramoglu et al. [6]	Biko et al. [12]	Blumfield et al. [13]	Caro-Dominguez et al. [14]	Hameed et al. [15]	Lu et al. [16]	Oterino Serrano et al. [8]	Palabiyik et al. [4]
Q1: Was the study question or objective clearly stated?	YES	YES	YES	YES	YES	YES	YES	YES
Q2: Was the study population clearly and fully described, including a case definition?	YES	YES	YES	YES	YES	YES	YES	YES
Q3: Were the cases consecutive?	YES	YES	NR	NR	NR	NR	NR	NR
Q4: Were the subjects comparable?	NO	NO	NO	NO	NO	NO	NO	NO
Q5: Was the intervention (i.e., imaging modality) clearly described?	YES	YES	YES	YES	NO	YES	YES	YES
Q6: Were the outcome measures clearly defined, valid, reliable, and implemented consistently across all study participants?	YES	YES	YES	YES	NO	YES	YES	YES
Q7: Was the length of follow-up adequate?	NA	NA	NA	NA	NA	NA	NA	NA
Q8: Were the statistical methods well-described?	YES	YES	NO	NO	NO	NR	YES	YES
Q9: Were the results well-described?	YES	YES	YES	YES	YES	YES	YES	YES
Quality Rating: Reviewer 1	GOOD	GOOD	FAIR	FAIR	FAIR	FAIR	GOOD	GOOD
Quality Rating: Reviewer 2	GOOD	GOOD	FAIR	FAIR	FAIR	FAIR	GOOD	GOOD

NA—not applicable; NR—not reported.

2.4. Data Extraction

Data extraction was performed independently by the primary reviewer using a data extraction tool adapted from the Cochrane Collaboration [17]. This form has been developed by adopting and customizing the "Data collection form for intervention review-RCT's and non-RCT's" of the Cochrane Collaboration. All information was collected and transcribed onto an Excel spreadsheet. Data that was inserted into the Excel spreadsheet was then reviewed separately by the second reviewer. As previously stated, if any disagreements arose, they were resolved by discussion, and if necessary via a third reviewer.

3. Results

3.1. Selection of Articles

Following the initial search, a total of 45 papers were identified from the four databases previously mentioned. After removing 25 duplicates, a total of 20 publications were included for the screening process. Manual screening of the title and abstract of these 20 papers resulted in 11 papers being included for the full-text review. From the full-text review, a total of eight papers met the inclusion criteria and were included in this systematic review. The PRISMA flowchart representing the search results is illustrated in Figure 1. The two independent reviewers agreed with the study selection and no discrepancies were found during the research process

3.2. Methodological Quality

The quality assessment resulted in four of the articles receiving an overall scoring of "good", with the remaining four receiving a score of "fair". Further details on the methodological quality assessment of the included studies is presented in Table 1. Improvements in the reporting of the statistical analysis of the studies included would have increased the quality grading of the four 'fair' rated studies.

Table 2 provides a summary of the key features of the studies included. All eight included studies were retrospective in enrolment. The enrolment period for the studies commenced between January 2020 and April 2020 and was completed between February 2020 and May 2020. The country of origin varied in six out of eight studies and were predominantly in the US, China and Europe. Six out of the eight studies were conducted in a single centre and the other two studies were multi-centre. The mechanism of selection of the participants was consecutive for two studies, the remaining studies (n = 6) failed to describe the selection mechanism.

Table 2. Summary of studies characteristics.

Article:	Bayramoglu et al. [6]	Biko et al. [12]	Blumfield et al. [13]	Caro-Dominguez et al. [14]	Hameed et al. [15]	Lu et al. [16]	Oterino Serrano et al. [8]	Palabiyik et al. [4]
Patient enrolment:	Retrospective	Retrospective	Retrospective	Retrospective	Retrospective	Retrospective	Retrospective	Retrospective
Country :	Istanbul	Philadelphia	New York (Bronx)	The Netherlands European Society of Paediatric Radiology	London	China	Spain	Istanbul
Enrolment beginning:	10 March 2020	17 March 2020	25 February 2020	12 March 2020	14 April 2020	22 January 2020	13 March 2020	11 March 2020
Enrolment ending:	31 May 2020	21 May 2020	1 May 2020	8 April 2020	9 May 2020	9 February 2020	6 April 2020	20 April 2020
Type of Study:	Single Centre	Multi Centre	Single Centre	Multi-centre	Single Centre	Single Centre	Single Centre	Single Centre
Consecutive/ Random selection:	Consecutive	Consecutive	Not Reported	Not Reported	Not Reported	Not Reported	Not Reported	Not Reported

Table 3 presents the patient demographics from the eight selected papers. The number of children studied in each of the papers varied greatly and not every child required CXR. In total, there were 762 children included in this systematic review of which 367 required a CXR, (209/367 [57%] were abnormal). All reports considered both male and female patients, but the median age of all patients varied but was still within the inclusion criteria of 0–18 years. All eight papers documented that all patients received a positive PCR test, but it is unclear which of these had a diagnosis of COVID-19 on CXR or with PCR testing. Seven out of eight studies stated the number of patients that were symptomatic or asymptomatic. But only three of the papers stated whether their patients had comorbidities (n = 166) before contracting coronavirus. It would be important to be aware of comorbidities as the related radiological appearances could be misread or misdiagnosed as COVID-19. Finally, all eight papers did document the number of normal CXR (n = 158) that were obtained, and they also stated the number of abnormal CXRs (n = 209), but the eight papers did not document specific details with regards to the sensitivity or the specificity of the CXR against PCR testing.

Table 3. Summary of patient demographics.

Article:	Bayramoglu et al. [6]	Biko et al. [12]	Blumfield et al. [13]	Caro-Dominguez et al. [14]	Hameed et al. [15]	Lu et al. [16]	Oterino Serrano et al. [8]	Palabiyik et al. [4]
Number of patients diagnosed with COVID-19	74	313	19	91	35	9	44	177
Number of patients requiring CXR	69	51	19	81	35	9	44	59

Table 3. *Cont.*

Article:	Bayramoglu et al. [6]	Biko et al. [12]	Blumfield et al. [13]	Caro-Dominguez et al. [14]	Hameed et al. [15]	Lu et al. [16]	Oterino Serrano et al. [8]	Palabiyik et al. [4]
Total number (median age, years)								
Male:	36 (11)	164 (6.6)	10 (8)	49 (6.1)	27 (11)	5 (7.8)	29 (6.6)	34 (9)
Female:	38 (12)	149 (9.4)	9 (8)	42 (6.1)	8 (11)	4 (7.8)	15 (6.6)	25 (9)
Symptomatic Asymptomatic	NR	92 221	19	85 6	35	8 1	44	59
Comorbidities:	0	41(74.5%)	12 (63.2%)	30 (33%)	NR	0 (0%)	NR	NR
Number of Normal CXR:	56 (81.1%)	34 (66.6%)	1 (5.2%)	10 (12.3%)	16 (45.7%)	5 (55.6%)	4 (9%)	32 (54.2%)
Number of Abnormal CXR:	13 (18.8%)	17 (33.3%)	18 (94.8%)	71 (87.7%)	19 (54.3%)	4 (44.4%)	40 (90.9%)	27 (45.8%)
Received PCR Test:	YES	YES	YES	YES	YES	YES	YES	YES
Sensitivity:	NR	NR	NR	NR	NR	NR	NR	NR
Specificity:	NR	NR	NR	NR	NR	NR	NR	NR

3.3. Chest Radiography Appearances of COVID-19 in Children:

The CXR COVID-19 appearances from the eight papers are shown in Table 4 below. Opacification was present in all eight studies, followed by pleural effusion which was present in six studies. Consolidation and peri-bronchial thickening features was found in four out of the eight studies. Less common features such as cardiomegaly, congestive heart failure, ARDS, pneumothorax, atelectasis, and mediastinal widening were present in one—two studies. The location of the features was documented in two out of the eight papers, with one study seeing 4% unilateral and 4% bilateral and the other study seeing 25% unilateral and 20% bilateral. Distribution of the features was documented in seven studies, six of the these showed that the distribution is predominantly in the perihilar or central regions of the lungs.

Table 4. Summary of chest radiographic features.

Article:	Bayramoglu et al. [6]	Biko et al. [12]	Blumfield et al. [13]	Caro-Dominguez et al. [14]	Hameed et al. [15]	Lu et al. [16]	Oterino Serrano et al. [8]	Palabiyik et al. [4]
Consolidation:			13 (68.4%)	28.3 (35%)	5 (14.2%)		8 (18.1%)	
Opacifications:	6 (8.6%)	30 (58.8%)	15 (78.9%)	28.4 (35%)	11 (31.4%)	4 (44.4%)	32 (72.7%)	27 (45.8%)
Peri bronchial Thickening:	7 (10.1%)			47 (58%)	12 (34.3%)		38 (86.3%)	
Pleural effusion:	1 (1.4%)	5 (9.8%)	4 (21%)	6 (7.4%)	4 (11.4%)		4 (9.1%)	
Cardiomegaly:			7 (36.8%)					
Congestive heart failure:			7 (36.8%)					
ARDS:			2 (10.5%)					
Pneumothorax:				2 (2.4%)				
Atelectasis:				2 (2.4%)	7 (20%)			
Mediastinal widening:							2 (4.5%)	
Location of Features:		NR	NR	NR	NR	NR	NR	
Unilateral:	3 (4.4%)							15 (25.4%)
Bilateral:	3 (4.4%)							12 (20.3%)
Distribution of features:				NR				
Perihilar (central):	3 (4.4%)	2 (6.6%)	11 (73.3%)		11 (31.4%)	4 (44.4%)	17 (38.6%)	
Peripheral:	3 (4.4%)	3 (10%)	1 (6.6%)				5 (11.4%)	31 (22%)
Diffused:		14 (46.6%)	5 (33.3%)				37 (84%)	16 (27.1%)
Lower lobes:			9 (60%)					
Scattered:		3 (10%)						
Not well-defined:		2 (6.6%)						

Table 5 sets out the common COVID-19 features. All eight studies reported opacifications. This was sub-divided into common types of opacities i.e., consolidation, ground glass opacities, interstitial, alveolar and hazy. Consolidation was the most common and was evident in half of the studies, followed by both glass opacities and interstitial opacities was seen in three out of the eight studies.

Table 5. Summary of common COVID-19 features.

Article:	Bayramoglu et al. [6]	Biko et al. [12]	Blumfield et al. [13]	Caro-Dominguez et al. [14]	Hameed et al. [15]	Lu et al. [16]	Oterino Serrano et al. [8]	Palabiyik et al. [4]
Peri-bronchial Thickening:	7 (10.1%)			47 (58%)	12 (34.3%)			
Opacities:	5 (7.2%)	30 (58.8%)	15 (78.9%)	56 (70.4%)	16 (45.7%)	4 (44.4%)	40 (90.9%)	27 (45.8%)
Ground Glass Opacities	ü 5 (7.2%)			ü 15 (18.9%)			ü 22 (50.0%)	
Interstitial		ü 16 (31.4%)	ü 6 (31.6%)	ü 12 (15.1%)				
Alveolar		ü 14 (27.4%)						
Consolidation			ü 13 (68.4%)	ü 28 (35.2%)	ü 5 (14.3%		ü 8 (18.2%)	
Hazy			ü 8 (42.1%)					

4. Discussion

This review of the literature utilizing a systematic methodology has provided a comprehensive evaluation of the published literature to date which have considered the CXR features of COVID-19 in children. This systematic review includes children from new-borns to adulthood (18 years old), with positive PCR testing confirming a COVID-19 infection.

The study enrolment on all eight studies, was retrospective which introduces a lower risk of bias to this systematic review. But all studies examined were at the initial stages of the pandemic between January–May 2020 and covered a short time of between 0.5–2.5 months. The limited number of publications available for inclusion and supports the initial findings that there are only a few studies carried out on the use of CXR and its related imaging appearances of COVID-19 in children in contrast to those available for adults.

It is important to note that not all children that test positive will require or should undergo a CXR or CT examination. In the systematic review, all eight studies stated the number of children that tested positive and the number of children that required CXR. In two of the eight studies less than half of the children required CXR whereas six out of the eight studies noted that greater than half or all the children required CXR. However, due to the lack of information regarding the severity of the symptoms and clinical status of the children (comorbidities), it is difficult to determine the justification for the high percentage of children requiring CXR.

Seven out of the eight studies documented whether the child was symptomatic or asymptomatic with six of these reporting that the children were symptomatic, only Biko et al. [12] reported that most of the children included in their study were asymptomatic. Given the lack of detailed information, it is difficult to determine whether and if so why asymptomatic paediatric patients underwent CXR.

Six case studies showed that where children required imaging, CXR was the preferred method. This is in line with a number of case studies and guidelines [9,11] where it has been cited that in paediatric patients, it is vital to use the lowest radiation doses possible for a diagnosis which would be in accordance with the ALARA principle. However, it should also be noted that imaging should only be undertaken in specific circumstances if symptoms worsen or are persistent.

Of the eight studies reviewed, only five studies stated their patients' comorbidity status. Three studies reported comorbidities in their patients whereas two studies [6,16] reported no comorbidities with any of their patients. Of the studies that reported comorbidities, Biko et al. [12] and Blumfield et al. [13] highlighted that more than half of their patients had comorbidities before acquiring a COVID-19 infection, whereas the study by Caro-

Dominquez et al. [14] reported a third of their patients had comorbidities before becoming infected. The type of comorbidity a patient may have prior to contracting COVID-19 may dictate the clinical presentation of the patient, which in turn could influence the radiological appearances on their CXR and may lead to misinterpretation or misdiagnoses of COVID-19. Given the potential for misdiagnosis, it is important that neither CXR nor chest CT is used to screen for COVID-19 or as a first-line of investigation to diagnose symptomatic COVID-19 [6]. However, in children presenting with moderate or severe symptoms and those with underlying risk factors, it has been reported that CXR can be useful in establishing an imaging baseline as well as assessing for alternative diagnosis [8].

Overall, seven out of the eight studies noted greater than 50% of the CXRs taken were abnormal however the lack of information regarding the severity of the symptoms makes it problematic when determining the reason behind the high numbers of abnormal CXRs.

In this review, all eight studies had one common clinical finding, which was the presence of opacifications. Both peri-bronchial thickening and pleural effusion were reported in six out of the eight studies, where consolidation was reported in four out of the eight studies. Finally, there were a number of infrequent features reported in paediatric patients including: atelectasis which was reported in two studies and cardiomegaly, congestive heart failure, ARDS, pneumothorax and mediastinal widening which were reported in one study each.

Study reviewers further assessed features that may be specific to COVID-19: including peri-bronchial thickening, ground glass opacities, consolidation [6] as well assessing CXRs for the distribution and type of pulmonary opacities, i.e., interstitial, hazy and consolidation [13]. All eight studies reported opacities on their CXRs, these opacities included consolidation. This is similar to adults where the most common radiographic features are airspace opacities, which are most commonly described as consolidation and less commonly as ground glass opacities [15,16]. Peri-bronchial thickening was a feature in three out of the eight studies in this review. This contrasts to the common radiographic findings for adults where peri-bronchial thickening was uncommon and nonspecific for COVID-19 [6,14].

5. Limitations

Firstly, only a small number of case studies were included in this systematic review. Furthermore, some of these studies were limited in terms of sample size. This could have potentially introduced bias. Secondly, the review was limited to publications written in English.

All the studies examined were carried out during the initial months of the pandemic, when there were many unknowns. It is possible that more recent studies on COVID-19 may provide additional findings. It would have been useful if imaging appearances could have been correlated against the time of presentation/day of hospitalization. It is highly probable that the time since the onset of infection would influence the frequency and severity of the imaging findings. This would, therefore, affect the results of this systematic review and readers should consider this context when interpreting our findings. Further sub-analysis of data could also be introduced, and this could consider the coronavirus strain togetherwith differences in the sex and age of the child and the presence of comorbidities.

Lastly, the reviewer noted a lack of detailed data and information regarding the patients' ages, symptoms, including symptom severity. In the absence of this information, the reviewer was unable to compare potential features associated with certain age groups specific and include symptoms that the patients presented with. Furthermore, the reviewer was not able to understand and develop patterns between the number of patients who were positive for a COVID-19 infection and who had abnormal CXRs and the linkage of this with the chest radiographic features and common COVID-19 features.

6. Conclusions

This systematic review provides a detailed evaluation of the currently available literature on the CXR appearances of COVID-19 in paediatrics. This review demonstrated seven studies where greater than 50% of their cohort had abnormal CXRs. Opacification was the number one feature reported in the studies, with consolidation, ground glass and interstitial opacities the main opacifications reported. Peri-bronchial thickening is one radiographic finding seen in the paediatric population but this is not typically seen in adults. Given the time elapsed since the first reported COVID-19 case there will be further experiences and data on the effects on children. Work is needed to identify any specific patient characteristics that may influence disease severity and progression, such factors may include sex, age and existing comorbidities.

Author Contributions: Conceptualization, M.F.M. and N.B.; methodology, M.F.M. and N.B.; writing—original draft preparation, N.B., N.M., S.D., M.F.M. and A.E.; writing—review and editing, A.E.; supervision, M.F.M. and N.M. All authors have read and agreed to the published version of the manuscript.

Funding: This research received no external funding.

Institutional Review Board Statement: Not applicable.

Informed Consent Statement: Not applicable.

Conflicts of Interest: The authors declare no conflict of interest.

References

1. Coronavirus Disease (COVID-19)–World Health Organization. Available online: https://www.who.int/emergencies/diseases/novel-coronavirus-2019 (accessed on 7 August 2021).
2. Swann, O.V.; Holden, K.A.; Turtle, L.; Pollock, L.; Fairfield, C.J.; Drake, T.M.; Seth, S.; Egan, C.; Hardwick, H.E.; Halpin, S.; et al. Clinical characteristics of children and young people admitted to hospital with COVID-19 in United Kingdom: Prospective multicentre observational cohort study. *BMJ* **2020**, *370*, m3249. [CrossRef] [PubMed]
3. Ludvigsson, J.F. Systematic review of COVID-19 in children shows milder cases and a better prognosis than adults. *Acta Paediatr.* **2020**, *109*, 1088–1095. [CrossRef] [PubMed]
4. Palabiyik, F.; Kokurcan, S.O.; Hatipoglu, N.; Cebeci, S.O.; Inci, E. Imaging of COVID-19 pneumonia in children. *Br. J. Radiol.* **2020**, *93*, 20200647. [CrossRef] [PubMed]
5. Rubin, G.D.; Ryerson, C.J.; Haramati, L.B.; Sverzellati, N.; Kanne, J.; Raoof, S.; Schluger, N.W.; Volpi, A.; Yim, J.-J.; Martin, I.B.K.; et al. The role of chest imaging in patient management during the COVID-19 pandemic: A multinational consensus statement from the fleischner society. *Radiology* **2020**, *296*, 172–180. [CrossRef] [PubMed]
6. Bayramoglu, Z.; Canıpek, E.; Comert, R.G.; Gasimli, N.; Kaba, O.; Yanartaş, M.S.; Torun, S.H.; Somer, A.; Erturk, S.M. Imaging features of pediatric COVID-19 on chest radiography and chest ct: A retrospective, single-center study. *Acad. Radiol.* **2020**, *28*, 18–27. [CrossRef] [PubMed]
7. Nino, G.; Zember, J.; Sanchez-Jacob, R.; Gutierrez, M.J.; Sharma, K.; Linguraru, M.G. Pediatric lung imaging features of COVID-19: A systematic review and meta-analysis. *Pediatr. Pulmonol.* **2020**, *56*, 252–263. [CrossRef] [PubMed]
8. Serrano, C.O.; Alonso, E.; Andrés, M.; Buitrago, N.M.; Vigara, A.P.; Pajares, M.P.; López, E.C.; Moll, G.G.; Espin, I.M.; Barriocanal, M.B.; et al. Pediatric chest x-ray in COVID-19 infection. *Eur. J. Radiol.* **2020**, *131*, 109236. [CrossRef] [PubMed]
9. ACR Recommendations for the Use of Chest Radiography and Computed Tomography (CT) for Suspected COVID-19 Infection. Available online: https://www.acr.org/Advocacy-and-Economics/ACR-Position-Statements/Recommendations-for-Chest-Radiography-and-CT-for-Suspected-COVID19-Infection (accessed on 7 August 2021).
10. PRISMA 2009 Flow Diagram. Available online: http://prisma-statement.org/documents/PRISMA%202009%20flow%20diagram.pdf (accessed on 7 August 2021).
11. Study Quality Assessment Tools | NHLBI, NIH. Available online: https://www.nhlbi.nih.gov/health-topics/study-quality-assessment-tools (accessed on 7 August 2021).
12. Biko, D.M.; Ramirez-Suarez, K.I.; Barrera, C.A.; Banerjee, A.; Matsubara, D.; Kaplan, S.L.; Cohn, K.A.; Rapp, J.B. Imaging of children with COVID-19: Experience from a tertiary children's hospital in the United States. *Pediatr. Radiol.* **2021**, *51*, 239–247. [CrossRef] [PubMed]
13. Blumfield, E.; Levin, T.L. COVID-19 in Pediatric Patients: A Case Series from the Bronx, NY. *Radiology* **2020**, *50*, 1369–1374. Available online: https://einstein.pure.elsevier.com/en/publications/covid-19-in-pediatric-patients-a-case-series-from-the-bronx-ny (accessed on 7 August 2021). [CrossRef] [PubMed]
14. Caro-Dominguez, P.; Shelmerdine, S.C.; Toso, S.; Secinaro, A.; Toma, P.; Damasio, M.B.; Navallas, M.; Riaza-Martin, L.; Gomez-Pastrana, D.; Mahani, M.G.; et al. Thoracic imaging of coronavirus disease 2019 (COVID-19) in children: A series of 91 cases. *Pediatr. Radiol.* **2020**, *50*, 1354–1368. [CrossRef] [PubMed]

15. Hameed, S.; Elbaaly, H.; Reid, C.E.L.; Santos, R.M.F.; Shivamurthy, V.; Wong, J.; Jogeesvaran, K.H. Spectrum of imaging findings at chest radiography, US, CT, and MRI in multisystem inflammatory syndrome in children associated with COVID-19. *Radiology* **2021**, *298*, E1–E10. [CrossRef] [PubMed]
16. Lu, Y.; Wen, H.; Rong, D.; Zhou, Z.; Liu, H. Clinical characteristics, and radiological features of children infected with the 2019 novel coronavirus. *Clin. Radiol.* **2020**, *75*, 520–525. [CrossRef] [PubMed]
17. Data Extraction Forms. Available online: https://dplp.cochrane.org/data-extraction-forms (accessed on 7 August 2021).

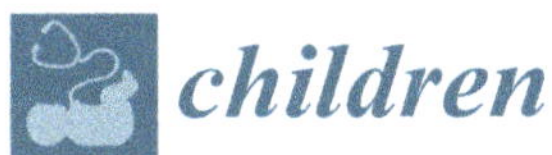

Review

Pictorial Review of MRI Findings in Acute Neck Infections in Children

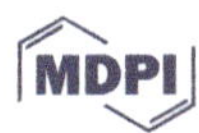

Janne Nurminen [1,*], Jaakko Heikkinen [1], Tatu Happonen [1], Mikko Nyman [1], Aapo Sirén [1], Jari-Pekka Vierula [1], Jarno Velhonoja [2], Heikki Irjala [2], Tero Soukka [3], Lauri Ivaska [4], Kimmo Mattila [1] and Jussi Hirvonen [1]

1   Department of Radiology, University of Turku and Turku University Hospital, 20520 Turku, Finland; jaheik4@gmail.com (J.H.); tatu.j.happonen@utu.fi (T.H.); mikko.nyman@varha.fi (M.N.); aapo.siren@varha.fi (A.S.); jari-pekka.vierula@varha.fi (J.-P.V.); kimmo.mattila@varha.fi (K.M.); jussi.hirvonen@utu.fi (J.H.)
2   Department of Otorhinolaryngology-Head and Neck Surgery, University of Turku and Turku University Hospital, 20520 Turku, Finland; jarno.velhonoja@varha.fi (J.V.); heikki.irjala@varha.fi (H.I.)
3   Department of Oral and Maxillofacial Surgery, University of Turku, 20014 Turku, Finland; tero.soukka@varha.fi
4   Department of Paediatrics and Adolescent Medicine, InFLAMES Research Flagship Center, University of Turku and Turku University Hospital, 20520 Turku, Finland; lauri.ivaska@varha.fi
*   Correspondence: janne.nurminen@varha.fi

Abstract: Pediatric neck infections and their complications, such as abscesses extending to deep neck compartments, are potentially life-threatening acute conditions. Medical imaging aims to verify abscesses and their extensions and exclude other complications. Magnetic resonance imaging (MRI) has proven to be a useful and highly accurate imaging method in acute neck infections in children. Children and adults differ in terms of the types of acute infections and the anatomy and function of the neck. This pictorial review summarizes typical findings in pediatric patients with neck infections and discusses some difficulties related to image interpretation.

Keywords: magnetic resonance imaging; infection; neck; emergency medicine; pediatric

Citation: Nurminen, J.; Heikkinen, J.; Happonen, T.; Nyman, M.; Sirén, A.; Vierula, J.-P.; Velhonoja, J.; Irjala, H.; Soukka, T.; Ivaska, L.; et al. Pictorial Review of MRI Findings in Acute Neck Infections in Children. *Children* **2023**, *10*, 967. https://doi.org/10.3390/children10060967

Academic Editor: Curtise Ng

Received: 5 May 2023
Revised: 23 May 2023
Accepted: 24 May 2023
Published: 29 May 2023

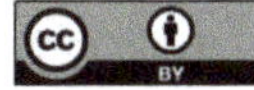

1. Introduction

Most conventional neck infections can be managed conservatively. However, deep neck infections possess a high risk for serious complications, such as abscess formation, mediastinitis, airway compromise, and venous thrombosis due to the infection spreading along the fascial planes and potential face and neck spaces. These complications are potentially lethal [1]. In children, prompt surgical treatment may be necessary, including cervical incision, intraoral incision, immediate tonsillectomy, or rarely, dental extraction [2]. Large abscesses and a younger age seem to predict surgical intervention [3,4].

Pediatric acute neck infections arise from common infections originating in the ears, nose, or throat and have the potential to disseminate to the deep neck spaces through direct continuity or lymphatic drainage to the lymph nodes [5]. When adequate cultivation procedures are utilized, anaerobic bacteria can be identified from most abscesses. Untreated abscesses can spontaneously rupture into the pharynx, resulting in fatal aspiration [6]. Neck swelling can initially be imaged with ultrasound, which has a high resolution for superficial structures. The main indication for cross-sectional imaging (as elaborated below) is the suspicion of a surgically drainable abscess in deep neck spaces for which ultrasound is insufficient.

In clinical practice, these infections have typically been imaged with contrast-enhanced computed tomography (CECT) [7,8], which has limited ability to differentiate abscess from lymphadenitis, cellulitis, and pathological masses [7] or to predict surgical drainage [9]. Of late, magnetic resonance imaging (MRI) has been acknowledged as a feasible and highly accurate primary imaging method in the emergency setting in both the general population [10] and specifically in children [11]. The apparent advantages of MRI over CECT are its superior diagnostic accuracy [12] and lack of ionizing radiation. The distribution of deep neck infections and MRI findings differ between adults and children [11]. These differences are partly due to the varying proportional distribution and function of lymph nodes in different age groups [13]. Due to these differences, the interpretation of pediatric neck MRI studies requires specific knowledge and attention.

The purpose of the current pictorial review is to present typical neck infection MRI findings in children, including the most useful edema patterns and typical abscesses, and underline the potential caveats and complications associated with deep neck infections. We focus on the soft tissue of the neck above and below the hyoid bone. Pediatric non-traumatic emergencies of the orbits, nose, and ear have recently been covered elsewhere [14].

2. MRI Protocol and Practical Performance

We utilized the Philips Ingenia 3 Tesla scanner (Philips Healthcare, Best, The Netherlands). Our routine neck infection protocol comprises seven sequences and lasts approximately 30 min [15]. We use the same sequences for adults and children. The sequences are T2 Dixon (axial and coronal planes), T1 SE (axial), DWI (axial), and contrast-enhanced T1 Dixon sequences (axial, coronal, and sagittal) (Table 1). A gadolinium-based contrast agent (Dotarem®; Guerbet, Villepinte, France) is routinely used. T2-weighted imaging is useful in assessing the anatomy: fat and water have a bright signal, lymphoid tissue has an intermediate signal, muscles have a low signal, and cortical bone has no signal. Specific edema patterns can be appreciated as bright areas in the fat-suppressed, T2-weighted images. We prefer the Dixon method for fat suppression because it reliably yields homogenous images even with large fields of view. The T1-weighted axial sequence is used to reference post-contrast Dixon sequences and to detect bone marrow fat obliteration in odontogenic neck infections. Pre-contrast T1-weighted sequences are also useful in assessing postoperative hematomas and chronic fluid collections, which may have a high T1 signal intensity. Together with diffusion-weighted imaging (DWI), contrast-enhanced sequences are used for diagnosing and characterizing abscesses. These sequences are important for assessing cystic masses, tumors, and necrotic lymph nodes [15]. The careful assessment of potential lymph node pathology is critical, especially in children. The DWI sequence is produced using standard echo-planar imaging (EPI) with a b-value of 1000 s/mm^2. In the context of neck infections, the DWI serves two functions. First, it is used for demonstrating or excluding diffusion restriction related to purulence in abscesses, and second, it is used for detecting lymphoid tissue in tonsils and lymph nodes. Our MRI protocol is consistent with the protocol suggested by a recent multicenter international consensus paper [16].

MRI has been proven feasible in pediatric patients with suspected neck infections [11]. In our previous validation cohort of 45 children, 16 (36%) were sedated with spontaneous breathing, and only 3 patients (7%) required general anesthesia [11]. The risk of ionizing radiation for CT and the potential adverse effects associated with sedation/anesthesia for MRI are frequently discussed in the literature [17]. Further, related to feasibility, MRI scanning can cause fear and anxiety in children which needs to be recognized and minimized. Potentially useful methods for mitigating anxiety include ambient surroundings, colors, music, and other audiovisual pastimes, a "scan buddy", and a mini-sized toy scanner [18].

Table 1. Practical approach to routine neck infection MRI protocol.

Phenomenon	Sequence	Findings	Suggestions	Notices
Soft tissue edema	T2 Dixon (water) post-contrast T1W Dixon (water)	Abnormal high signal	Radiologic evidence of an infection; specific edema patterns suggest a more severe course of disease.	All kinds of inflammation

Table 1. *Cont.*

Phenomenon	Sequence	Findings	Suggestions	Notices
Abscess	T1 SE T2 Dixon (water) DWI post-contrast T1 Dixon (water)	Non-enhancing collection with low ADC values enclosed in abnormally enhancing soft tissue edema.	Detection of an abscess usually requires operative consideration and exact abscess location, and extensions are useful in operative planning.	Abscesses may have an intermediate T2 signal content; blood products and/or postoperative status may complicate abscess assessment; necrotic lymph nodes may be misinterpreted as suppurative lymphadenitis.
Bone marrow edema	T1 SE T2 Dixon (water) post-contrast T1 Dixon (water)	Low signal in T1 and high signal in T2 Dixon (water) and post-contrast T1 Dixon.	Bone marrow edema may confirm odontogenic origin and point to the affected tooth.	Recent dental operations cause similar reactive findings; MRI artifacts may complicate assessment.
Complications	Whole protocol	Abscess extending to multiple deep neck spaces, mediastinis, venous thrombosis, and airway compromise.	Detection of potentially life-threatening conditions.	Magnetic resonance angiography (MRA) or CECT may be needed to diagnose venous thrombosis; defining airway compromise is difficult.
Cystic masses and potential neoplasms	Whole protocol	Identification of cystic component vs. neoplastic tissue, both with or without signs of infection.	Relevant differential diagnostics; exclusion of findings requiring immediate interventions.	Differential diagnosis may be limited and needs clinical correlation; biopsy may be required.

Image quality can be deteriorated by artifacts induced by patient motion or metallic foreign bodies, but the proportion of non-diagnostic MRI scans is low (about 1%) even in the acute setting [10]. Especially in pediatric patients, the dental hardware related to orthodontics can easily complicate the assessment of the DWI, hampering radiological diagnostics if odontogenic infections are suspected. Luckily, odontogenic infections are rare in small children [11].

3. Anatomical Considerations, MRI Terminology, and Edema Patters

3.1. Neck Anatomy and Key Areas of Scrutiny

The normal anatomy of the pediatric oropharynx is presented in Figure 1. MRI accurately demonstrates lymphoid tissue in the tonsils, which may be quite prominent in small children and teenagers. The differences between children and adults in proportional neck anatomy and disease processes also create the framework for image findings and interpretation [11]. These include the differing distribution of lymph nodes in the neck, as nodes located in the retropharyngeal space tend to be affected by the infectious processes more often in children than in adults [10,11]. The lymph nodes are normally larger in children than in adults as lymph nodes can undergo atrophy and diminish in physical activity [13] (Figures 2 and 3). No new lymph nodes develop with age. Children's lymph nodes, both in the retropharyngeal space and laterally, are challenged by antigen exposure and presentation for the first time in these individuals' lives, and when the nodes encounter a new antigen, they can become enlarged. In adult life, when challenged with a specific antigen, the immunological memory generates an antibody without the need for a new recognition response [13].

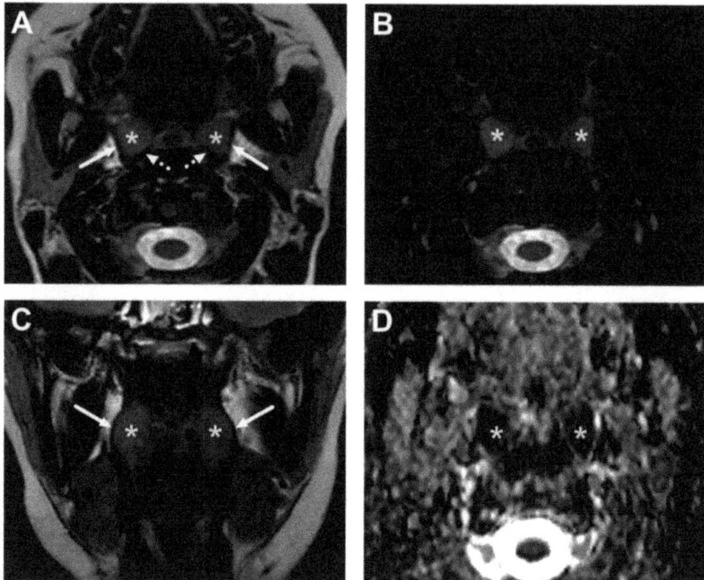

Figure 1. Normal MRI anatomy of the oropharynx in a 12-year-old. Axial T2-weighted (**A**), fat-suppressed T2-weighted (**B**), and coronal T2-weighted (**C**) images and an ADC map (**D**) demonstrate the palatine tonsils (white asterisk) bounded laterally by the superior constrictor muscle (arrows) and posteriorly by the palatopharyngeus muscle (dotted arrows).

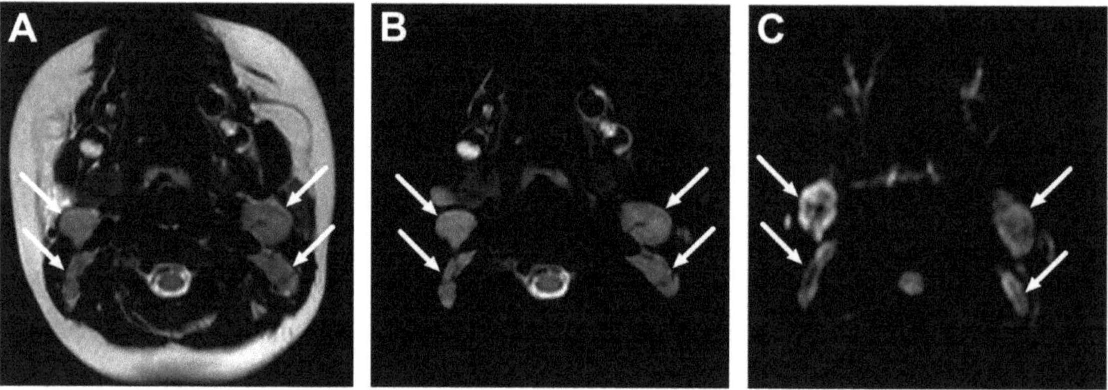

Figure 2. Normal level II lymph nodes in a 2-year-old on axial T2-weighted (**A**), fat-suppressed T2-weighted (**B**), and diffusion trace (**C**) images (arrows).

Viral or bacterial infections are the most common causes of acute lymphadenopathy in children [19]. The lymph nodes in viral cervical lymphadenitis are often soft, small, bilateral, mobile, and non-tender, whereas in bacterial-associated lymphadenitis, the nodes are usually unilateral, tender, and of acute onset. In non-viral cases, an empiric oral antibiotic is often prescribed as early as possible [20]. Large, reddened, and worsening lymph nodes may require hospitalization for parenteral antibiotics and occasionally surgical removal. Cervical lymphadenitis caused by nontuberculous mycobacteria is relatively common in children and may require surgical intervention; however, treatment strategies vary between countries and institutions [21–23].

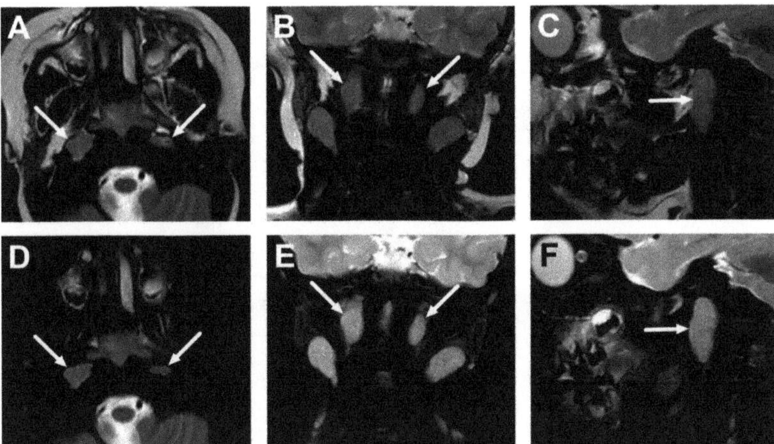

Figure 3. Normal lateral retropharyngeal lymph nodes (of Rouvière) in a 2-year-old on axial (**A**), coronal (**B**), and sagittal (**C**) T2-weighted images and axial (**D**), coronal (**E**), and sagittal (**F**) fat-suppressed T2-weighted images (arrows).

As lateral lymphadenitis is common in children, the careful analysis of the lymph nodes is essential in looking for suppurative lymphadenitis (intranodal abscess) which may require surgery or drainage [11]. Children also tend to have more retropharyngeal deep neck infections than adults; thus, scrutinizing the retropharyngeal space anatomy and disease processes is necessary [11]. In children, severe deep neck infections may spread caudally into the mediastinum. We encourage extending at least one axial pre-contrast T2-weighted Dixon sequence and one axial post-contrast T1-weighted Dixon sequence down to the level of lung hilum in order to determine or exclude disease processes such as anterior or posterior mediastinal edema, pleural fluid collections, and mediastinal abscesses.

The thymus can often be seen in children as a homogenous mass with smooth margins in the upper mediastinum (Figure 4) and should not be mistaken for pathology. The superior part of the thymus often extends cranially, immediately below the left thyroid gland. Another normal structure that is usually easily visible in children on fat-suppressed T2-weighted images is the thoracic duct (Figure 5).

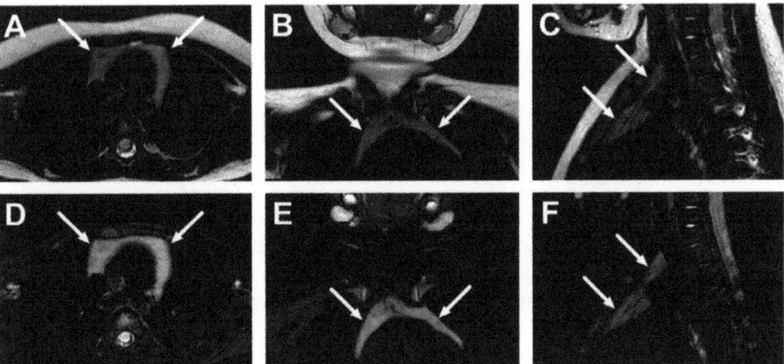

Figure 4. Normal thymus in the upper mediastinum in a 2-year-old on axial (**A**), coronal (**B**), and sagittal (**C**) T2-weighted images, and axial (**D**), coronal (**E**), and sagittal (**F**) fat-suppressed T2-weighted images (arrows).

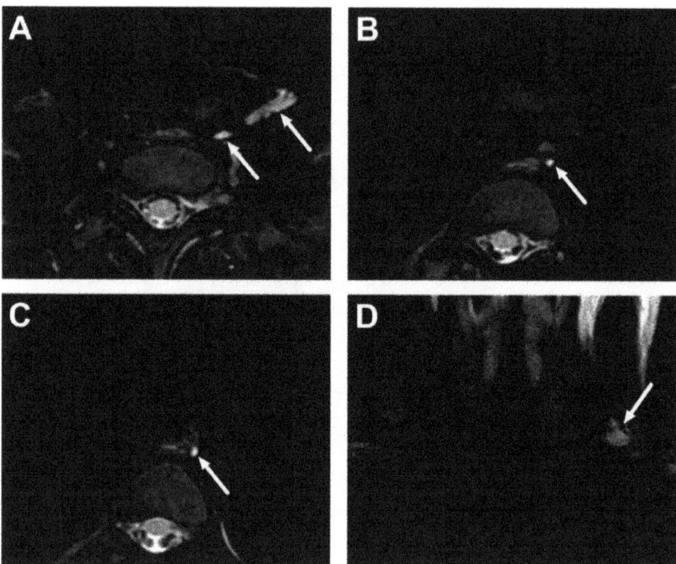

Figure 5. Normal thoracic duct (arrows) in a 15-year-old on three consecutive axial fat-suppressed T2-weighted images (**A–C**, superior to inferior) and a coronal fat-suppressed T2-weighted image (**D**).

3.2. Terminology of Pathology

In MRI, we define infection as (1) an abnormal, high signal indicating edema in fat-suppressed T2-weighted sequences or (2) a high signal in fat-suppressed post-contrast T1-weighted sequences indicating pathological tissue enhancement. Abscess MRI criteria include an abnormal isointense or hyperintense collection on T2-weighted sequences with low ADC values and no central enhancement, as well as enhancement surrounding this collection on T1-weighted Dixon post-contrast sequences [15]. In diagnosing abscesses, all sequences should be carefully scrutinized together because lesions that have a low ADC value may be interpreted as either suppurative fluid or solid tissue with high cellularity, depending on the pattern upon contrast enhancement.

3.3. Edema Patterns

Reactive, non-suppurative soft tissue edema is common in acute neck infections [15]. While areas of soft tissue edema do not necessarily contain abscesses or other targets for surgically treatable fluid collections, they indicate the severity of the infection [15].

In children, two of the most useful edema patterns are retropharyngeal edema (RPE) (Figure 6), and mediastinal edema (ME) (Figure 7). RPE is seen in about half of the patients with acute neck infections [24–26]. The retropharyngeal space is bordered by the buccopharyngeal fascia and the superior constrictor muscle anteriorly and the prevertebral fascia posteriorly. The alar fascia further divides this compartment into the "true" retropharyngeal space anteriorly and the "danger space" posteriorly. The distinction between the true retropharyngeal space and the so-called "danger space" cannot be made on radiological grounds; thus, the term "retropharyngeal" is radiologically sufficiently adequate to denote both anatomical entities. RPE is as common in children as in adults and is a significant predictor of the need for treatment in the intensive care unit (ICU) [26].

ME is seen in about one-quarter of patients with acute neck infections and can be divided into two categories: anterior and posterior. Anterior ME is commonly a continuum of edema from the visceral and/or anterior cervical spaces, whereas posterior ME is a continuation of RPE caudally. Similar to RPE, ME is encountered as often in children as in adults and is a significant predictor of the length of hospital stay [26].

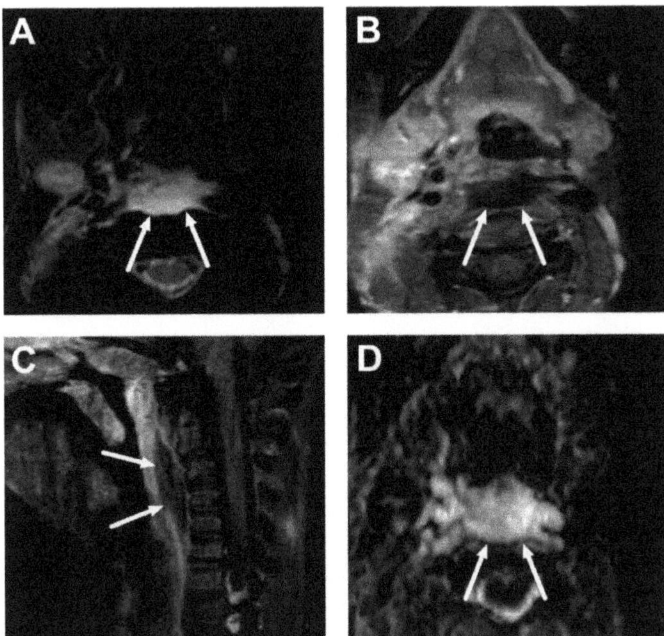

Figure 6. Reactive, non-suppurative edema (arrows) in the retropharyngeal space (RPE) in a 3-year-old child with lateral lymphadenitis. Images are axial fat-suppressed T2-weighted (**A**), fat-suppressed post-contrast axial (**B**), and sagittal (**C**) T1-weighted and an ADC map (**D**). The high signal in the ADC maps confirms that this non-enhancing fluid collection is not purulent but reactive. Surgical drainage is not required.

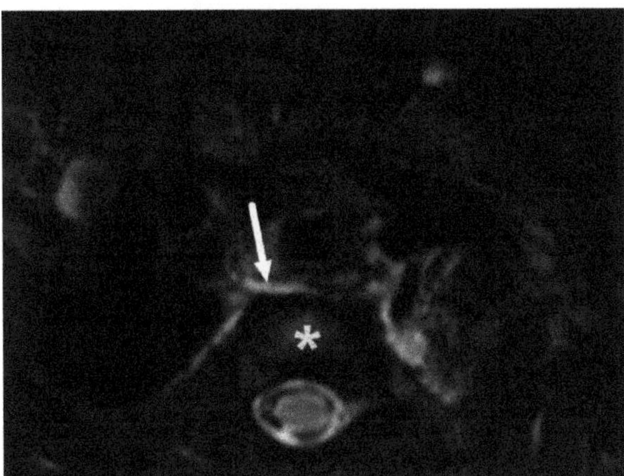

Figure 7. Reactive, non-suppurative edema in the mediastinum (ME) in a 3-year-old child with lateral lymphadenitis on an axial fat-suppressed T2-weighted image (arrow) at the level of the first thoracic vertebra (asterisk).

4. Typical Pediatric Deep Neck Infections

4.1. Tonsillitis, Peritonsillar Abscesses, and Parapharyngeal Abscesses

Tonsillitis (pharyngotonsillitis) is a common oropharyngeal infection. In our previous validation cohort, these types of infections were proportionally less common in children than in adults [11]. MRI findings in tonsillitis include edema and the post-contrast enhancement of the palatine tonsils and surrounding oropharyngeal mucosa. Due to high cellularity, the tonsils display innately restricted diffusion (Figure 1). Post-contrast imaging sequences are beneficial in distinguishing intrinsic diffusion restriction from peritonsillar abscesses (PTA) that exhibit pathological diffusion restriction [15]. PTAs form in the oropharyngeal mucosal space, the potential space between the tonsillar capsule and the superior constrictor muscles [27] (Figure 8) and are the most common type of abscess found in many cohorts [28]. They are usually treated without imaging, and conservative treatment with antibiotics is sufficient. As local incision and drainage are usually not applicable due to lack of cooperation, immediate tonsillectomy in general anesthesia is a good treatment option. However, if a complicated course of illness is suspected, such as parapharyngeal swelling or an unsuccessful local incision in older children, patients may benefit from MRI from which the true extension of the PTA and possible complications can be determined. PTAs are frequently located superiorly or caudally from the craniocaudal midpoint and may thus be unreachable if simple ambulatory needle drainage is attempted. PTAs may be bilateral, and this can result in airway compromise. If the abscess breaches through the superior constrictor muscle and the buccopharyngeal fascia laterally, it may reach the parapharyngeal space [27] (Figure 9). Large parapharyngeal abscesses are likely to require surgical drainage or at least close surveillance [29].

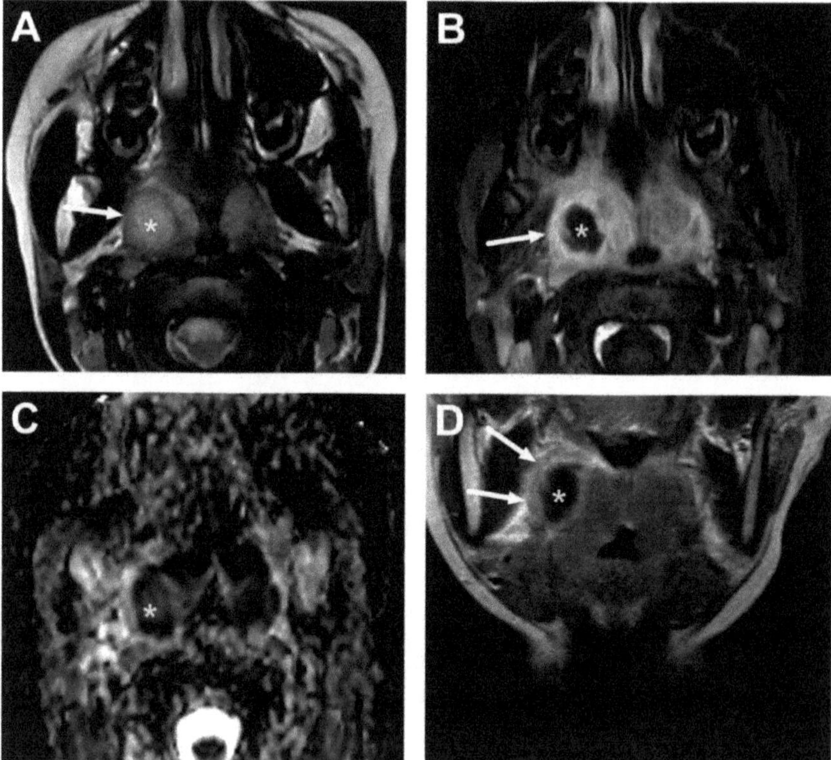

Figure 8. A peritonsillar abscess (PTA) (asterisk) in a 10-year-old on axial T2-weighted (**A**) and fat-suppressed post-contrast T1-weighted images (**B**), an ADC map (**C**), and a coronal post-contrast T1-weighted image (**D**). The abscess can be seen confined in the pharyngeal mucosal space, surrounded by the edematous superior constrictor muscle (arrows).

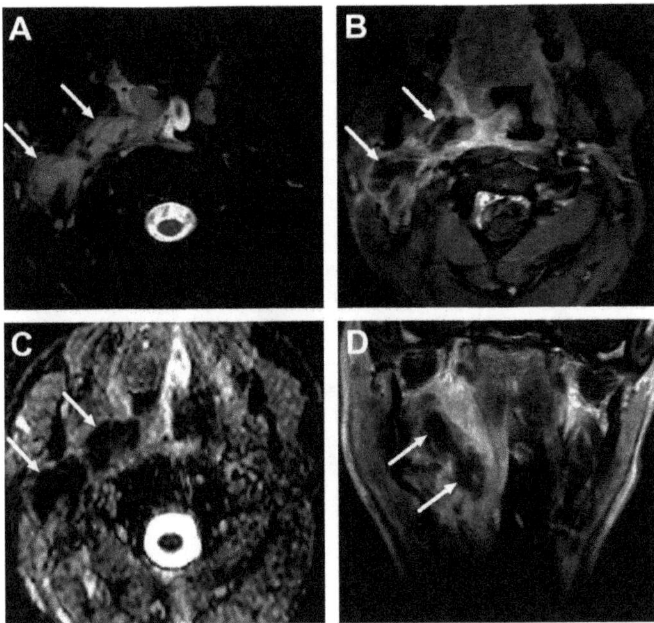

Figure 9. Parapharyngeal space abscess (arrows) in a 15-year-old teenager. Images are axial fat-suppressed T2-weighted (**A**) and fat-suppressed post-contrast axial T1-weighted (**B**) images, an ADC map (**C**), and a coronal post-contrast T1-weighted image (**D**). Notice that the abscess extends laterally, far beyond the border of the superior constrictor muscle. In image (**D**), the abscess can be seen extending caudally in the submandibular space, which communicates freely with the parapharyngeal space superiorly. Note that the abscess extends laterally beyond the internal carotid artery. Purulence was found during surgery, and *Fusobacterium necrophorum* was found in the pus culture.

4.2. Retropharyngeal Abscesses and Suppurative Lymphadenitis

Retropharyngeal infections tend to occur in young children [30]. In our previous validation cohort, all but one of the patients under the age of seven had a primary neck infection located in the retropharyngeal space or the lymph nodes; conversely, no patients aged 8–17 years had retropharyngeal infections [11]. Upon close inspection, most retropharyngeal infections actually represent suppurative lymphadenitis. They typically originate from the lateral retropharyngeal lymph nodes of Rouvière (Figures 10 and 11) but can rarely originate from the midline nodes (Figure 12). Quite often, the lateral retropharyngeal nodal abscess extends laterally into the post-styloid parapharyngeal space (carotid space)—these two spaces communicate freely (Figures 10 and 11). A "true" retropharyngeal abscess between the fascial planes also exists but is less commonly encountered [11] (Figure 13). In addition to suppurative lymphadenitis in the retropharyngeal space, lymph nodes containing purulence are found more laterally and superficially in the neck [11]. Lateral lymphadenitis may be diagnosed well with ultrasound. In these cases, MRI may be useful to confirm purulence (intranodal abscess formation) with DWI and to exclude any deep extension of abscesses. Ultrasound has been found to be an equally sensitive and specific method compared to CT in lateral neck abscesses in children [31]. Smaller children with *Staphylococcus aureus* infections tend to present with lateral lymphadenitis with large infectious mass-like lesions accompanied by widespread soft tissue edema, and careful assessment of both DWI and fat-saturated post-contrast T1-weighted sequences is crucial (Figure 14). Large abscesses and those not responding to medical treatment may require surgery, preferably via a transoral route, if the abscess does not extend lateral to the carotid arteries [32,33] (Figures 9–11).

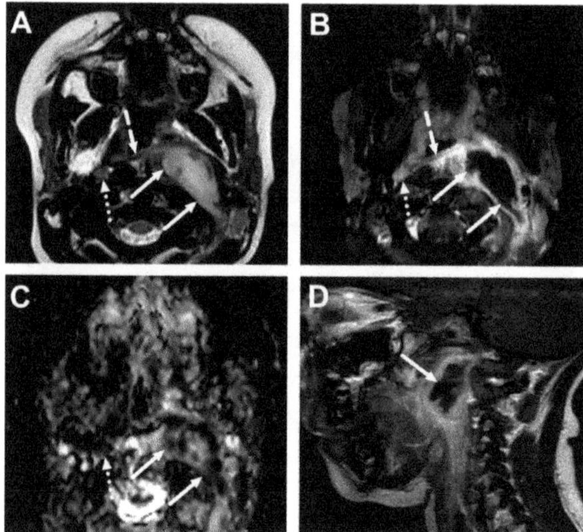

Figure 10. Suppurative lymphadenitis in the lateral retropharyngeal space in a 3-year-old child on axial T2-weighted (**A**) and fat-suppressed post-contrast T1-weighted images (**B**), an ADC map (**C**), and a sagittal post-contrast T1-weighted image (**D**). A large abscess (arrows) is posterior to the superior constrictor muscle (dashed arrows), confirming retropharyngeal location, and extends laterally to the post-styloid parapharyngeal (carotid) space. A normal retropharyngeal lymph node can be seen on the right side (dotted arrows). The abscess extends laterally slightly beyond the internal carotid artery. Purulence was found during surgery, and *Streptococcus pyogenes* was identified in the pus culture.

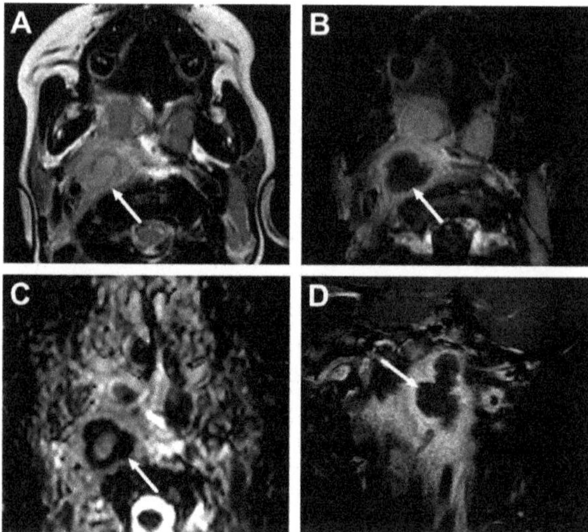

Figure 11. Suppurative lymphadenitis in the lateral retropharyngeal space in another 3-year-old child on axial T2-weighted (**A**) and fat-suppressed post-contrast T1-weighted images (**B**), an ADC map (**C**), and a sagittal fat-suppressed post-contrast T1-weighted image (**D**). A large abscess (arrows) extends laterally to the post-styloid parapharyngeal (carotid) space. Note that the abscess does not extend laterally beyond the internal carotid artery. Purulence was found during surgery, and *Streptococcus mitis* was identified in the pus culture.

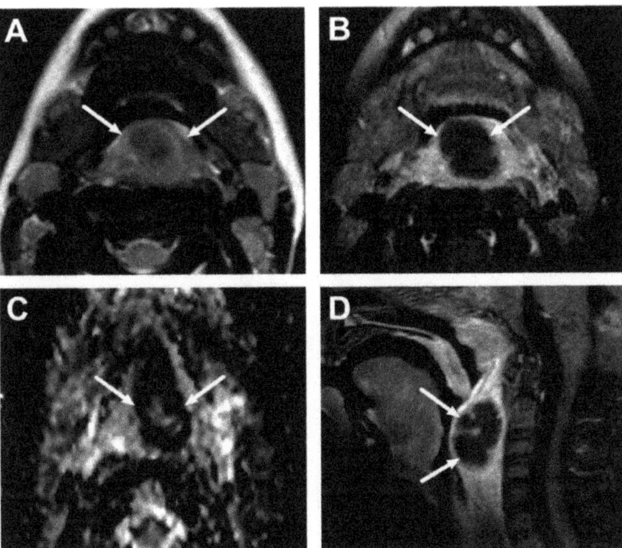

Figure 12. Suppurative lymphadenitis in the midline retropharyngeal space in another 3-year-old child on axial T2-weighted (**A**) and fat-suppressed post-contrast T1-weighted images (**B**), an ADC map (**C**), and a sagittal fat-suppressed post-contrast T1-weighted image (**D**). A large abscess (arrows) extends laterally to the post-styloid parapharyngeal (carotid) space. Purulence was found during transoral surgery.

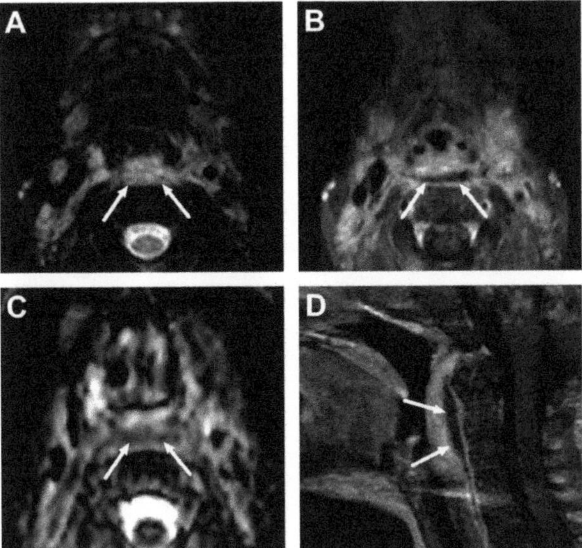

Figure 13. True retropharyngeal abscess in a 10-month-old infant on axial fat-suppressed T2-weighted (**A**) and fat-suppressed post-contrast axial T1-weighted (**B**) images, an ADC map (**C**), and a sagittal post-contrast T1-weighted image (**D**). A linear-shaped abscess (arrows) can be seen between the fasciae. Low ADC values (**C**) suggest purulence and not simply reactive edema.

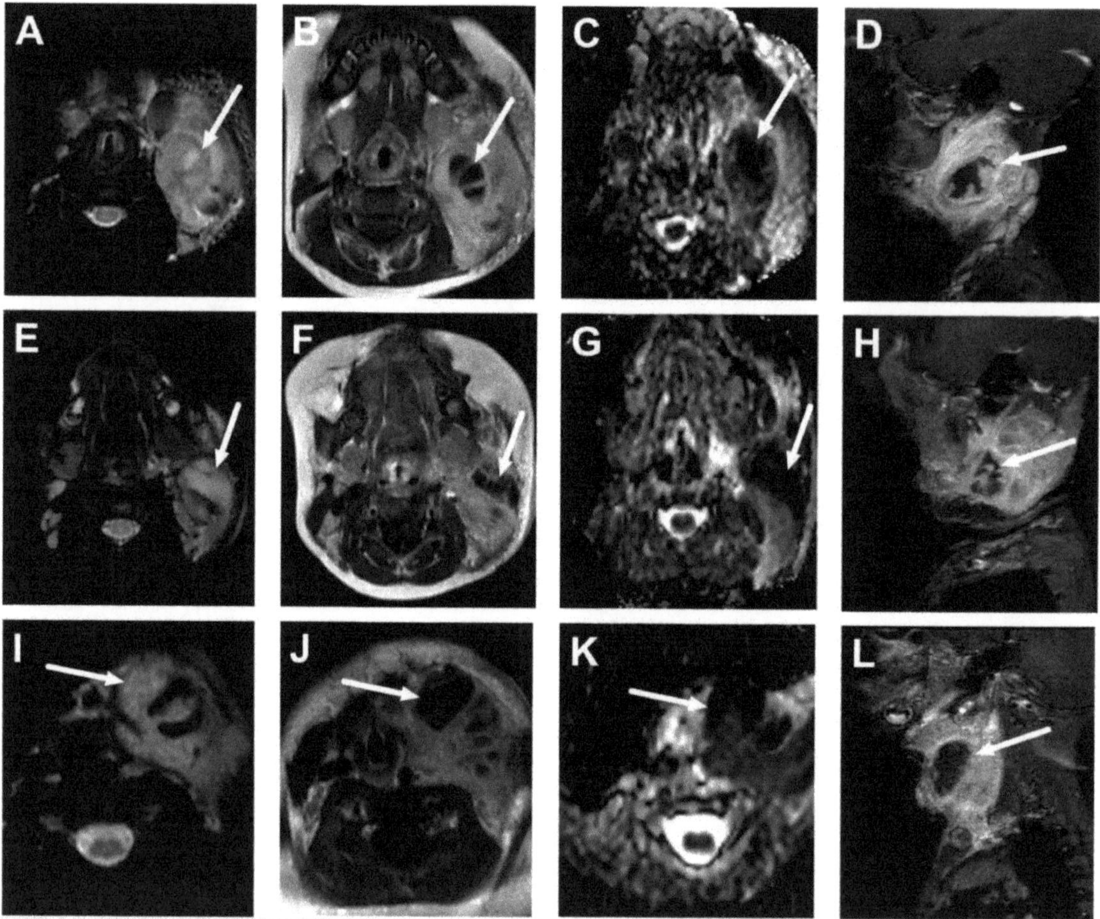

Figure 14. Lateral suppurative lymphadenitis in three infants less than 1 year of age (**A–L**). Images are axial fat-suppressed T2-weighted (**A,E,I**), post-contrast T1-weighted (**B,F,J**), ADC maps (**C,G,K**), and sagittal fat-suppressed T1-weighted (**D,H,L**). Note the large masses with surrounding edema and non-enhancing areas with low ADC values, which are indicative of intranodal abscesses (arrows). All patients underwent surgical drainage, and *Staphylococcus aureus* was found in the pus cultures.

4.3. Oral Cavity

Teeth are the most common cause of infection in the oral cavity. Luckily, they are rare in children [11] but may be encountered in teenagers with tooth infections. In children with primary teeth and thus many unerupted permanent teeth, clinical diagnosis and exploration may be complicated because of honeycombed anatomy, especially of the mandible. Odontogenic neck infections can be accurately described using MRI [15]. The typical locations for odontogenic abscesses are the sublingual and submandibular spaces (Figure 15). In our clinical practice, we do not use the historical term "Ludwig's angina" because it is vague and does not capture actionable imaging outcomes: etiology and surgically drainable abscesses.

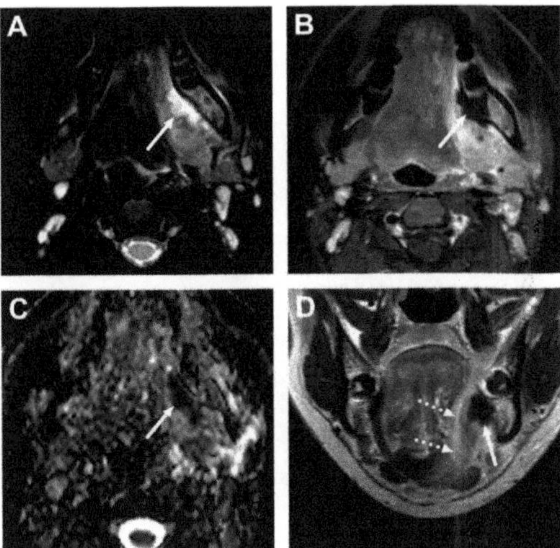

Figure 15. Odontogenic subperiosteal abscess (arrows) in the submandibular space following root canal treatment in a 15-year-old teenager. Images are axial fat-suppressed T2-weighted (**A**) and fat-suppressed post-contrast (**B**) images, an ACD map (**C**), and coronal post-contrast T1-weighted (**D**). An abscess is in the submandibular space, inferior to the edematous mylohyoid muscle (dotted arrows).

4.4. Sialadenitis

Infections of the salivary glands (sialadenitis) in children may be bacterial or viral [34]. In acute sialadenitis, MRI demonstrates a swollen salivary gland with edematous surroundings (Figures 16 and 17). Abscesses can be identified using DWI and post-contrast T1-weighted images. In obstructive sialadenitis, sialoliths may be seen as foci of the signal void [15].

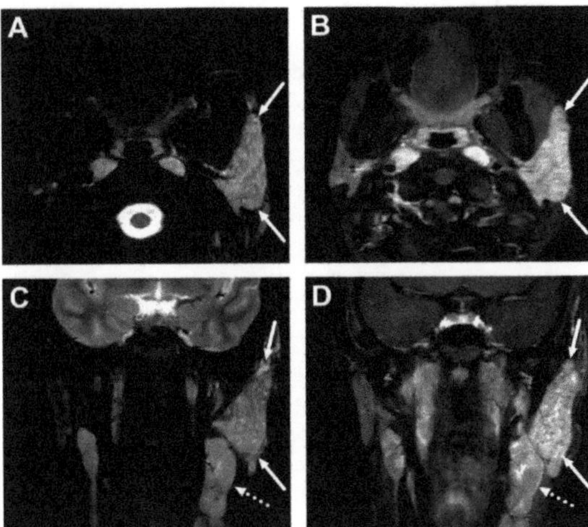

Figure 16. Acute parotitis of the left parotid gland (arrows) in a 16-year-old teenager. Images are axial (**A**) and coronal (**C**) fat-suppressed T2-weighted images and axial (**B**) and coronal (**D**) post-contrast T1-weighted images. The left parotid gland is swollen, edematous, and enhancing. No abscesses are seen. Note the slightly enlarged level II lymph nodes on the coronal images (dotted arrows).

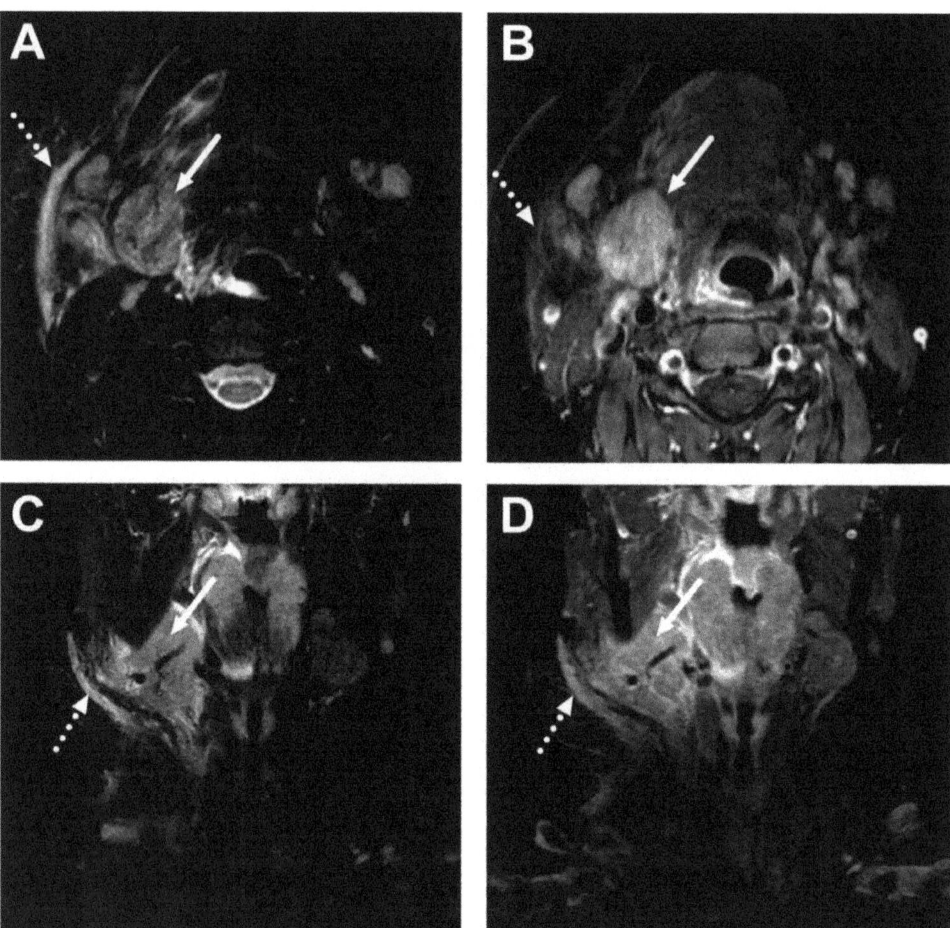

Figure 17. Acute sialadenitis of the right submandibular salivary gland (arrows) in a 13-year-old teenager. Images are axial (**A**) and coronal (**C**) fat-suppressed T2-weighted images and axial (**B**) and coronal (**D**) post-contrast T1-weighted images. The submandibular gland is swollen, edematous, and enhancing, but no abscesses exist. Note the considerable surrounding edema and enhancement in the adjacent soft tissues (dotted arrows).

5. Challenging MRI Findings and Pitfalls

5.1. Lymphadenitis with Purulence vs. Necrosis

In early lymphadenitis, the lymph node may be necrotic but not yet abscessed. It may be difficult to differentiate between a non-enhancing lymph node with restricted diffusion (a low ADC because of purulence, indicating intranodal abscess) and a lymph node with delayed enhancement accompanied by restricted diffusion (a low ADC because of high cellularity of lymphoid tissue, indicating necrotic or near-necrotic lymphadenitis) (Figure 18). Indeed, necrotic lymph nodes may enhance slower than normal nodes, and the enhancement may not be noticed if later scans (about 10 min after contrast administration) are not carefully scrutinized. Therefore, necrosis and slow enhancement may be confused for non-enhancement in early scans.

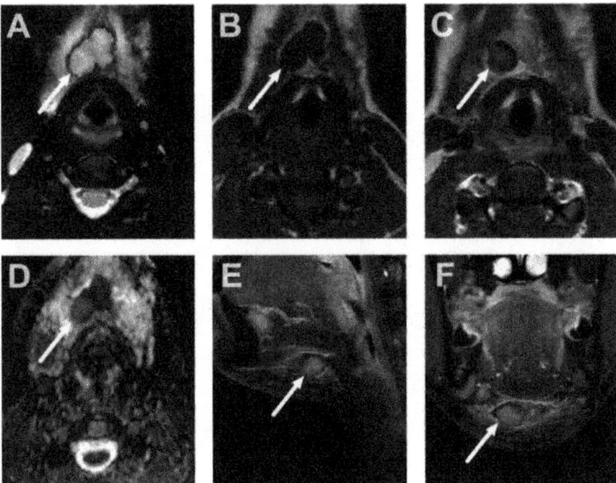

Figure 18. Necrotic lymphadenitis misinterpreted as suppurative lymphadenitis in a 15-year-old adolescent. Lymphadenitis is suggested on the axial fat-suppressed T2-weighted image (**A**) and poor enhancement on the post-contrast T1-weighted image (**C**) compared with the pre-contrast image (**B**) (arrows). The ADC demonstrates restricted diffusion (**D**) (arrow). The finding was initially misinterpreted as suppurative lymphadenitis (intranodal abscess formation); however, in post-contrast images taken at later time points, some delayed enhancement is seen (**E,F**) (arrows), ruling out suppuration. Consequent surgery found necrosis but no purulence. Image adapted from Ref. [15] under the Creative Commons Attribution License (CC BY 4.0).

5.2. Cystic Masses

Cystic masses, such as branchial cleft cysts, thyroglossal duct cysts, and vascular malformations, comprise the majority of congenital neck masses in children [35]. Some cystic lesions, such as lymphatic malformations, can grow rapidly during an acute neck infection. In general, the secondary infection of a cystic mass is suggested by a thick enhancement of the cyst wall and edema of the surrounding soft tissues (Figures 19–21). ADC maps from DWI are useful in detecting or ruling out purulence of the cyst fluid (Figures 20 and 21).

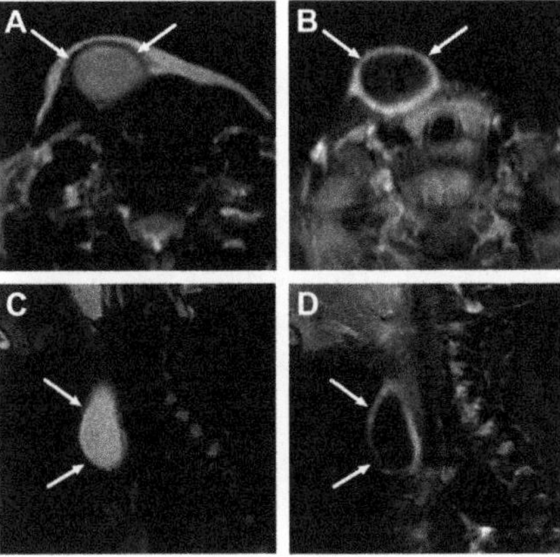

Figure 19. Second branchial cleft cyst (histologically confirmed) (arrows) in an 11-month-old infant on axial T2-weighted (**A**) and fat-suppressed post-contrast T1-weighted (**B**); and sagittal fat-suppressed T2-weighted (**C**), and post-contrast T1-weighted images (**D**). The thick rim enhancement suggests an acute infection; unfortunately, the ADC map was non-diagnostic in this case because of artifacts. The patient was managed medically in the acute phase.

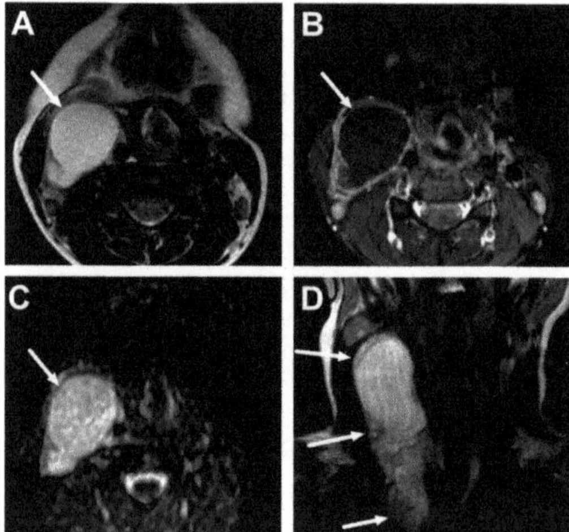

Figure 20. A large cystic mass (arrows) anteromedial to the sternocleidomastoid muscle in an 8-year-old child. Images are axial T2-weighted (**A**) and fat-suppressed post-contrast axial T1-weighted (**B**) images, an ADC map (**C**), and a coronal T2-weighted image (**D**). Acute enlargement and thick rim enhancement suggest an acute infection, but the ADC values are high, suggesting no purulence in the cyst. The patient was managed conservatively, and the cyst disappeared completely during follow-up, so no histopathological proof was obtained. The cyst extended caudally into the mediastinum (**D**), which is unlikely for a second branchial cleft cyst, suggesting the possibility of a thymic cyst, although these are rare and more commonly found on the left side.

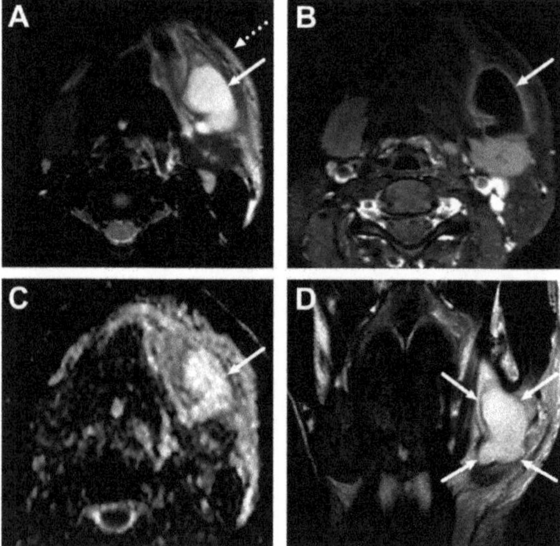

Figure 21. Lymphatic malformation with secondary infection in a 15-year-old teenager on axial T2-weighted (**A**) and fat-suppressed post-contrast axial T1-weighted (**B**) images, an ADC map (**C**), and a coronal T2-weighted image (**D**) (arrows). The coronal image (**D**) confirms the typical location in the submandibular space. Widespread edema of the surrounding soft tissues (dotted arrow in (**A**)) suggests an acute infection, but ADC values are high, suggesting no purulence in the malformation. The patient was later successfully treated with sclerotherapy.

5.3. Artifacts

Gas can be difficult to detect from MRI because the signal void may not be easily distinguished from other areas of low signal [15]. All sequences should be carefully evaluated for a complete and consistent signal void (Figure 22). Metallic braces can cause a significant signal loss in the oral cavity in children and teenagers (Figure 22).

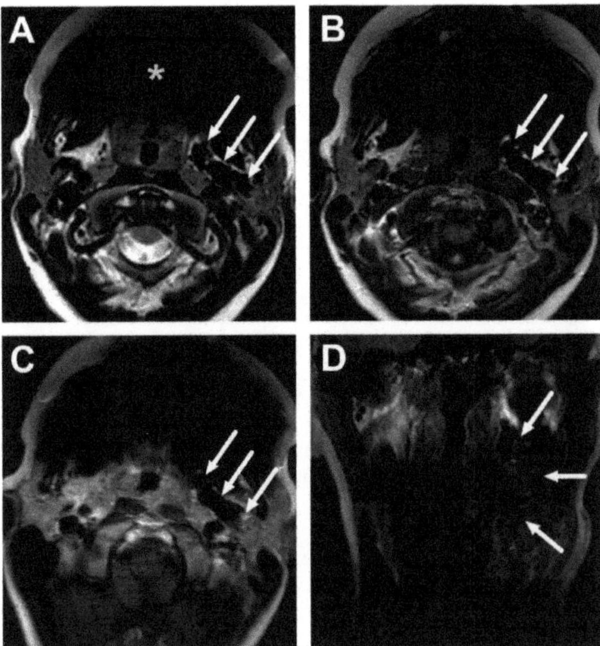

Figure 22. Neck pain and swelling after tonsillectomy in an 11-year-old child. Gas is shown as areas of signal void (arrows) in all sequences in the left parapharyngeal and submandibular spaces. Images are axial T2-weighted (**A**), pre-contrast T1-weighted (**B**), post-contrast T1-weighted (**C**) images, and a coronal post-contrast T1-weighted image (**D**). The anterior signal void (asterisk) is an artifact due to braces.

6. Complications

6.1. Mediastinitis

A mediastinal extension is related to a more severe course of illness in both children and adults [15] (Figure 23). The infection usually extends caudally from a primary neck infection site via the retropharyngeal route [11]. In order to screen for mediastinal disease, at least fat-saturated T2-weighted and post-contrast T1-weighted sequences in the axial plane should be extended to the upper mediastinum. If the whole mediastinum is to be imaged, the MRI protocol needs to be adjusted accordingly because of potential motion and susceptibility artifacts. Sometimes, a CT study is performed to confirm mediastinal findings (Figure 23).

MRI findings of mediastinal extension include anterior or posterior edema and/or abscess formation and pleural fluid accumulation (Figure 23). Minor edema findings are likely reactive (Figure 7) and should not be diagnosed as actual evidence of infection spread. On the contrary, extensive edema and especially abscess formation warrants acute clinical assessment for operative treatment and intensive care [15].

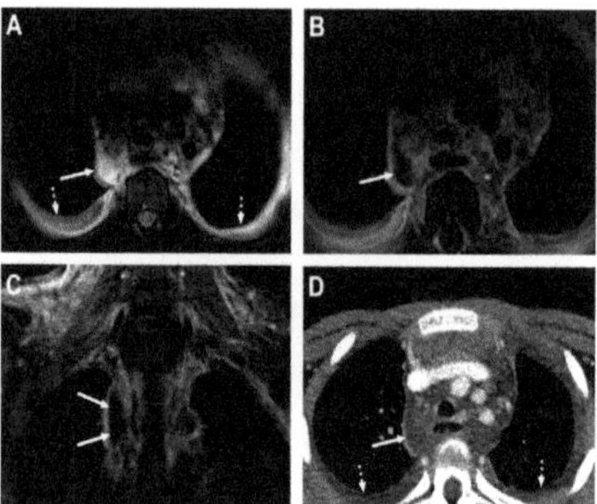

Figure 23. Descending mediastinitis in a 9-year-old child with widespread abscesses originating from the throat. The mediastinum was originally imaged with MRI; axial fat-suppressed T2-weighted (**A**) and post-contrast T1-weighted images (**B**); and a coronal post-contrast T1-weighted image (**C**). Imaging was consequently supplanted with CECT (**D**). Images show a mediastinal abscess (arrows) and pleural effusions (dotted arrows). The patient underwent surgery, and *Streptococcus pyogenes* was found in the pus cultures.

6.2. Venous Thrombosis

When venous thrombosis in the context of deep neck infection is diagnosed, the eponym *Lemierre's syndrome* has historically been used. With internal jugular vein thrombophlebitis, this syndrome also encompasses bacteremia (typically *Fusobacterium necrophorum*) secondary to current oropharyngeal infection, resulting in septic emboli [36,37]. Lemierre's syndrome has been associated with multiorgan failure and increased mortality risk [36] and thus requires prompt action. Luckily, this state is rare, but a moderate increase in incidence has been noticed in the past decades [38]. The syndrome does not always appear in its classical form, and a variant course of illness has been described [39].

Diagnosing thrombophlebitis is not always simple in MRI, as the thrombus may not be separable from a flow void in T1-weighted sequences (Figure 24). The lack of a flow void can also be indicative, and post-contrast sequences must be closely evaluated. In this context, MR angiography or a CECT of the head, neck, and thorax are alternative strategies to MRI to exclude possible complications, such as intracranial venous sinus thrombosis. Compared to CECT, the MRI scanning of multiple body parts is time-consuming, but MRI is more accurate in evaluating intracranial and epidural pathology in this setting.

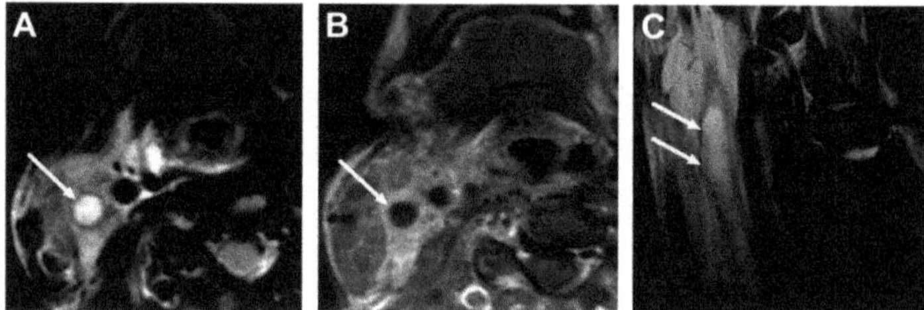

Figure 24. Thrombosed internal jugular vein (arrows) related to Lemierre's syndrome in a 15-year-old adolescent with a throat infection and septicemia, demonstrated on axial fat-suppressed T2-weighted (**A**) and post-contrast T1-weighted (**B**) images, and a coronal T2-weighted image (**C**). Excluding thrombosis may be challenging on standard MRI sequences. In this case, the lack of flow void is seen on the T2-weighted images (**A,C**), whereas the hypointense thrombus is difficult to separate from the flow void on the T1-weighted image (**B**). *Fusobacterium necrophorum* was found in blood cultures. Image partially adapted from Ref. [15] under the Creative Commons Attribution License (CC BY 4.0).

7. Conclusions

Emergency MRI has been proven to be a feasible imaging method in children with acute deep neck infections. MRI has superior diagnostic accuracy compared to CECT, encouraging more widespread use, especially in younger individuals. The differences between children and adults in anatomic proportions and the distribution of infectious diseases in the neck result in distinctive MRI findings. The subtleties in MRI findings of pediatric deep neck infections require careful assessment and knowledge.

To summarize the MRI findings: all acute neck infections cause varying degrees of edema, which is characterized as an abnormally high T2 signal on fat-suppressed images and enhancement shown as a high signal in fat-suppressed post-contrast T1-weighted sequences. For example, edema and post-contrast enhancement of the palatine tonsils and surrounding oropharyngeal mucosa are typical MRI findings in tonsillitis. Abscesses, such as those in peritonsillar, parapharyngeal, and retropharyngeal spaces, exhibit peripheral enhancement and a central, non-enhancing collection of pus, which can be effectively visualized with DWI as low ADC values. The location or extension of the abscess through various anatomical structures (e.g., parapharyngeal abscess extending from the peritonsillar space lateral to the superior constrictor muscle) can then be used for proper classification. Careful examination of all MRI sequences is important to avoid various pitfalls. For example, necrotic lymph nodes may be difficult to distinguish from purulent lymphadenitis. Early scans may confuse necrosis and delayed enhancement for non-enhancement, and both can show low ADC values, indicating high cellularity or purulence.

Author Contributions: Conceptualization, J.H. (Jussi Hirvonen) and J.N.; methodology J.H. (Jussi Hirvonen); software, validation, formal analysis and investigation, J.H. (Jussi Hirvonen), J.H. (Jaakko Heikkinen), J.N., A.S. and J.-P.V.; resources and data curation, J.H. (Jussi Hirvonen) and J.N.; writing—original draft preparation, J.N. and J.H. (Jussi Hirvonen); writing—review and editing, J.N., J.H. (Jaakko Heikkinen), T.H., M.N., A.S., J.-P.V., J.V., H.I., T.S., L.I., K.M. and J.H. (Jussi Hirvonen); visualization, supervision, project administration and funding acquisition, J.N. and J.H. (Jussi Hirvonen). All authors have read and agreed to the published version of the manuscript.

Funding: J.H. (Jussi Hirvonen) received a research grant from the Sigrid Jusélius Foundation. This funding had no role in the study design, data acquisition, analysis or interpretation, or article writing.

Institutional Review Board Statement: The national legislation in Finland requires no Institutional Review Board approval or waiver in retrospective studies of existing data.

Informed Consent Statement: Images of the current study are published under study permission granted by the Hospital District of Southwestern Finland. Informed consent was waived due to the retrospective nature of this study.

Data Availability Statement: Data availability is not applicable to this article as no new data were created or analyzed in the study.

Conflicts of Interest: The authors declare no conflict of interest.

References

1. Boscolo-Rizzo, P.; Stellin, M.; Muzzi, E.; Mantovani, M.; Fuson, R.; Lupato, V.; Trabalzini, F.; Da Mosto, M.C. Deep neck infections: A study of 365 cases highlighting recommendations for management and treatment. *Eur. Arch. Oto-Rhino-Laryngol.* **2012**, *269*, 1241–1249. [CrossRef] [PubMed]
2. Velhonoja, J.; Lääveri, M.; Soukka, T.; Hirvonen, J.; Kinnunen, I.; Irjala, H. Early surgical intervention enhances recovery of severe pediatric deep neck infection patients. *Int. J. Pediatr. Otorhinolaryngol.* **2021**, *144*, 110694. [CrossRef] [PubMed]
3. Cheng, J.; Elden, L. Children with Deep Space Neck Infections: Our Experience with 178 Children. *Otolaryngol. Head Neck Surg.* **2013**, *148*, 1037–1042. [CrossRef]
4. Donà, D.; Gastaldi, A.; Campagna, M.; Montagnani, C.; Galli, L.; Trapani, S.; Pierossi, N.; De Luca, M.; D'Argenio, P.; Tucci, F.M.; et al. Deep Neck Abscesses in Children: An Italian Retrospective Study. *Pediatr. Emerg. Care* **2021**, *37*, e1358–e1365. [CrossRef] [PubMed]
5. Garca, M.F.; Budak, A.; Demir, N.; Cankaya, H.; Kiroglu, A.F. Characteristics of Deep Neck Infection in Children According to Weight Percentile. *Clin. Exp. Otorhinolaryngol.* **2014**, *7*, 133–137. [CrossRef]

6. Brook, I. Microbiology and management of peritonsillar, retropharyngeal, and parapharyngeal abscesses. *J. Oral Maxillofac. Surg.* **2004**, *62*, 1545–1550. [CrossRef]

7. Elden, L.M.; Grundfast, K.M.; Vezina, G. Accuracy and Usefulness of Radiographic Assessment of Cervical Neck Infections in Children. *J. Otolaryngol.* **2001**, *30*, 082–089. [CrossRef]

8. Vural, C.; Gungor, A.; Comerci, S. Accuracy of computerized tomography in deep neck infections in the pediatric population. *Am. J. Otolaryngol.* **2003**, *24*, 143–148. [CrossRef]

9. Malloy, K.M.; Christenson, T.; Meyer, J.S.; Tai, S.; Deutsch, E.S.; Barth, P.C.; O'reilly, R.C. Lack of association of CT findings and surgical drainage in pediatric neck abscesses. *Int. J. Pediatr. Otorhinolaryngol.* **2008**, *72*, 235–239. [CrossRef]

10. Nurminen, J.; Velhonoja, J.; Heikkinen, J.; Happonen, T.; Nyman, M.; Irjala, H.; Soukka, T.; Mattila, K.; Hirvonen, J. Emergency neck MRI: Feasibility and diagnostic accuracy in cases of neck infection. *Acta Radiol.* **2021**, *62*, 735–742. [CrossRef]

11. Nurminen, J.; Heikkinen, J.; Happonen, T.; Velhonoja, J.; Irjala, H.; Soukka, T.; Ivaska, L.; Mattila, K.; Hirvonen, J. Magnetic resonance imaging findings in pediatric neck infections—A comparison with adult patients. *Pediatr. Radiol.* **2022**, *52*, 1158–1166. [CrossRef]

12. Hagelberg, J.; Pape, B.; Heikkinen, J.; Nurminen, J.; Mattila, K.; Hirvonen, J. Diagnostic accuracy of contrast-enhanced CT for neck abscesses: A systematic review and meta-analysis of positive predictive value. *PLoS ONE* **2022**, *17*, e0276544. [CrossRef]

13. Ogura, I.; Kaneda, T.; Kato, M.; Mori, S.; Motohashi, J.; Lee, K. MR study of lateral retropharyngeal lymph nodes at different ages. *Oral Surg. Oral Med. Oral Pathol. Oral Radiol. Endodontology* **2004**, *98*, 355–358. [CrossRef]

14. D'arco, F.; Lee, P.; Siddiqui, A.; Nash, R.; Ugga, L. Radiologic diagnosis of non-traumatic paediatric head and neck emergencies. *Pediatr. Radiol.* **2023**, *53*, 768–782. [CrossRef]

15. Hirvonen, J.; Heikkinen, J.; Nyman, M.; Happonen, T.; Velhonoja, J.; Irjala, H.; Soukka, T.; Mattila, K.; Nurminen, J. MRI of acute neck infections: Evidence summary and pictorial review. *Insights Imaging* **2023**, *14*, 5. [CrossRef]

16. D'arco, F.; Mertiri, L.; de Graaf, P.; De Foer, B.; Popovič, K.S.; Argyropoulou, M.I.; Mankad, K.; Brisse, H.J.; Juliano, A.; Severino, M.; et al. Guidelines for magnetic resonance imaging in pediatric head and neck pathologies: A multicentre international consensus paper. *Neuroradiology* **2022**, *64*, 1081–1100. [CrossRef]

17. Callahan, M.J.; Cravero, J.P. Should I irradiate with computed tomography or sedate for magnetic resonance imaging? *Pediatr. Radiol.* **2022**, *52*, 340–344. [CrossRef]

18. Runge, S.B.; Christensen, N.L.; Jensen, K.; Jensen, I.E. Children centered care: Minimizing the need for anesthesia with a multi-faceted concept for MRI in children aged 4–6. *Eur. J. Radiol.* **2018**, *107*, 183–187. [CrossRef]

19. Rosenberg, T.L.; Nolder, A.R. Pediatric Cervical Lymphadenopathy. *Otolaryngol. Clin. North Am.* **2014**, *47*, 721–731. [CrossRef]

20. Block, S.L. Managing Cervical Lymphadenitis—A Total Pain in the Neck! *Pediatr. Ann.* **2014**, *43*, 390–396. [CrossRef]

21. Kontturi, A.; Soini, H.; Ollgren, J.; Salo, E. Increase in Childhood Nontuberculous Mycobacterial Infections after Bacille Calmette-Guérin Coverage Drop: A Nationwide, Population-Based Retrospective Study, Finland, 1995–2016. *Clin. Infect. Dis.* **2018**, *67*, 1256–1261. [CrossRef]

22. Lyly, A.; Kontturi, A.; Salo, E.; Nieminen, T.; Nokso-Koivisto, J. Childhood nontuberculous mycobacterial lymphadenitis-observation alone is a good alternative to surgery. *Int. J. Pediatr. Otorhinolaryngol.* **2020**, *129*, 109778. [CrossRef] [PubMed]

23. Zimmermann, P.; Tebruegge, M.; Curtis, N.; Ritz, N. The management of non-tuberculous cervicofacial lymphadenitis in children: A systematic review and meta-analysis. *J. Infect.* **2015**, *71*, 9–18. [CrossRef] [PubMed]

24. Hoang, J.K.; Branstetter, B.F., IV; Eastwood, J.D.; Glastonbury, C.M. Multiplanar CT and MRI of Collections in the Retropharyngeal Space: Is It an Abscess? *Am. J. Roentgenol.* **2011**, *196*, W426–W432. [CrossRef] [PubMed]

25. Tomita, H.; Yamashiro, T.; Ikeda, H.; Fujikawa, A.; Kurihara, Y.; Nakajima, Y. Fluid collection in the retropharyngeal space: A wide spectrum of various emergency diseases. *Eur. J. Radiol.* **2016**, *85*, 1247–1256. [CrossRef]

26. Heikkinen, J.; Nurminen, J.; Velhonoja, J.; Irjala, H.; Happonen, T.; Soukka, T.; Mattila, K.; Hirvonen, J. Clinical and prognostic significance of emergency MRI findings in neck infections. *Eur. Radiol.* **2022**, *32*, 1078–1086. [CrossRef]

27. Esposito, S.; De Guido, C.; Pappalardo, M.; Laudisio, S.; Meccariello, G.; Capoferri, G.; Rahman, S.; Vicini, C.; Principi, N. Retropharyngeal, Parapharyngeal and Peritonsillar Abscesses. *Children* **2022**, *9*, 618. [CrossRef]

28. Côrte, F.C.; Firmino-Machado, J.; Moura, C.P.; Spratley, J.; Santos, M. Acute pediatric neck infections: Outcomes in a seven-year series. *Int. J. Pediatr. Otorhinolaryngol.* **2017**, *99*, 128–134. [CrossRef]

29. Wong, D.K.; Brown, C.; Mills, N.; Spielmann, P.; Neeff, M. To drain or not to drain—Management of pediatric deep neck abscesses: A case–control study. *Int. J. Pediatr. Otorhinolaryngol.* **2012**, *76*, 1810–1813. [CrossRef]

30. Woods, C.R.; Cash, E.D.; Smith, A.M.; Smith, M.J.; Myers, J.A.; Espinosa, C.M.; Chandran, S.K. Retropharyngeal and Parapharyngeal Abscesses Among Children and Adolescents in the United States: Epidemiology and Management Trends, 2003–2012. *J. Pediatr. Infect. Dis. Soc.* **2016**, *5*, 259–268. [CrossRef]

31. Collins, B.; Stoner, J.A.; Digoy, G.P. Benefits of ultrasound vs. computed tomography in the diagnosis of pediatric lateral neck abscesses. *Int. J. Pediatr. Otorhinolaryngol.* **2014**, *78*, 423–426. [CrossRef]

32. Hoffmann, C.; Pierrot, S.; Contencin, P.; Morisseau-Durand, M.-P.; Manach, Y.; Couloigner, V. Retropharyngeal infections in children. Treatment strategies and outcomes. *Int. J. Pediatr. Otorhinolaryngol.* **2011**, *75*, 1099–1103. [CrossRef]

33. Kirse, D.J.; Roberson, D.W. Surgical Management of Retropharyngeal Space Infections in Children. *Laryngoscope* **2001**, *111*, 1413–1422. [CrossRef]

34. Friedman, E.; Patiño, M.O.; Udayasankar, U.K. Imaging of Pediatric Salivary Glands. *Neuroimaging Clin.* **2018**, *28*, 209–226. [CrossRef]
35. Buch, K.; Reinshagen, K.L.; Juliano, A.F. MR Imaging Evaluation of Pediatric Neck Masses: Review and Update. *Magn. Reson. Imaging Clin.* **2019**, *27*, 173–199. [CrossRef]
36. Gore, M.R. Lemierre Syndrome: A Meta-analysis. *Int. Arch. Otorhinolaryngol.* **2020**, *24*, e379–e385. [CrossRef]
37. Osowicki, J.; Kapur, S.; Phuong, L.K.; Dobson, S. The long shadow of Lemierre's syndrome. *J. Infect.* **2017**, *74*, S47–S53. [CrossRef]
38. Ramirez, S.; Hild, T.G.; Rudolph, C.N.; Sty, J.R.; Kehl, S.C.; Havens, P.; Henrickson, K.; Chusid, M.J. Increased Diagnosis of Lemierre Syndrome and Other *Fusobacterium necrophorum* Infections at a Children's Hospital. *Pediatrics* **2003**, *112*, e380. [CrossRef]
39. George, E.; Callen, A.L.; Glastonbury, C.M. Atypical thrombophlebitis patterns in head and neck infections. *Neuroradiol. J.* **2023**. [CrossRef]

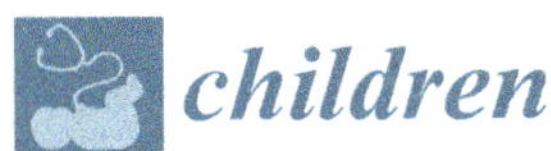

Article

Can Shear Wave Elastography Help Differentiate Acute Tonsillitis from Normal Tonsils in Pediatric Patients: A Prospective Preliminary Study

Bunyamin Ece [1] and **Sonay Aydin** [2,*]

1   Department of Radiology, Kastamonu University, Kastamonu 37150, Turkey; bunyaminece@hotmail.com
2   Department of Radiology, Erzincan University, Erzincan 24100, Turkey
*   Correspondence: sonay.aydin@erzincan.edu.tr

Abstract: Shear wave elastography (SWE) is a non-invasive imaging technique used to quantify the elasticity/stiffness of any tissue. There are normative SWE studies on tonsils in healthy children in the literature. The purpose of this study is to analyze the palatine tonsils in children with acute tonsillitis using ultrasound and SWE. In this prospective study, pediatric patients aged 4–18 years diagnosed with acute tonsillitis and healthy children were included. Those with antibiotic use, chronic tonsillitis, adenoid hypertrophy, and having chronic disease, immunodeficiency, and autoimmune disease, or any rheumatological disease were excluded. The volume and elasticity of palatine tonsil were measured via ultrasound and SWE. The study included 81 (46 female, 35 male) acute tonsillitis patients, and 63 (38 female, 25 male) healthy children between the ages of 4 and 18. Elasticity (kPa) values of tonsils were found significantly higher in the tonsillitis group (SWE-R: 25.39 ± 4.64, SWE-L: 25.01 ± 4.17) compared to the normal group (SWE-R: 9.71 ± 2.37, SWE-L: 9.39 ± 2.19) ($p < 0.001$). In the tonsillitis group, a significant positive correlation was found between tonsil volume and elasticity (r: 0.774, p: 0.002). In conclusion, in pediatric patients with acute tonsillitis, higher kPa values were obtained with SWE in the palatine tonsils.

Keywords: acute tonsillitis; shear wave elastography; stiffness; children; ultrasonography; pediatric

Citation: Ece, B.; Aydin, S. Can Shear Wave Elastography Help Differentiate Acute Tonsillitis from Normal Tonsils in Pediatric Patients: A Prospective Preliminary Study. *Children* **2023**, *10*, 704. https:// doi.org/10.3390/children10040704

Academic Editor: Curtise Ng

Received: 28 February 2023
Revised: 4 April 2023
Accepted: 6 April 2023
Published: 10 April 2023

1. Introduction

Palatine tonsils are lymphoepithelial tissues that are part of the mucosal immune system, and in the lateral oropharyngeal wall, they lie within the tonsillar fossa, which is bounded anteriorly and posteriorly by the mucosal arches containing the palatoglossus and palatopharyngeus muscles, respectively [1]. The palatine tonsil contains 10–30 tubular branched crypts that extend through the entire thickness of the organ and expand the surface of the tonsils [2]. They are located in a strategic area where the respiratory and digestive tracts meet to provide continuous lymphoid stimulation. They perform a significant function in the protection against foreign infections because of their locations [3].

Palatine tonsils grow rapidly in the first years of life due to their immunological function. Although the exact growth mechanism is unknown, it is thought to occur when external antigen presentation triggers/catalyzes lymphoid hyperplasia and tonsil parenchyma enlargement. Tonsil size is most prominent in childhood and is directly linked to bacterial load and the amount of B and T lymphocytes. Later, depending on age, tonsillar involution can be seen [2].

Tonsillitis occurs if the proliferation of pathogens in the lymphoid tissue exceeds the protective power of activated lymphoid and immunoglobulin-producing cells [2]. Acute tonsillitis is an acute inflammatory condition that affects the tonsillar tissues of the oropharynx and is most common in school-aged children. It affects nearly all children at least once in their lives. Infection typically starts as a superficial infection and can only progress through peritonsillar cellulitis to the endpoint of a potentially life-threatening peritonsillar abscess [4]. Due to the possibility for airway obstruction, acute tonsillar enlargement is especially important [5]. It is critical to recognize and treat acute tonsillitis because of the complications that might emerge in untreated individuals.

The evaluation of tonsillitis for most patients involves a physical examination, risk classification using scoring systems, and consideration of fast antigen testing or throat culture. However, it is important to begin with a complete history and physical exam before conducting any evaluation. This data can then be used to calculate a Centor Score, which takes into account the presence of a fever, tonsillar enlargement, and/or exudates, tender cervical lymphadenopathy, and the absence of a cough. Each finding is worth one point, but the criterion has been updated to include an age adjustment: patients aged 3 to 15 years receive an extra point, while patients aged 45 and older have one point deducted from their score [6,7].

Patients with a score of 0 to 1 generally do not require further testing or antibiotics. For those with a score of 2 to 3 points, rapid strep testing and throat culture are possible options. However, clinicians should consider testing and prescribing empiric antibiotics for patients with scores of 4 or above. Throat culture can be used alone or in combination with fast antigen testing to screen for Group A Beta-hemolytic Streptococcus. It is worth noting that although the fast antigen test is specific (88% to 100%), it is not very sensitive (61% to 95%), which means false negatives are possible [8].

In cases of complex illnesses, such as patients with unstable vital signs, a toxic appearance, difficulty swallowing or tolerating oral intake, or trismus, a more thorough evaluation may be necessary. This may include neck imaging and laboratory testing, such as a complete blood count and basic metabolic panel to check renal function [9].

A lateral neck X-ray is a cheap and easily accessible diagnostic tool that holds clinical value for tonsil and neck soft tissue evaluation. It can be used as a first-line investigation to assess whether there is an increase in the width of the soft tissues in front of the vertebrae, and it may also detect the presence of gas or an air-fluid level [10,11]. Additionally, for more detailed evaluation, magnetic resonance imaging (MRI) and computed tomography (CT) are commonly used methods to radiologically evaluate pathologies related to the palatine tonsil. However, these imaging methods have some disadvantages, including high costs, the necessity for sedation in children, and exposure to ionizing radiation. Recently, ultrasound (US) has been increasingly used to diagnose peritonsillar infections and to evaluate tonsils' morphological and volumetric changes [12–14].

Shear wave elastography (SWE) is a non-invasive imaging technique used to quantify the elasticity/stiffness of any tissue. SWE is a useful technique, particularly for children, due to its low operator dependence, ease of use, and reproducibility [15]. The literature includes SWE studies of different organs, such as the liver [16], testis [17], breast [18], thymus [19], parotid [20], kidney, and spleen [21] in children and adolescents. In the palatine tonsils, the literature includes studies showing normal values with SWE in healthy children and adolescents [14,22]. However, to our knowledge, there are no reports in the literature of a SWE study evaluating tissue elasticity/stiffness in cases of acute tonsillitis. In this respect, our study is the first to examine SWE values in patients with acute tonsillitis.

The purpose of this study is to use US and SWE to analyze the palatine tonsils in children with acute tonsillitis, examine the effect of tonsillar infection on tissue stiffness, and compare to the normal population.

2. Materials and Methods

Ethics committee approval was obtained from the hospital's local ethics committee for this prospective study (ethics committee no: E-457297017-3902100.137). In addition, informed consent was obtained from the parents before the transcervical US and SWE examinations. Data for the study were collected between January 2021 and April 2022.

2.1. Patient Selection

Tonsillitis group: Pediatric patients between the ages of 4 and 18 who were diagnosed with acute tonsillitis and volunteered to participate in the study were included in the tonsillitis group. We selected patients with acute tonsillitis from our hospital's pediatric outpatient clinic, family physician, or pediatric emergency department, and all patients were examined at the same state university hospital. There was no private service or a paid inspection. The diagnosis of acute tonsillitis was primarily based on the patient's medical history and physical examination findings. During a physical exam, a clinician decided to diagnose acute tonsillitis by examining the throat for signs of inflammation, such as redness, swelling, and the presence of pus or white spots on the tonsils and enlarged lymph nodes.

Healthy control group: Healthy child participants without active disease and between the ages of 4 and 18 were included. Healthy individuals without any known disease or signs of infection or fever during the examination were included in the control group.

The exclusion criteria were determined as follows: Being younger than 4 years old or older than 18 years old, having a history of tonsillectomy, having started antibiotic treatment before or using antibiotics for an existing disease, having any chronic disease, having known adenoid/tonsillar hypertrophy, having peritonsillar abscess and collection, having immunodeficiency or cancer, and having an autoimmune disease or any rheumatological disease that may affect the tonsils. In addition, patients with recurrent acute tonsillitis and chronic tonsillitis characterized by persistent inflammation and infection of the tonsils were excluded from the study.

As a result, bilateral tonsils of 81 patients in the tonsillitis group and 63 patients in the healthy control group were evaluated.

The patients' age, sex, BMI, height, and weight were all recorded in order to look for possible correlations between these parameters and tonsil dimensions, volumes, and SWE stiffness values (kPa).

2.2. Ultrasound and Shear Wave Elastography Assessment

The tonsil US examination was conducted with the patient lying down in the supine position, with their head tilted back slightly. The patient's neck was in extension and their head was turned towards the side being examined. After applying a clear gel to the patient's neck over the area where the tonsils are located, then ultrasound examination started using high-frequency linear-array transducers (L12-3, 3–12 MHz).

First the submandibular gland was discovered, then the palatine tonsil was visualized as a well-circumscribed hypoechoic structure just deep within the submandibular gland. Longitudinal and transverse plane imaging was performed according to the extension of the tonsil. During the ultrasound, the practitioner sometimes asked the patient to swallow to observe the movement of the tonsils. The diameters of both the right and left tonsils were measured in the anteroposterior, transverse, and longitudinal planes (Figure 1).

The volume of tonsils was automatically calculated using the US machine utilizing three simple measurements. Tonsil elastography measurements were determined automatically by the SWE feature of the machine (Figure 2). It was important to avoid applying pressure to the probe and to keep the practitioner's hand stable throughout ultrasonographic imaging. Elasticity values were measured in kilopascals (kPa). Elasticity values of the lesions were measured three times using three different ROIs of 1 cm^2 from the different areas by the same observer, and the average of these measurements was recorded as the final data. The US and SWE examinations were conducted by a radiologist with ten years of experience.

On the day of presentation to the outpatient clinic, patients underwent US and SWE examinations without having to wait for a separate appointment. After the patients were examined in the outpatient clinic, they were directed to the radiology department for imaging. The majority of patients sought medical attention within the first 2–3 days of symptom onset when their symptoms were most severe. Chronic cases and recurrent acute cases were excluded from the study with as much care as possible.

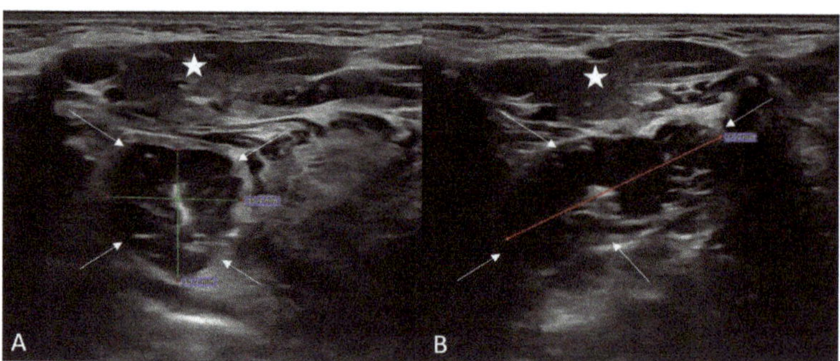

Figure 1. Ultrasonographic evaluation and measurements of the palatine tonsil in a healthy participant (Asterisk: Submandibular gland, Arrows: Palatine tonsil). (**A**): Transverse plane, (**B**): Longitudinal plane.

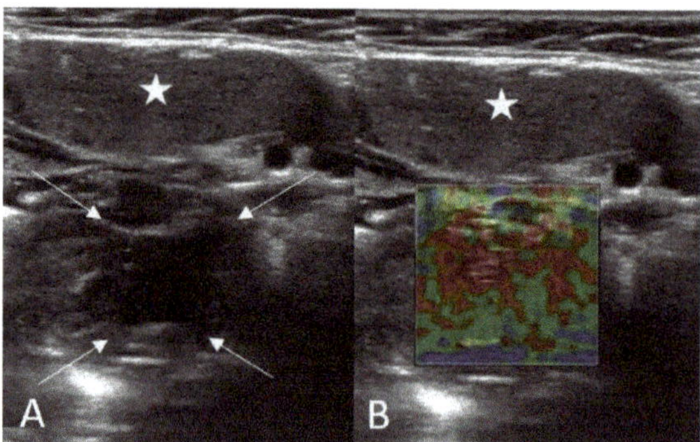

Figure 2. Shear wave elastography (SWE) evaluation of the palatine tonsil (**A**,**B**): Asterisk: Submandibular gland, Arrows: Palatine tonsil).

2.3. Statistical Analysis

Data analysis was performed using the SPSS software for social sciences (version 20) for Windows (IBM SPSS Inc., Chicago, IL, USA). To determine if the data had a normal distribution, the Kolmogorov–Smirnov test was utilized. Mean and standard deviation were used to present numerical variables with a normal distribution, while variables with a non-normal distribution were reported as medians with minimum and maximum values. Categorical variables were reported using numbers and percentages. Fisher's chi-square test was used to compare the percentages of sexes between the normal and acute tonsillitis groups. Tonsil elasticity and volume parameters were compared between groups using the Mann–Whitney U and Student's t tests, and compared based on gender using the Mann–Whitney U test. The Wilcoxon test was utilized to compare the parameters on the right and left sides. To explore potential relationships between tonsil elasticity and age, height, and weight values, Spearman correlation analysis was utilized. Logistic regression analysis was used to examine potential relationships between tonsil elasticity and sex. A two-tailed value of $p < 0.05$ was considered statistically significant.

3. Results

In the study, 144 (84 females, 60 males) participants aged 4–18 years were included. Of these, 81 (46 females, 35 males) were in the tonsillitis group and 63 (38 females, 25 males) were in the control group. The age and sex data of the tonsillitis group and the control group are shown in detail in Table 1. In terms of mean age and sex, there was no significant difference between the tonsillitis and control groups ($p > 0.05$) (Table 1).

Table 1. Age and sex distribution of the participants.

	Tonsillitis Group (n = 81)	Control Group (n = 63)	*p* Value
Age * (year) (Mean $\pm$ SD)	10.9 $\pm$ 2.8	11.5 $\pm$ 3.2	0.442
Sex ** (Female/Male), n(%)	46(57)/35(43)	38(60)/25(40)	0.748

* Student's *t* test, ** Fisher's Chi-square test, SD: Standard deviation.

The mean kPa values obtained from the right and left palatine tonsils by SWE and the mean volume values of the right and left palatine tonsils are shown in detail in Table 2. Accordingly, in the comparisons made separately for the right and left tonsils, kPa values were found to be significantly higher in the tonsillitis group compared to the control group ($p < 0.001$, for the right and left tonsils). The volume measurements obtained for the right and left tonsils were statistically significantly higher in the tonsillitis group compared to the control group ($p = 0.026$, $p = 0.021$ for the right and left tonsils, respectively) (Table 2).

Table 2. Data in the tonsillitis and healthy control groups, and comparison between groups.

	Tonsillitis Group (n = 81)	Control Group (n = 63)	*p* Value
SWE-R * (kPa) (Mean $\pm$ SD)	25.39 $\pm$ 4.64	9.71 $\pm$ 2.37	<0.001
SWE-L * (kPa) (Mean $\pm$ SD)	25.01 $\pm$ 4.17	9.39 $\pm$ 2.19	<0.001
Volume-R * (mm^3) (Mean $\pm$ SD)	2.90 $\pm$ 0.63	1.71 $\pm$ 1.20	0.026
Volume-L * (mm^3) (Mean $\pm$ SD)	2.97 $\pm$ 0.51	1.69 $\pm$ 0.80	0.021

* Student's *t* test, SWE: Shear Wave Elastography, kPa: Kilopascal, SD: Standard Deviation.

In the correlation analyses performed separately in the tonsillitis group, control group and total study group, no significant statistical correlation was found between the elasticity (kPa) with sex, height, weight, body mass index (BMI), and tonsil volume ($p > 0.05$) (Table 3). In the tonsillitis group, a statistically significant positive correlation was found between tonsil volume and elasticity (Table 3).

Table 3. Correlation analyses between elasticity and sex, weight, height, body mass index (BMI), tonsil volume (r = correlation coefficient; *p* = statistical significance).

	Tonsillitis Group (n = 81)		Control Group (n = 63)		Total Study Group (n = 144)	
	r	*p*	r	*p*	r	*p*
Sex/Elasticity *	0.452	0.163	0.313	0.396	0.423	0.260
Weight/Elasticity **	0.834	0.402	0.532	0.590	0.317	0.428
Height/Elasticity **	0.253	0.725	0.454	0.534	0.135	0.615
BMI/Elasticity **	0.345	0.243	0.318	0.712	0.192	0.533
Tonsil Volume/Elasticity **	0.774	0.002	0.160	0.663	0.065	0.618

* Logistic regression test, ** Spearman correlation test, BMI: Body Mass Index.

4. Discussion

In our study, we aimed to investigate the changes in elasticity and volume in acute tonsillitis by comparing palatine tonsil volume and SWE measurements with normal values in acute tonsillitis, which is one of the common pathologies in the pediatric patient group. For this, we applied SWE for quantitative evaluation immediately after the gray scale examination. According to the results of our study, a significant increase was found in tissue stiffness and tissue volume in the palatine tonsil compared to the normal group in pediatric patients with acute tonsillitis.

Ultrasonography is not typically the primary imaging modality used for assessing tonsils. However, given the limitations of CT and MRI, ultrasound can be a useful supplementary tool. In addition to being simple, noninvasive, and affordable, ultrasound can also be performed at the patient's bedside. Moreover, previous studies have shown that ultrasound is a helpful tool for evaluating tonsils and that volume measurements obtained through ultrasound are consistent with actual values [23–25]. As a matter of fact, Asimakopoulos et al. [26] found that US is a suitable objective method for determining tonsil volume in pediatric patients. There is an inherent existence of some form of signal-dependent noise in ultrasound imaging systems. Speckle noise is inherently present in ultrasound images. Its inherent presence occurs during the image acquisition phase. This noise can make it difficult to identify structures and can also degrade the image quality. Despeckling is an important preprocessing step in ultrasound imaging and can improve the accuracy of diagnosis and treatment planning. Despeckling techniques are used to reduce or eliminate this noise while preserving the underlying information. Much research has been completed in this field to remove speckle noise while preserving medical information in the image. The ultrasound devices which were used in the current study have this technology, so that we can acquire clear US and SWE images, and a successful sonographic imaging and study [27–30].

Shear wave elastography is a new method used to test tissue stiffness in a variety of tissues and organs, most notably the liver, breast, and thyroid [31,32]. SWE has been increasingly used in recent years to noninvasively identify normal and malignant cervical lymph nodes, usually by measuring lymph node stiffness [32,33]. Unlike other imaging techniques, it has been stated in the literature that SWE is noninvasive, inexpensive, convenient and reproducible, and that it can be performed in real time to monitor the stiffness of tissues [33].

In the literature, there are studies that evaluate the measurement of tonsil volume using ultrasound and evaluate normal kPa values of the palatine tonsils with elastography. In the first published study by Asumakopoulos et al. [26], they compared tonsil volume measured by ultrasound with the actual volume obtained from tonsillectomy in 52 tonsils from 26 children with adenotonsillar hypertrophy, aged 2–6 years. The study found that the mean tonsil volume measured by ultrasound was 3.6–3.9 mL, which was similar to the actual volume. In a study comparing obesity and hepatosteatosis with tonsillar volume, Ozturk et al. [34] found mean tonsillar volumes ranging between 3.18 mL and 4.45 mL in 97 children with a mean age of 13–14. In another study by Ozturk et al. [35], the mean tonsil volumes were found to be 2.03 mL in the chronic tonsillitis group and 5.36 mL in the obstructive sleep apnea syndrome (OSAS) group among 67 pediatric patients with a mean age of 10 years. Aydin et al. [36] conducted a normative study on 274 healthy children with a mean age of 7 years and found a mean tonsil volume of 1.5 mL. Mengi et al. [37] in their study of 85 patients with recurrent tonsillitis and OSAS, of which 50 were children with a mean age of 5.7 years, found the mean actual and ultrasound volumes in children as 3.5 mL and 3.67 mL, respectively. In our study, we found the mean tonsil volume as 2.90–2.97 mL in the acute tonsillitis group with a mean age of 10.9 years, and 1.69–1.71 mL in the healthy control group. When compared to studies in the literature that included adenotonsillar hypertrophy cases and OSAS patients, the tonsillar volume results of our study were lower. This may be because we excluded cases of tonsillar hypertrophy, recurrent tonsillitis, and chronic tonsillitis from our study. Tonsil volume measurements in normal healthy children in the literature and the measurements in our healthy control group were similar. The palatine tonsil volume in the tonsillitis group was found to be higher compared to the healthy control group in our study. These data demonstrate an increase in tonsil volume in cases of acute inflammation, suggesting that ultrasonography can detect this. As far as we are aware, there are two study [14,22] in the English literature that examine the normal elasticity values (kPa) of palatine tonsils using SWE, with similar results to ours.

Our study focused on the evaluation with SWE in patients with acute tonsillitis of the palatine tonsil. In our investigation, the mean elasticity values in the tonsillitis group were found to be statistically significantly higher when compared to the healthy control group. Our study provides first and preliminary findings regarding the SWE elasticity values of tonsillitis; hence, we cannot compare our findings to those of earlier research. However, we can compare it with the studies in the literature on several infective-inflammatory disorders. Accordingly, similar to our study, Qin Qin et al. [33] reported an increase in SWE values in acute bacterial cervical lymphadenitis. Lee JM et al. [38], in their study on Kikuchi patients, diagnosed with the acoustic radiation force impulse (ARFI) elastography method, found an increase in ARFI elastography values in Kikuchi patients and reactive hyperplasic lymph nodes compared to normal lymph nodes, similar to our study. Yoğurtçuoğlu et al. [39] found significantly higher mean elastography values than normal healthy kidneys in their ARFI study in patients with acute glomerulonephritis. According to our study and the findings in the literature, we conclude that there is an increase in the elasticity values of the tissues and tension and stiffening in the tissues in cases of infection-inflammation. This could be related to the fact that inflammatory cell infiltration and tissue liquefaction [40] in the palatine tonsil cause a significantly increased tension in the palatine tonsil in acute tonsillitis, resulting in high kPa values.

Studies in the literature have indicated that they evaluate shear wave flexibility in the hardest region of the lymph nodes due to the substantial regional variation in the distribution of lymphatic vessels in the SWE examination of the lymph nodes [41,42]. In our study, we performed measurements from solid areas while avoiding cryptic areas during SWE measurements in tonsils with increased volume. Similar to the literature, we think that tonsil flexibility can be evaluated more accurately in tonsils without heterogeneous internal structure.

Kamel et al. [43], in their study evaluating thyroid gland elasticity in pediatric patients with autoimmune thyroid disease, found thyroid SWE values to be significantly higher in children with autoimmune thyroiditis compared to healthy children due to parenchymal stiffness caused by lymphocytic infiltration and interstitial fibrosis. In the literature, a proportionally higher increase in tissue stiffness values has been found in autoimmune thyroiditis. However, when we look at our results, there is a moderate increase in proportion. One reason for this may be that fibrosis is not expected due to the pathophysiology of acute tonsillitis [5]. In addition, it is known that SWE may weaken while passing through the tissues due to its technical nature, and because the palatine tonsils are located relatively deeper than the thyroid tissue and lymph nodes, the push pulse may also weaken while passing through the tissues [44]. To compare the changes in the acute and chronic phases, there is a need for prospective longitudinal studies comparing acute tonsillitis and chronic tonsillitis and tonsillar hypertrophy patients in terms of tissue stiffness values.

Our study had some limitations. One of the limitations is the relatively small patient population. Therefore, the results may not be representative of the general population. Larger sample groups and multicenter studies are needed. Another limitation of our study is that patients with tonsillitis were not differentiated between viral or bacterial tonsillitis. Additional studies are needed to determine whether there will be a difference in SWE values in viral or bacterial tonsillitis. The major concern with US examinations is the high operator dependency variability, especially for quantitative SWE measurements. Another limitation is that the sonographic measurements were performed by only one physician. We opted to do so because extended examination times and reexamination were causing heightened discomfort and agitation among pediatric patients. Due to this situation, we were unable to assess the reproducibility of our measurements, and additional studies involving large patient groups and multiple practitioners are required to investigate the reproducibility of these measurements. Although this is a limitation of our study, the fact that all measurements were taken by a single physician ensured standardization between measurements in our study. Furthermore, although we determined cases with chronic tonsillitis and recurrent tonsillitis as exclusion criteria during patient selection, it was difficult to provide this strictly. It is challenging to assert that all patients are nonrecurrent and that this is the initial sickness. As a result, it is possible that we were unable to completely eliminate fibrotic changes during some tonsil evaluations.

5. Conclusions

The results of our study show that pediatric patients with acute tonsillitis exhibit higher kPa values in the palatine tonsils compared to the normal population, indicating increased stiffness. Additionally, we observed an increase in tonsil volume in acute tonsillitis. To the best of our knowledge, this is the first study to use SWE among patients with acute tonsillitis, and further prospective studies with larger populations are necessary to confirm these findings.

Author Contributions: Methodology, B.E. and S.A.; investigation, B.E and S.A.; resources, S.A.; writing—original draft preparation, B.E. and S.A.; writing—review and editing, S.A. and B.E.; visualization, S.A. and B.E.; supervision, S.A. All authors have read and agreed to the published version of the manuscript.

Funding: This research received no external funding.

Institutional Review Board Statement: The study was conducted in accordance with the Declaration of Helsinki and approved by the Institutional Review Board (or Ethics Committee) of Erzincan University (Ebyu-kaek-no: E-457297017-3902100.137)" for studies involving humans.

Informed Consent Statement: Written informed consent has been obtained from the patient(s) to publish this paper.

Data Availability Statement: The data that support the findings of this study are available from the corresponding author upon reasonable request.

Conflicts of Interest: The authors declare no conflict of interest.

References

1. Fossum, C.C.; Chintakuntlawar, A.; Price, D.L.; Garcia, J.J. Characterization of the oropharynx: Anatomy, histology, immunology, squamous cell carcinoma and surgical resection. *Histopathology* **2017**, *70*, 1021–1029. [CrossRef]
2. Nave, H.; Gebert, A.; Pabst, R. Morphology and immunology of the human palatine tonsil. *Anat. Embryol.* **2001**, *204*, 367–373. [CrossRef]
3. Brandtzaeg, P. Immunology of tonsils and adenoids: Everything the ENT surgeon needs to know. *Int. J. Pediatr. Otorhinolaryngol.* **2003**, *67* (Suppl. S1), S69–S76. [CrossRef]
4. Banarkar, A.N.; Adeyiga, A.O.; Fordham, M.T.; Preciado, D.; Reilly, B.K. Tonsil ultrasound: Technical approach and spectrum of pediatric peritonsillar infections. *Pediatr. Radiol.* **2015**, *46*, 1059–1067. [CrossRef] [PubMed]
5. Sidell, D.; Shapiro, N.L. Acute tonsillitis. *Infect. Disord. Drug Targets* **2012**, *12*, 655–660. [CrossRef] [PubMed]
6. McIsaac, W.J.; Kellner, J.D.; Aufricht, P.; Vanjaka, A.; Low, D.E. Empirical validation of guidelines for the management of pharyngitis in children and adults. *JAMA* **2004**, *291*, 1587–1595. [CrossRef]
7. ESCMID Sore Throat Guideline Group; Pelucchi, C.; Grigoryan, L.; Galeone, C.; Esposito, S.; Huovinen, P.; Little, P.; Verheij, T. Guideline for the management of acute sore throat. *Clin. Microbiol. Infect.* **2012**, *18*, 1–28. [CrossRef] [PubMed]
8. Georgalas, C.C.; Tolley, N.S.; Narula, P.A. Tonsillitis. *BMJ Clin. Evid.* **2014**, *2014*, 0503.
9. Anderson, J.; Paterek, E. Tonsillitis. [Updated 2022 September 18]. In *StatPearls [Internet]*; StatPearls Publishing: Treasure Island, FL, USA, 2023. Available online: https://www.ncbi.nlm.nih.gov/books/NBK544342/ (accessed on 25 March 2023).
10. Sao Pedro, T.; Scolnik, D.; Traubici, J.; Stephens, D. Utility of Soft Tissue Lateral Neck Radiographs in the Emergency Department: The 5-Year Experience of a Large Tertiary Care Pediatric Hospital. *Pediatr. Emerg. Care* **2020**, *36*, e254–e257. [CrossRef]
11. Virk, J.S.; Pang, J.; Okhovat, S.; Lingam, R.K.; Singh, A. Analysing lateral soft tissue neck radiographs. *Emerg. Radiol.* **2012**, *19*, 255–260. [CrossRef]
12. Secko, M.; Sivitz, A. Think ultrasound first for peritonsillar swelling. *Am. J. Emerg. Med.* **2015**, *33*, 569–572. [CrossRef] [PubMed]
13. Ding, J.; Cheng, H.; Ning, C.; Huang, J.; Zhang, Y. Quantitative measurement for thyroid cancer characterization based on elastography. *J. Ultrasound Med.* **2011**, *30*, 1259–1266. [CrossRef] [PubMed]
14. Öztürk, M.; Çaliskan, E.; Bayramoglu, Z.; Adaletli, I. Quantitative Assessment of Palatine Tonsils in Healthy Children and Adolescents With Shear-Wave Elastography. *Ultrasound Q.* **2018**, *34*, 213–218. [CrossRef] [PubMed]
15. Uysal, E.; Öztürk, M. Quantitative Assessment of Thyroid Glands in Healthy Children With Shear Wave Elastography. *Ultrasound Q.* **2019**, *35*, 297–300. [CrossRef] [PubMed]

16. Schenk, J.P.; Alzen, G.; Klingmuller, V.; Teufel, U.; El Sakka, S.; Engelmann, G.; Selmi, B. Measurement of real-time tissue elastography in a phantom model and comparison with transient elastography in pediatric patients with liver diseases. *Diagn. Interv. Radiol.* **2013**, *20*, 90–99. [CrossRef]

17. Bayramoglu, Z.; Kandemirli, S.G.; Comert, R.G.; Akpinar, Y.E.; Caliskan, E.; Yilmaz, R.; Oktar, T.M.; Cetin, B.; Cingoz, M.; Adaletli, I. Shear wave elastography evaluation in pediatric testicular microlithiasis: A comparative study. *J. Med. Ultrasound* **2017**, *45*, 281–286. [CrossRef]

18. Balleyguier, C.; Ciolovan, L.; Ammari, S.; Canale, S.; Sethom, S.; Al Rouhbane, R.; Vielh, P.; Dromain, C. Breast elastography: The technical process and its applications. *Diagn. Interv. Imaging* **2013**, *94*, 503–513. [CrossRef]

19. Bayramoğlu, Z.; Öztürk, M.; Çalışkan, E.; Ayyıldız, H.; Adaletli, İ. Normative values of thymus in healthy children; stiffness by shear wave elas-tography. *Diagn. Interv. Radiol.* **2020**, *26*, 147–152. [CrossRef]

20. Güngör, G.; Yurttan, N.; Bilal, N.; Menzicioglu, M.S.; Duymus, M.; Avcu, S.; Citil, S. Evaluation of Parotid Glands With Real-time Ultrasound Elastography in Children. *J. Ultrasound Med.* **2016**, *35*, 611–615. [CrossRef]

21. Palabiyik, F.B.; Inci, E.; Turkay, R.; Bas, D. Evaluation of Liver, Kidney, and Spleen Elasticity in Healthy Newborns and Infants Using Shear Wave Elastography. *J. Ultrasound Med.* **2017**, *36*, 2039–2045. [CrossRef]

22. Aydin, S.; Senbil, D.C.; Karavas, E.; Kadirhan, O.; Kantarci, M. Shear-Wave Elastography of Palatine Tonsils: A Normative Study in Children. *J. Med. Ultrasound* **2023**. epub ahead of print. Available online: http://www.jmuonline.org/preprintarticle.asp?id=367923 (accessed on 25 March 2023).

23. Hosokawa, T.; Yamada, Y.; Takahashi, H.; Tanami, Y.; Sato, Y.; Hosokawa, M.; Oguma, E. Size of the Tonsil on Ultrasound in Children Without Tonsil-Associated Symptoms. *Ultrasound Q.* **2020**, *36*, 24–31. [CrossRef]

24. Nightingale, K.; Soo, M.S.; Nightingale, R.; Trahey, G. Acoustic radiation force impulse imaging: In vivo demonstration of clinical feasibility. *Ultrasound Med. Biol.* **2002**, *28*, 227–235. [CrossRef]

25. Coquia, S.F.; Hamper, U.M.; Holman, M.E.; DeJong, M.R.; Subramaniam, R.M.; Aygun, N.; Fakhry, C. Visualization of the Oropharynx With Transcervical Ultrasound. *Am. J. Roentgenol.* **2015**, *205*, 1288–1294. [CrossRef]

26. Asimakopoulos, P.; Pennell, D.J.; Mamais, C.; Veitch, D.; Stafrace, S.; Engelhardt, T. Ultrasonographic assessment of tonsillar volume in children. *Int. J. Pediatr. Otorhinolaryngol.* **2017**, *95*, 1–4. [CrossRef] [PubMed]

27. Liu, F.; Chen, L.; Qin, P.; Xu, S.; Dong, Z.; Zhao, X.; Wan, X.; Chen, X.; Qin, B. Is despeckling necessary for deep learning based ultrasound image segmentation? *TechRxiv* **2023**, 1–16. [CrossRef]

28. Guo, Y.; Lu, Y.; Liu, R.W.; Zhu, F. Blind Image Despeckling Using Multi-Scale Attention-Guided Neural Network. *IEEE Trans. Artif. Intell.* **2023**, 1–12. [CrossRef]

29. Singh, P.; Diwakar, M.; Singh, S.; Kumar, S.; Tripathi, A.; Shankar, A. A homomorphic non-subsampled contourlet transform based ultrasound image des-peckling by novel thresholding function and self-organizing map. *Biocybern. Biomed. Eng.* **2022**, *42*, 512–528. [CrossRef]

30. Singh, P.; Diwakar, M. Total variation-based ultrasound image despeckling using method noise thresholding in non-subsampled contourlet transform. *Int. J. Imaging Syst. Technol.* **2023**. [CrossRef]

31. Evans, A.; Whelehan, P.; Thomson, K.; McLean, D.; Brauer, K.; Purdie, C.; Baker, L.; Jordan, L.; Rauchhaus, P.; Thompson, A. Invasive breast cancer: Relationship between shear-wave elastographic findings and histologic prognostic factors. *Radiology* **2012**, *263*, 673–677. [CrossRef]

32. Wong, V.W.-S.; Vergniol, J.; Wong, G.L.-H.; Foucher, J.; Chan, H.L.-Y.; Le Bail, B.; Choi, P.C.-L.; Kowo, M.; Chan, A.W.-H.; Merrouche, W.; et al. Diagnosis of fibrosis and cirrhosis using liver stiffness measurement in nonalcoholic fatty liver disease. *Hepatology* **2009**, *51*, 454–462. [CrossRef] [PubMed]

33. Qin, Q.; Wang, D.; Xu, L.; Lan, Y.; Tong, M. Evaluating Lymph Node Stiffness to Differentiate Bacterial Cervical Lymphadenitis and Lymph Node–First Presentation of Kawasaki Disease by Shear Wave Elastography. *J. Ultrasound Med.* **2020**, *40*, 1371–1380. [CrossRef]

34. Ozturk, M. Ultrasonographic Measurement of Palatine Tonsil Size and Its Correlation with Body-Mass Index and Hepatoste-atosis in Adolescents. *Ann. Med. Res.* **2021**, *24*, 0253–0257.

35. Ozturk, M.; Kilinc, T. Sonographic measurement of palatine tonsil volume in children and comparison with actual volume. *Med. Sci.* **2017**, *6*, 685-8. [CrossRef]

36. Aydin, S.; Uner, C. Normal palatine tonsil size in healthy children: A sonographic study. *Radiol. Med.* **2020**, *125*, 864–869. [CrossRef]

37. Mengi, E.; Sağtaş, E.; Kara, C.O. Assessment of Tonsil Volume With Transcervical Ultrasonography in Both Children and Adults. *J. Ultrasound Med.* **2019**, *39*, 529–534. [CrossRef] [PubMed]

38. Lee, J.-M.; Hwang, J.-Y.; Bae, J.-H.; Kim, M.R.; Kim, Y.-W.; Park, S.E.; Yeom, J.A.; Roh, J. Acoustic radiation force impulse imaging of biopsy-proven Kikuchi disease: Initial experiences for evaluating feasibility in pediatric patients. *Ultrasonography* **2019**, *38*, 58–66. [CrossRef]

39. Yoğurtçuoğlu, B.; Damar, Ç. Renal elastography measurements in children with acute glomerulonephritis. *Ultrasonography* **2021**, *40*, 575–583. [CrossRef]

40. Wells, R.G. Tissue mechanics and fibrosis. *Biochim. Biophys. Acta* **2013**, *1832*, 884–890. [CrossRef]

41. Lo, W.-C.; Hsu, W.-L.; Wang, C.-T.; Cheng, P.-W.; Liao, L.-J. Incorporation of shear wave elastography into a prediction model in the assessment of cervical lymph nodes. *PLoS ONE* **2019**, *14*, e0221062. [CrossRef]

42. Skerl, K.; Vinnicombe, S.; Giannotti, E.; Thomson, K.; Evans, A. Influence of region of interest size and ultrasound lesion size on the performance of 2D shear wave elastography (SWE) in solid breast masses. *Clin. Radiol.* **2015**, *70*, 1421–1427. [CrossRef] [PubMed]

43. Kamel, S.M.; ElKhashab, K.M.; Bhagat, S.; Elzayat, W.A. Shear wave elastography as a quantitative method for thyroid gland elasticity assessment in pediatrics patients with autoimmune-related thyroid disease, diagnostic utility and laboratory correlation. *Egypt. J. Radiol. Nucl. Med.* **2022**, *53*, 1–8. [CrossRef]

44. Barr, R.G. Elastography in clinical practice. *Radiol. Clin. N. Am.* **2014**, *52*, 1145–1162. [CrossRef] [PubMed]

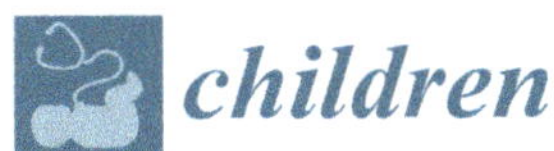

Case Report

Contrast-Enhanced Ultrasound (CEUS) as an Ancillary Imaging Test for Confirmation of Brain Death in an Infant: A Case Report

Peter Slak [1,2], Luka Pušnik [2] and Domen Plut [1,2,*]

1 Clinical Radiology Institute, University Medical Centre Ljubljana, Ljubljana 1000, Slovenia
2 Faculty of Medicine, University of Ljubljana, Ljubljana 1000, Slovenia
* Correspondence: plut.domen@gmail.com

Abstract: The practices for determining brain death are based on clinical criteria and vary immensely across countries. Cerebral angiography and perfusion scintigraphy are the most commonly used ancillary imaging tests for brain death confirmation in children; however, they both share similar shortcomings. Hence, contrast-enhanced ultrasound (CEUS) as a relatively inexpensive, easily accessible, and easy-to-perform technique has been proposed as an ancillary imaging test for brain death confirmation. CEUS has established itself as a favourable and widely used diagnostic imaging method in many different areas, but its application in delineating brain pathologies still necessities further validation. Herein, we present a case report of a 1-year-old polytraumatised patient in whom CEUS was applied as an ancillary imaging test for confirmation of brain death. As CEUS has not been validated as an ancillary test for brain death confirmation, the diagnosis was additionally confirmed with cerebral perfusion scintigraphy.

Keywords: contrast-enhanced ultrasound; head ultrasound; brain death; infants; ancillary test

Citation: Slak, P.; Pušnik, L.; Plut, D. Contrast-Enhanced Ultrasound (CEUS) as an Ancillary Imaging Test for Confirmation of Brain Death in an Infant: A Case Report. *Children* **2022**, *9*, 1525. https://doi.org/10.3390/children9101525

Academic Editor: Curtise Ng

Received: 19 September 2022
Accepted: 3 October 2022
Published: 5 October 2022

Publisher's Note: MDPI stays neutral with regard to jurisdictional claims in published maps and institutional affiliations.

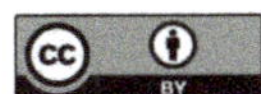

1. Introduction

Brain death is characterised by the complete and irreversible loss of brain functions, defined by the cessation of cortical and brainstem activities. The clinical criteria for the diagnosis in children were set in 1987, then updated in 2011 [1]. For the confirmation of brain death, the clinician must identify the underlying causes and determine their irreversibility. Conditions such as intoxication, hypotension, hypothermia, and metabolic/electrolyte disorders that could affect the neurologic examination have to be corrected before making the diagnosis. There is no global consensus regarding confirmatory tests [2]. The confirmation is typically made by verifying three criteria: unconsciousness, the absence of brainstem reflexes, and the apnoea test. As the latest is normally more difficult to implement in infants and can potentially cause harm in circulatory unstable patients, there is a variety of ancillary imaging tests that can assist in making the diagnosis [3].

The gold standard as an ancillary imaging test is cerebral angiography, as it confirms the cessation of cerebral circulatory blood flow. Nonetheless, this technique has several shortcomings: it is cumbersome, not always readily available, and potentially harmful, as it can exacerbate patients' hemodynamics. Cerebral angiography, along with radionuclide scanning, remain the most used ancillary imaging tests in infants. They both, however, require trained professionals to interpret the results and can be challenging to perform in a patient who needs to be transported from an intensive care unit [4]. An additional imaging test to confirm cerebral circulatory arrest is Doppler ultrasonography (US). With Doppler US, the blood flow through intracranial and extracranial arteries can be evaluated. This method can be performed at the bedside, is cost-efficient, and poses less risk than angiography. The major setback of this technique can be transmission problems, as inadequate penetration of US beams through the temporal bone in some subjects does not always allow a reliable evaluation of intracranial vessels [5,6].

Contrast-enhanced ultrasound (CEUS) is a relatively new technique with emerging application potential that is performed with a US scanner and requires the administration of US contrast agents. US contrast agents are extremely safe, with no cardio-, hepato-, or nephrotoxic effects and with a low incidence of side effects [7]. The most widely utilised contrast agents are made up of inert gas microbubbles that are stabilised by protein or lipid shells, with a size smaller than the red blood cells. In response to the exposition to the US beam, the microbubbles resonate—that is, enlarge and shrink—and, with that, send nonlinear signals back to the transducer. Intravenously administered US contrast agents remain confined within the blood pool without diffusion into the interstitial space, including in the setting of intracranial imaging. The US scanner detects circulating microbubbles as strong echoes moving within the vessels in real-time, providing micro- and macrovascular information used to assess vascular perfusion of the whole brain [8,9]. Therefore, CEUS allows better visualisation of the cerebral vasculature in comparison to Doppler US and the evaluation of cerebral perfusion [7,10,11]. Studies in adult populations have shown that the rate of nonconclusive Doppler US examinations for determining cerebral circulatory arrest significantly reduces if CEUS is performed [6,12]. Herein, we present a case of a 1-year-old polytraumatised patient in whom CEUS was used as an ancillary imaging test for confirmation of brain death.

2. Case Report

A 1-year-old girl, involved in a traffic collision, was found asystolic with dilatated and nonreactive pupils. The paramedics immediately initiated cardiopulmonary resuscitation, and the patient was transferred to the nearest hospital. At arrival, the girl was still unconscious and asystolic. After 20 min, cardiac action was re-established. On physical examination, numerous wounds and contusions were found on the patient's head, and bleeds from the nose and ears were observed. Additional contusions were noted on the trunk and extremities. The girl did not react to painful stimuli and had a Glasgow coma scale assessment score of 3. A complete blood count showed low haemoglobin (80 g/L) with elevated serum lactate levels (14 mmol/L). Whole-body computed tomography (CT) was performed forthwith. A head CT disclosed several fractures of the frontal and occipital bones, bilateral subarachnoid haemorrhage in the frontal region, and massive haemorrhage in the right maxillary sinus. No changes were noted in the cervical spine. CT of the chest and abdomen showed multiple contusions of the lungs and haematomas in the mediastinum and right inguinal region. For the treatment of severe hypotension (45/35 mmHg), the patient received blood transfusions, norepinephrine, and dopamine. The patient was transferred to a tertiary hospital centre. As intracranial hypertension (ICP = 40 mmHg) was persisting, treatment with mannitol and analgosedation was initiated. Therapeutic hypothermia was not induced due to the presence of coagulopathy. A follow-up CT scan of the head was performed approximately 12 h after the accident and showed marked cerebral oedema with completely displaced ventricles. The subarachnoid haemorrhage was more extensive, and pronounced transtentorial herniation through the foramen magnum was noted. CT brain angiography disclosed absent blood flow within the cerebral arteries (Figure 1). The patient's condition continuously deteriorated despite intensive treatment. Due to the poor prognosis, it was decided that further treatment was not feasible, and formal tests to confirm brain death were conducted.

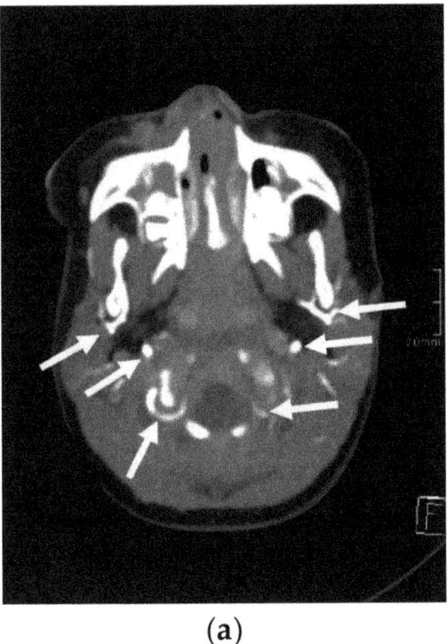 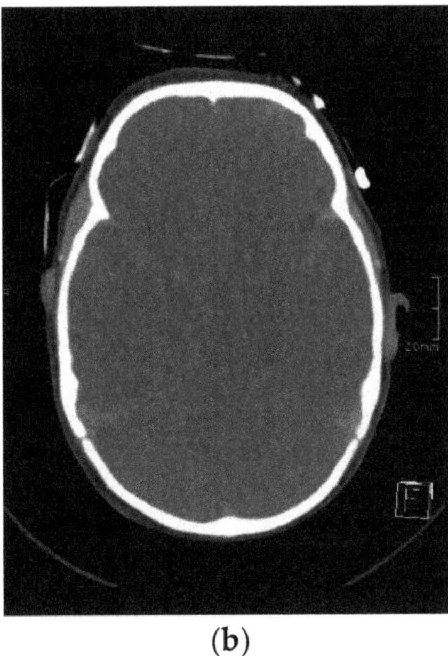

(a) **(b)**

Figure 1. Axial 3-mm-slab maximum intensity projection of the brain computed tomography angiography (CTA) of the 1-year-old infant. The CTA images (**a**,**b**) demonstrate absent contrast opacification of the intracranial arteries. Note the normal opacification of the extracranial arteries (arrows).

CEUS was performed as an ancillary imaging test for the confirmation of brain death. Before the examination, the details of the examination and the risks for the patient were explained to the child's guardian. Written informed consent was obtained from the child's guardian to perform the brain CEUS scan. The examination was performed by a paediatric radiologist with 2 years of subspecialty experience in paediatric brain imaging and 4 years of experience in performing CEUS examinations. For the examination, a Mindray M9 ultrasound scanner with a 1.4–5.1 MHz convex ultrasound transducer was used (Mindray, Shenzhen, China). SonoVue (Bracco, Milan, Italy) was used as the contrast agent. The anterior fontanelle was used as the acoustic window to scan the brain in the coronal and sagittal planes. Firstly, pre-contrast grey-scale imaging was performed to optimise the image. After that, a contrast-specific imaging mode and a low dynamic mechanical index (MI) of 0.06–0.07 was used for the scanning during the CEUS examination. To enable the simultaneous attachment of the US contrast agent and saline to the line, to avoid any delays in flushing the line with a saline flush, a three-way stopcock was connected to the existing peripheral intravenous line. At the start of the examination, 0.3 mL of US contrast agent, followed by a saline flush, was intravenously applied through a peripheral line. Only one bolus of US contrast agent was administered during the examination. For the first 60 s after the contrast administration, a continuous cine clip was obtained in the coronal plane at the level of the third ventricle, including the frontal horns of the lateral ventricles and heads of the caudate nuclei bilaterally. After that, intermittent images were obtained during the next 10 min in order to assess brain perfusion and avoid excessive contrast microbubble destruction from continuous imaging. The CEUS examination showed enhancement of the extracranial vessels and a lack of enhancement of the intracranial vessels (Figure 2). Only a scant amount of contrast microbubbles was observed within the left middle cerebral artery and pericallosal artery during the examination (Figure 3). After 10 min, we observed complete microbubble clearance and finished with the examination. The brain CEUS examination was performed in a paediatric intensive care unit at the bedside, and the whole procedure, including preparation, lasted approximately 15 min. No adverse effects were observed after the intravenous application of US contrast agent.

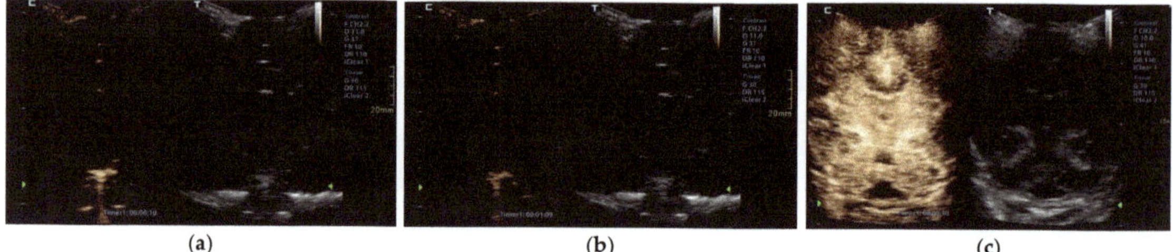

(a) (b) (c)

Figure 2. Midcoronal contrast-enhanced ultrasound images of a 1-year-old infant's brain obtained (**a**) 10 s and (**b**) 69 s after the contrast administration. Both images demonstrate a lack of enhancement of the intracranial vasculature and no brain perfusion. (**c**) Normal CEUS brain scan in another infant is shown as a comparison.

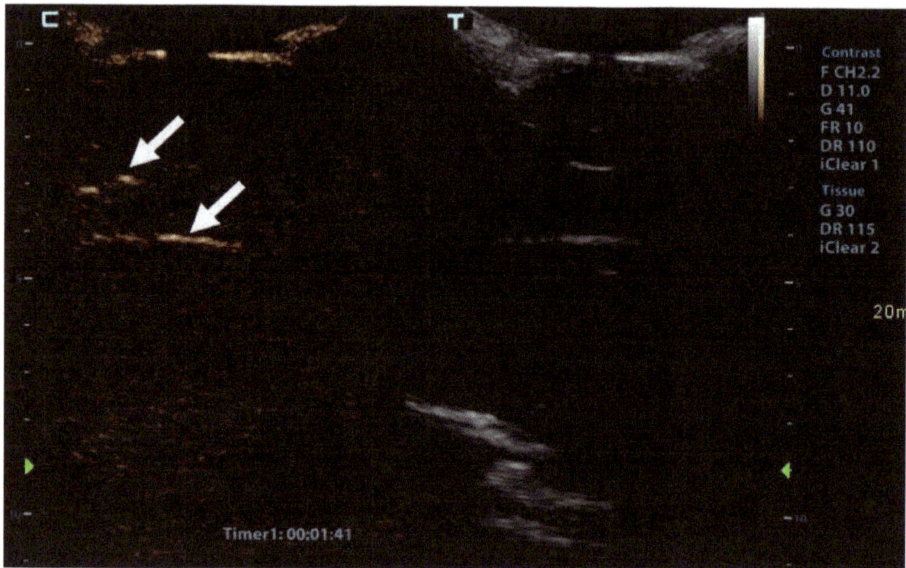

Figure 3. Sagittal contrast-enhanced ultrasound image of a 1-year-old infant's brain obtained 101 s after contrast administration. The image demonstrates a scant amount of contrast microbubbles within the pericallosal artery and its branch (arrows) and no brain perfusion.

After the US examination, cerebral perfusion scintigraphy was performed as a widely accepted ancillary imaging test for brain death confirmation. The perfusion scintigraphy showed no accumulation of the radionuclides in the brain or the brainstem (Figure 4).

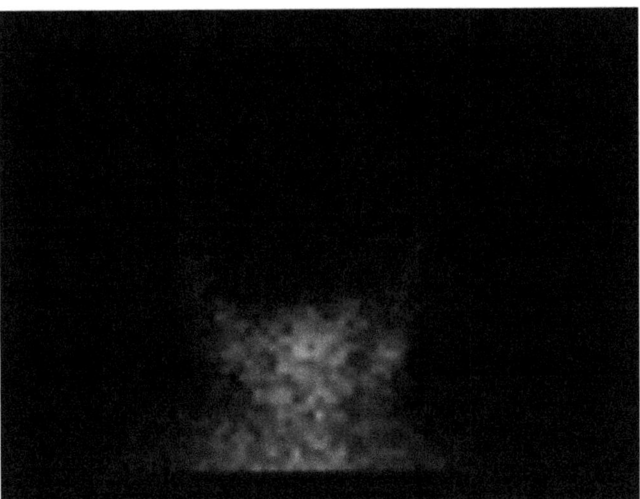

Figure 4. Radionuclide brain scan in the 1-year-old infant. Brain scintigraphy shows the absence of cerebral perfusion in supratentorial and infratentorial areas consistent with the diagnosis of brain death.

3. Discussion

We presented a case of a polytraumatised infant with foraminal herniation of the cerebellar tonsils in whom CEUS was employed as an ancillary imaging test for the confirmation of brain death. As CEUS is not a validated ancillary test for brain death conformation, the diagnosis was additionally confirmed with cerebral perfusion scintigraphy.

In recent years, CEUS has established itself as a beneficial and widely used diagnostic imaging method in many different areas, such as echocardiography, for the evaluation of vesicoureteral reflux and characterisation of liver neoplasms [10]. Due to a lack of clinical reports and safety studies, the use of CEUS for the assessment of brain pathology in children is, for now, still considered off-label [11,13]. Nevertheless, there has been an increasing number of reports on the use of CEUS in children for the assessment of hypoxic-ischemic injury, acute ischemic stroke, brain tumours, paediatric neurovascular diseases, epilepsy, and the confirmation of brain death [5,11,14,15]. These reports validate CEUS as a great method for the evaluation of the brain in children, especially the brain vasculature and vascular pathologic processes. We found only one report where CEUS was used as an ancillary imaging test for the confirmation of brain death in an infant. In this report by Hwang et al., the neonate passed away before they could confirm brain death with a formal radiologic evaluation. Therefore, in their case, the CEUS findings could not be compared to a validated imaging method [5]. In the case we presented, the absence of brain perfusion was confirmed by perfusion scintigraphy.

CEUS allows the observation of organ perfusion over a longer period of time, which makes it a great tool for the evaluation of organ perfusion. It takes up to 15 min for the contrast microbubbles to be metabolised and disappear from the vessels [16,17]. In our case, we observed the brain for 10 min. During this time, we did not observe any constant flow through any of the intracranial arteries. However, during the observation period, a scant of contrast microbubbles were observed within the left middle cerebral artery and pericallosal artery for a few seconds. It is important to note that, although we observed scant contrast microbubbles within the intracranial arteries, the perfusion scintigraphy showed no accumulation of the radionuclides in the brain. Therefore, we can assume that scant microbubbles within the intracranial arteries can be a finding on CEUS during the test for brain death confirmation and that this finding does not exclude a brain death diagnosis.

However, as this was the first such examination that we performed and no other similar reports exist in the literature, we cannot make any final conclusions. In the aforementioned case by Hwang et al., they reported "near absent perfusion of the intracranial vessels", which is similar to our case [5]. Further research will be needed to better delineate the extent and context of scant microbubbles within intracranial arteries for this kind of test.

The safety profile of US contrast agents has been documented in numerous studies in adult and paediatric populations. The US contrast is considered safe, with a comparable or lower risk of adverse events to the MRI contrast agents and almost 70-times lower risk compared to the iodinated CT contrast agents. Furthermore, it can be used in the case of impaired renal function, as it is not nephrotoxic [7]. An additional advantage of this technique is also that the administration of the US contrast agent can be repeated within the same setting if, for any reason, an examination fails or the results are not entirely clear after the first bolus. There is still limited data on the contrast safety in the paediatric population, with individual reports and questionnaire-based surveys reporting mild transitory adverse effects such as skin reactions, hypoventilation, altered taste, light-headedness, and transient tinnitus [18,19]. Nonetheless, in general, the US contrast is considered to have a favourable safety profile [20]. In our case, no adverse effects after intravenous application of the US contrast agent were observed.

In the adult population, the transcranial Doppler US is considered one of the main ancillary tests for the confirmation of brain death [21]. For the transcranial Doppler US, the thin temporal bone near the zygomatic arch bilaterally is usually used as the acoustic window (i.e., transtemporal window), although the suboccipital acoustic window can also be used. If a diastolic retrograde blood flow, systolic spikes, or completely absent blood flow in the main intracranial arteries are observed, this confirms the cerebral circulatory arrest [22]. Nevertheless, the transtemporal window does not always allow good visualisation of the intracranial arteries. Welschehold et al. recently demonstrated that transcranial Doppler US was not always feasible in approximately a quarter of their adult subjects [6]. Several researchers turned to CEUS with the transcranial Doppler US technique to achieve a better visualisation of intracranial arteries. These studies performed on the adult population show that the rate of nonconclusive transcranial Doppler US examinations for determining cerebral circulatory arrest significantly reduces if the US contrast agent is applied [6,12].

In our opinion, CEUS is approaching the ideal ancillary test for the confirmation of brain death in infants. The open anterior fontanelle in infants serves as an ideal acoustic window for the assessment of brain vasculature, much better than the transtemporal window in the adult population [5,8,17,23]. CEUS is also relatively inexpensive, easily accessible, safe, and available at the bedside, with the results not susceptible to sedative medications [4]. Nevertheless, further validation is still required before CEUS can be employed as an adjunct to other ancillary tests. Such a validation of the method would be valuable, as there is still a paucity of data regarding additional ancillary imaging tests for a brain death diagnosis in children, and only a scarce number of them have been validated in the paediatric population [24].

4. Conclusions

We presented a case of an infant in whom CEUS was employed as an ancillary imaging test for the confirmation of brain death. The case demonstrated CEUS as a reliable, rapid, non-invasive, easy-to-perform at the bedside, and feasible technique that could serve as an ancillary imaging test for brain death confirmation in infants. Further comparative studies on larger cohorts are required to confirm its potential.

Children **2022**, *9*, 1525

Author Contributions: Conceptualisation, P.S., D.P., and L.P.; data collection and assembly, P.S., D.P., and L.P.; data analysis and interpretation, P.S., D.P., and L.P.; writing of the manuscript, P.S., D.P., and L.P.; critical review and revision of the manuscript, D.P. and P.S.; and submission of the manuscript, D.P. All authors have read and agreed to the published version of the manuscript.

Funding: This research received no external funding.

Institutional Review Board Statement: Not applicable.

Informed Consent Statement: Written informed consent was obtained from the patient's guardian to perform the brain CEUS scan and, later, to publish this paper.

Data Availability Statement: The data supporting the findings of this study are private due to the protection of personal data.

Conflicts of Interest: The authors declare no conflict of interest.

References

1. Nakagawa, T.A.; Ashwal, S.; Mathur, M.; Mysore, M. Guidelines for the Determination of Brain Death in Infants and Children: An Update of the 1987 Task Force Recommendations. *Pediatrics* **2011**, *128*, e720–e740. [CrossRef] [PubMed]
2. Wijdicks, E.F.M. Brain Death Worldwide: Accepted Fact but No Global Consensus in Diagnostic Criteria. *Neurology* **2002**, *58*, 20–25. [CrossRef]
3. Dixon, T.D.; Malinoski, D.J. Devastating Brain Injuries: Assessment and Management Part I: Overview of Brain Death. *West J. Emerg. Med.* **2009**, *10*, 11–17. [PubMed]
4. Henderson, N.; McDonald, M. Ancillary Studies in Evaluating Pediatric Brain Death. *J. Pediatr. Intensive Care* **2017**, *6*, 234–239. [CrossRef]
5. Hwang, M.; Riggs, B.J.; Saade-Lemus, S.; Huisman, T.A.G.M. Bedside Contrast-Enhanced Ultrasound Diagnosing Cessation of Cerebral Circulation in a Neonate: A Novel Bedside Diagnostic Tool. *Neuroradiol. J.* **2018**, *31*, 578–580. [CrossRef]
6. Welschehold, S.; Geisel, F.; Beyer, C.; Reuland, A.; Kerz, T. Contrast-Enhanced Transcranial Doppler Ultrasonography in the Diagnosis of Brain Death. *J. Neurol. Neurosurg. Psychiatry* **2013**, *84*, 939–940. [CrossRef]
7. Sidhu, P.; Cantisani, V.; Deganello, A.; Dietrich, C.; Duran, C.; Franke, D.; Harkanyi, Z.; Kosiak, W.; Miele, V.; Ntoulia, A.; et al. Role of Contrast-Enhanced Ultrasound (CEUS) in Paediatric Practice: An EFSUMB Position Statement. *Ultraschall Med.-Eur. J. Ultrasound* **2016**, *38*, 33–43. [CrossRef]
8. Hwang, M.; Back, S.J.; Didier, R.A.; Lorenz, N.; Morgan, T.A.; Poznick, L.; Steffgen, L.; Sridharan, A. Pediatric Contrast-Enhanced Ultrasound: Optimization of Techniques and Dosing. *Pediatr. Radiol.* **2021**, *51*, 2147–2160. [CrossRef]
9. Gumus, M.; Oommen, K.C.; Squires, J.H. Contrast-Enhanced Ultrasound of the Neonatal Brain. *Pediatr. Radiol.* **2022**, *52*, 837–846. [CrossRef] [PubMed]
10. Freeman, C.W.; Hwang, M. Advanced Ultrasound Techniques for Neuroimaging in Pediatric Critical Care: A Review. *Children* **2022**, *9*, 170. [CrossRef]
11. Hwang, M.; Barnewolt, C.E.; Jüngert, J.; Prada, F.; Sridharan, A.; Didier, R.A. Contrast-Enhanced Ultrasound of the Pediatric Brain. *Pediatr. Radiol.* **2021**, *51*, 2270–2283. [CrossRef] [PubMed]
12. Llompart-Pou, J.A.; Abadal, J.M.; Velasco, J.; Homar, J.; Blanco, C.; Ayestarán, J.I.; Pérez-Bárcena, J. Contrast-Enhanced Transcranial Color Sonography in the Diagnosis of Cerebral Circulatory Arrest. *Transplant. Proc.* **2009**, *41*, 1466–1468. [CrossRef] [PubMed]
13. Squires, J.H.; McCarville, M.B. Contrast-Enhanced Ultrasound in Children: Implementation and Key Diagnostic Applications. *Am. J. Roentgenol.* **2021**, *217*, 1217–1231. [CrossRef]
14. Prada, F.; del Bene, M.; Saini, M.; Ferroli, P.; DiMeco, F. Intraoperative Cerebral Angiosonography with Ultrasound Contrast Agents: How I Do It. *Acta Neurochir.* **2015**, *157*, 1025–1029. [CrossRef] [PubMed]
15. Kanno, H.; Ozawa, Y.; Sakata, K.; Sato, H.; Tanabe, Y.; Shimizu, N.; Yamamoto, I. Intraoperative Power Doppler Ultrasonography with a Contrast-Enhancing Agent for Intracranial Tumors. *J. Neurosurg.* **2005**, *102*, 295–301. [CrossRef] [PubMed]
16. Schneider, M. Characteristics of SonoVue™. *Echocardiography* **1999**, *16*, 743–746. [CrossRef] [PubMed]
17. European Medicines Agency: Summary of Product Characteristics. SonoVue. Available online: https://www.ema.europa.eu/en/documents/product-information/sonovue-epar-product-information_en.pdf (accessed on 10 July 2022).
18. Coleman, J.L.; Navid, F.; Furman, W.L.; McCarville, M.B. Safety of Ultrasound Contrast Agents in the Pediatric Oncologic Population: A Single-Institution Experience. *Am. J. Roentgenol.* **2014**, *202*, 966–970. [CrossRef]
19. Riccabona, M. Application of a Second-Generation US Contrast Agent in Infants and Children—A European Questionnaire-Based Survey. *Pediatr. Radiol.* **2012**, *42*, 1471–1480. [CrossRef]
20. Ntoulia, A.; Anupindi, S.A.; Back, S.J.; Didier, R.A.; Hwang, M.; Johnson, A.M.; McCarville, M.B.; Papadopoulou, F.; Piskunowicz, M.; Sellars, M.E.; et al. Contrast-Enhanced Ultrasound: A Comprehensive Review of Safety in Children. *Pediatr. Radiol.* **2021**, *51*, 2161–2180. [CrossRef] [PubMed]

21. Walter, U.; Schreiber, S.J.; Kaps, M. Doppler and Duplex Sonography for the Diagnosis of the Irreversible Cessation of Brain Function (Brain Death): Current Guidelines in Germany and Neighboring Countries. *Ultraschall Med.-Eur. J. Ultrasound* **2016**, *37*, 558–578. [CrossRef]
22. Ducrocq, X.; Hassler, W.; Moritake, K.; Newell, D.W.; von Reutern, G.-M.; Shiogai, T.; Smith, R.R. Consensus Opinion on Diagnosis of Cerebral Circulatory Arrest Using Doppler-Sonography. *J. Neurol. Sci.* **1998**, *159*, 145–150. [CrossRef]
23. Hwang, M. Introduction to Contrast-Enhanced Ultrasound of the Brain in Neonates and Infants: Current Understanding and Future Potential. *Pediatr. Radiol.* **2019**, *49*, 254–262. [CrossRef] [PubMed]
24. Fainberg, N.; Mataya, L.; Kirschen, M.; Morrison, W. Pediatric Brain Death Certification: A Narrative Review. *Transl. Pediatr.* **2021**, *10*, 2738–2748. [CrossRef] [PubMed]

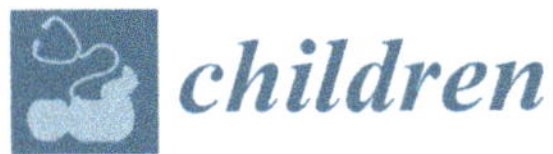

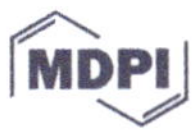

Systematic Review

Diagnostic Efficacy of Advanced Ultrasonography Imaging Techniques in Infants with Biliary Atresia (BA): A Systematic Review and Meta-Analysis

Simon Takadiyi Gunda [1], Nonhlanhla Chambara [1], Xiangyan Fiona Chen [1], Marco Yiu Chung Pang [2] and Michael Tin-cheung Ying [1],*

1   Department of Health Technology and Informatics, The Hong Kong Polytechnic University, Hung Hom, Kowloon, Hong Kong SAR 999077, China
2   Department of Rehabilitation Sciences, The Hong Kong Polytechnic University, Hung Hom, Kowloon, Hong Kong SAR 999077, China
*   Correspondence: michael.ying@polyu.edu.hk; Tel.: +852-3400-8566

Abstract: The early diagnosis of biliary atresia (BA) in cholestatic infants is critical to the success of the treatment. Intraoperative cholangiography (IOC), an invasive imaging technique, is the current strategy for the diagnosis of BA. Ultrasonography has advanced over recent years and emerging techniques such as shear wave elastography (SWE) have the potential to improve BA diagnosis. This review sought to evaluate the diagnostic efficacy of advanced ultrasonography techniques in the diagnosis of BA. Six databases (CINAHL, Medline, PubMed, Google Scholar, Web of Science (core collection), and Embase) were searched for studies assessing the diagnostic performance of advanced ultrasonography techniques in differentiating BA from non-BA causes of infantile cholestasis. The meta-analysis was performed using Meta-DiSc 1.4 and Comprehensive Meta-analysis v3 software. Quality Assessment of Diagnostic Accuracy Studies tool version 2 (QUADAS-2) assessed the risk of bias. Fifteen studies consisting of 2185 patients (BA = 1105; non-BA = 1080) met the inclusion criteria. SWE was the only advanced ultrasonography technique reported and had a good pooled diagnostic performance (sensitivity = 83%; specificity = 77%; AUC = 0.896). Liver stiffness indicators were significantly higher in BA compared to non-BA patients ($p < 0.000$). SWE could be a useful tool in differentiating BA from non-BA causes of infantile cholestasis. Future studies to assess the utility of other advanced ultrasonography techniques are recommended.

Keywords: biliary atresia; ultrasonography; diagnostic accuracy; intraoperative cholangiography (IOC); diagnostic performance; elastography

Citation: Gunda, S.T.; Chambara, N.; Chen, X.F.; Pang, M.Y.C.; Ying, M.T.-c. Diagnostic Efficacy of Advanced Ultrasonography Imaging Techniques in Infants with Biliary Atresia (BA): A Systematic Review and Meta-Analysis. *Children* **2022**, *9*, 1676. https://doi.org/10.3390/children9111676

Academic Editors: Curtise Ng and Ilias Tsiflikas

Received: 22 September 2022
Accepted: 27 October 2022
Published: 31 October 2022

Publisher's Note: MDPI stays neutral with regard to jurisdictional claims in published maps and institutional affiliations.

1. Introduction

Biliary atresia (BA) is a congenital, inflammatory, destructive cholangiopathy affecting infancy and is characterised by progressive fibrosis and obliteration of both the intrahepatic and extrahepatic bile ducts [1,2]. The continued obliteration of the bile ducts and failure to restore biliary drainage is reported to progress to cholestasis, hepatic fibrosis, cirrhosis, end-stage liver failure, and, eventually, death if no liver transplantation is performed [3,4]. Clinically, infants with BA present with cholestatic jaundice, pale stool and dark urine that goes beyond the neonatal period [5]. The worldwide incidence of BA is reported to vary across the geographic plain, ranging from 1.5 per 10,000 live births in Taiwan [6] to 1 per 18,400 live births in France [7], with high incidence in East Asian countries such as China and Japan [8]. Despite BA being an uncommon disease, it is associated with high morbidity and mortality if undiagnosed and if treatment is delayed.

The Kasai portoenterostomy (KPE) is the primary treatment option for biliary atresia [2], to which success of the KPE procedure minimises the need for liver transplantation up to adulthood [4]. The success of KPE is, however, age-dependent, with a 2-month age at KPE being observed to result in high biliary recanalization and stabilization success rates of (80%) [1] and jaundice disappearance [9,10]. To mitigate the detrimental effects of poor prognosis arising from delayed age at KPE and misdiagnosis that may prompt unwarranted KPE, there is a need for an early and accurate differential diagnosis of BA.

Biliary atresia is diagnosed using several methods at present, including, but not limited to, clinical history, liver biopsy, medical imaging techniques such as intraoperative cholangiography (IOC), endoscopic retrograde cholangiography (ERC), and ultrasonography [10]. According to Chen et al. [11], IOC is the current strategy for the accurate diagnosis of BA. However, it is invasive and less accessible and could lead to considerable morbidity. Ultrasonography is a non-invasive, non-ionising, reliable, readily available, and cost-effective imaging modality [12], which is used as a screening and diagnostic tool for paediatric cholestasis evaluation to exclude biliary atresia [13]. Although there are no ultrasounographic features that are definitive of the diagnosis of BA, the triangular cord sign, gallbladder length, gallbladder morphologic characteristics, absence of gallbladder, and the presence of hepatic subcapsular flow are among some of the traditional signs consistent with BA diagnosis at ultrasound [14,15]. Ultrasonography imaging techniques have advanced in recent years, with several emerging techniques such as elastography, three and four-dimension (3D/4D) ultrasound, contrast-enhanced ultrasound (CEUS), and artificial intelligence that enable improved structural, hemodynamic, and functional evaluations of various organs [16]. The clinical utility of these advanced ultrasonography techniques is reported in various conditions and patient groups. Three-dimensional ultrasound was demonstrated to be comparable to magnetic resonance urography in the assessment of renal parenchymal volume [17], whereas, in obstetrics [18], prostate, and breast imaging 3D ultrasound becomes part of routine practice in adult imaging with undebated diagnostic and patient management benefits [19]. The application of 3D ultrasound in neonatal ventricular volume assessment is also promising [20]. CEUS utilises intravascular microbubble agents to delineate perfusion abnormalities that are linked to different pathological conditions, such as tumors and brain ischemia, among others, for which conventional ultrasound is limited [21].

Despite the demonstration of the clinical performance of the recent advanced ultrasonography techniques in various subjects and conditions, their efficacy in the diagnosis of biliary atresia is, however, understudied. This systematic review and meta-analysis are, therefore, aimed at evaluating the efficacy of the recent technological advances in medical ultrasonography in the diagnosis of infantile biliary atresia. It is hypothesised that the current available evidence demonstrates the clinical utility of the recently developed ultrasonography imaging techniques for the diagnosis of infantile biliary atresia.

2. Materials and Methods

The study involved searching the following six electronic databases; Cumulative Index to Nursing and Allied Health Literature (CINAHL Complete via EbscoHost), Medline, PubMed, Google Scholar, Web of Science (core collection), and Embase. The Hong Kong Polytechnic University online library was used to access these databases, with the last search performed on the 11 October 2022. The study followed the Preferred Reporting Items for Systematic Review and Meta-analysis (PRISMA) 2020 guidelines, as informed by Page et al. [22].

2.1. Search Strategy

The search strategy adopted involved searching the databases for the four concepts derived from the PICO framework structured research question, where p (study population) = infants with biliary atresia; I (intervention) = ultrasonography imaging technique that includes advanced ultrasonography techniques such as shear wave elastography, artificial intelligence, and grayscale ultrasonography mode; C (comparison) = liver biopsy representing the gold standard by which the accuracy level was compared, or cholangiography; O (outcome) = indicators of diagnostic performance (diagnostic accuracy, sensitivity, and specificity). The concepts were searched using (1.) MeSH descriptors in Medline and Pubmed, Emtree terms in Embase and CINAHL subject headings, and (2.) keywords and their related terms (synonyms, hyponyms). The reference section of the selected articles was also searched for relevant studies. The boolean operator "OR" was used to search within each PICO element concept (MeSH or Emtree terms) and the related entry terms or synonyms, whereas "AND" was utilised to search the concepts of the three PICO framework elements (population, intervention, and outcome). The database search strings are shown in Table S1.

2.2. Inclusion and Exclusion Criteria

The studies included in the systematic review and meta-analysis were (1.) peer-reviewed studies involving humans and published in the English language from inception to 11 October 2022, (2.) studies assessing the diagnostic accuracy of advanced ultrasonography techniques such as shear wave elastography (SWE) in the differential diagnosis of biliary atresia from other causes of infantile cholestasis, (3.) studies assessing the diagnostic accuracy of algorithms combining the advanced ultrasonographic features such as shear wave velocity (SWV) with traditional diagnostic features from grayscale and color Doppler ultrasound such as the triangular cord sign, (4.) studies in which the measures of diagnostic performance are represented by the following diagnostic performance measures: overall accuracy, sensitivity, specificity, likelihood ratio, positive predictive values, negative predictive value and the area under the receiver operating curve (AUCROC) [23], (5.) studies in which parental consent and institutional ethical approval were obtained prior to data collection.

Exclusion criteria are studies with (1.) no gold standard used to compare diagnostic accuracy such as liver biopsy and surgical confirmation, (2.) inadequate information on study-population characteristics such as age and gender, (3.) inadequate information on the diagnostic performance outcome measures, (4.) conference proceedings, posters, case reports, reviews, editorial letters or commentaries, (5.) diagnostic accuracy measures of other imaging modalities and not ultrasonography, and (6.) non-English.

2.3. Data Extraction

Two reviewers, SG and NC, independently screened the title and abstract of the studies from the search strategy to exclude irrelevant articles and performed a full-text evaluation to check for eligible articles that were included in the systematic review and meta-analysis, whilst the third reviewer, MY, was responsible for resolving any disagreements. The data extraction form based on the PRISMA 2020 guidelines [22] was used to extract data on the authors, date of publication, study methodology (information for the assessment of the risk of bias, study settings, subject's characteristics, ultrasonography features assessed, the gold standard against which the index test was compared), and the measures of diagnostic accuracy among other items from the eligible studies. The random effects model was used to determine the sensitivity and specificity of each ultrasound characteristic.

2.4. Quality Assessment

The Quality Assessment of Diagnostic Accuracy Studies tool version 2 (QUADAS-2) was utilised to assess the risk of bias and the methodological quality. The risk of bias and applicability concerns in the eligible studies were assessed on the following four domains, mainly, the (1.) selection of the patients, (2.) index test (3.) reference standard and (4.) flow and timing. The risk of bias and applicability in these domains were categorised into high, low or unclear, and meta-analysis was performed in studies that exhibited a low risk of bias in the assessed four domains.

2.5. Statistical Analysis

The Comprehensive Meta-Analysis Software version 3.3.070 was used for the comparison of the liver stiffness measurements between BA and non-BA patients through computing the effect size and confidence intervals for both individual studies and meta-analyses. These were displayed in the forest plots. Inconsistences in the studies were assessed using the I-square value and Chi-squared statistics (Q) tests, together with the qualitative assessment of the forest plots, whereas publication bias was assessed using the same software and depicted as a Funnel plot of inverse standard error by standardized difference in means. The effect size was expressed as the standardised mean difference (SMD) for the two continuous liver stiffness measures of (SWV and SWE kPa) between the BA and non-BA patients using a random effect model based on the mean, standard deviation and sample size. Hozo et al. Hozo, Djulbegovic [24]'s formula was used to convert the median and interquartile range (IQR) values to the respective means and standard deviations (SD) for studies in which the outcome measure was reported as median and IQR values. The Meta-DiSc (version 1.4, the Unit of Clinical Biostatistics team of the Ramón y Cajal Hospital in Madrid (Spain) was used to perform the pooling of the sensitivity, specificity and other diagnostic performance measures, utilising the incorporated DerSimonian-Laird random effect model.

3. Results

3.1. Literature Search

The initial database search strategy retrieved a total of 1060 records, as follows: Pubmed (n = 384), Embase (n = 247), CINAHL-Medline (n = 195), Web of Science (n = 34) and Google Scholar (n = 200) as shown in Figure 1. A total of 542 duplicates were identified and removed, and the remaining 518 records underwent a title and abstract screening. The title and abstract screening process excluded a total of 412 articles based on several reasons with the majority of the studies being excluded for utilising imaging modalities other than ultrasonography for the diagnosis of BA. These imaging modalities included magnetic resonance imaging, scintigraphy, computed tomography angiography, and endoscopic retrograde cholangiopancreatography [25–27]. Studies involved non-imaging diagnostic tests, such as the duodenal tube test [28,29], anti-smooth muscle antibodies and liver enzymes biomarkers [30,31] were also excluded. A total of thirteen systematic reviews and meta-analysis studies were excluded as they did not meet the publication criteria of original research articles, with some studies reporting the wrong population and index items. These studies consisted of five meta-analyses [32–36], and eight combined systematic reviews and meta-analyses [37–44]. Three of the meta-analysis focused on summarising the evidence on the diagnostic performance of various conventional ultrasound parameters for the diagnosis of biliary atresia [33–35]. In addition, Sun et al. [36] systematic review and meta-analysis was excluded, as it focused on evaluating the utility of hepatic subcapsular flow using conventional color doppler ultrasonography techniques, whereas, in the study of Guo et al. [32], meta-analysis was excluded as it assessed the diagnostic accuracy of acoustic radiation impulse force in the staging of hepatic fibrosis, not in the diagnosis of BA. Despite assessing the diagnostic performance of shear-wave elastography in differentiating BA from non-BA cases of jaundice, two studies [45,46] were excluded as the full-text articles were not available.

The remaining 106 studies underwent full-text article review and a total of 52 studies were excluded as they did not assess the diagnostic accuracy of advanced ultrasound imaging techniques but focused on the conventional grayscale ultrasound and Doppler techniques, where parameters such as gallbladder abnormalities, triangular cord sign, and the presence or absence of hepatic subcapsular flow on color Doppler ultrasound were assessed as predictor variables in the diagnosis of BA. A total of eight studies that were excluded during the full article review, which assessed the diagnostic performance of the advanced ultrasonography technique of SWE, not for the preoperative diagnosis of BA but the preoperative diagnosis of hepatic fibrosis in children with BA [47–54], whereas one study assessed the preoperative diagnostic accuracy of 2D SWE for liver cirrhosis in BA patients [55]. The other excluded studies focused on the diagnosis of liver fibrosis among post-operative BA children using elastography techniques [54], whereas two studies were excluded due to wrong outcomes as they evaluated the accuracy of the elastography techniques in the diagnosis of liver fibrosis, and this was for participants outside the specified age-range of the present study, which focused on infants below 1 year of age [56,57]. A study by Zhou et al. [58] that utilized an ensembled deep learning model, which was reported to surpass human expertise in the diagnosis of BA, was, however, excluded from the study, as the model was based on conventional sonographic gallbladder images. Two studies were excluded as they assessed the diagnostic utility of the contrast-enhanced ultrasound technique in percutaneous ultrasound-guided cholecysto-cholangiography among infants with BA [59,60].

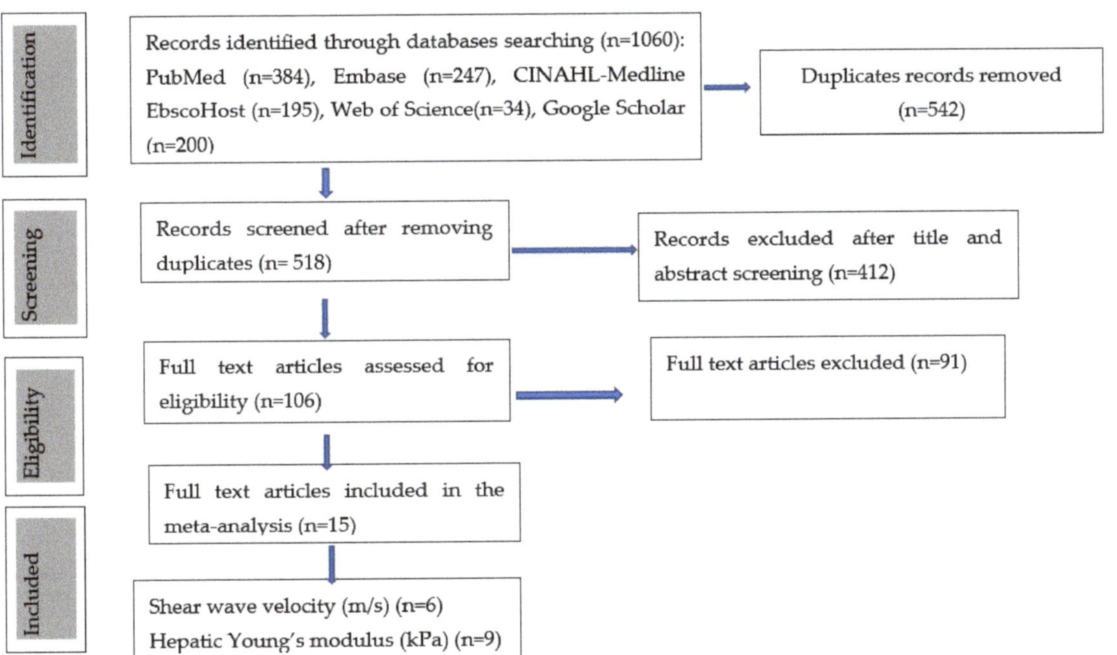

Figure 1. Study selection process (flow chart diagram).

Finally, a total of fifteen studies published in peer-reviewed journals, up to the 11 October 2022, met the eligibility criteria, in which the advanced ultrasonography technique of elastography was used for the diagnosis of BA among infants presenting with cholestasis (Figure 1).

3.2. Study Characteristics

The fifteen included studies were mainly single center, and consisted of twelve prospective cohort study designs [11,61–71], and four retrospective designs [11,72–74]. One study consisted of both prospective and retrospective study designs [11]. The total number of patients from the included studies was 2185, of which 50.6% of the patients were diagnosed with BA (n = 1105) whilst 49.4% were non-BA (n = 1080) patients. The main patient characteristics are presented in Table 1 and Figure 2.

Table 1. Main patient characteristics of the included studies.

Author(s), Year	Ref	Country	Type of Patient	Patients (n)			Age (Days)		
				Total (n = 2185)	BA (n = 1105)	Non-BA (n = 1080)	Overall Age	BA	Non-BA
Liu et al. (2021)	[61]	China	Infants with Cholestasis	59	26	33	NA	[a] 72.5 ± 29.0 (30–127)	[a] 81.3 ± 35.2 (25–141)
Boo et al. (2021)	[62]	Taiwan	Cholestatic infants	61	15	46	NA	[a] 45 (13–121); [b] 30 (22–63)	[b] 35.5 (24–51.3)
Chen et al. (2020)	[11]	China	Cholestatic infants	495 ([R] 308; [P] 187)	293 ([R] 186; [P] 107)	202 ([R] 122; [P] 80)	[a] 52.4 ± 19.5	[aR] 55.2 (19.7) [aP] 51.0 (18.8)	[aR] 51.9 (18.8) [aP] 45.8 (26.8)
Duan et al. (2019)	[63]	China	Cholestatic hepatitis	138	51	87	NA	[c] 43 (5–88) days	[c] 30 (5–90)
Wu et al. (2018)	[64]	Taiwan	Cholestatic infants	48	15	33	[a] 45.87 (9–87)	[b] 45 (34.5–60.5)	[b] 40 (27–56)
Dillman et al. (2019)	[65]	USA	Neonatal cholestasis	41	13	28	[b] 37 (24–52)		
Leschied et al. (2015)	[66]	USA	Infantile liver disease	11	6	5	[a] 107 (42–336)	[a] 79 (range 42–196)	[a] 140 (56–336)
Liu et al. (2022)	[72]	China	Infantile cholestasis	156	83	73	[b] 36 days (25–41)	NA	NA
Sandberg et al. (2021)	[67]	China	Cholestatic jaundice	318	212	106	NA	[a] 59.7 ± 18.8 (20–114)	[a] 65.7 ± 25.6 (9–186)
Shen et al. (2020)	[73]	China	Cholestatic jaundice	282	135	147	NA	[a] 59 ± 18.8	[a] 70 ± 20.4
Wang et al. (2016)	[68]	China	Cholestatic hepatitis	55	38	17	NA (16–140)	[a] 42	[a] 50
Zhou et al. (2017)	[69]	China	Cholestatic infants	172	97	75	NA	[a] 65.3 ± 20.5 (26–134)	[a] 62.4 ± 22.0 (2–140)
Zhou et al. (2022)	[70]	China	Cholestatic infants	35	22	13	NA	[b] 61 (45–75)	[b] 69 (50–87)
Wang et al. (2021)	[75]	China	Cholestatic infants	294 ([T] 150; [V] 144)	89 ([T] 150; [V] 144)	205 ([T] 150; [V] 144)	[a] 42.94 (4–67)	[bT] 46 (33–54) [bV] 50 (33–57)	[bT] 47 (33–54) [bV] 44 (33–57)
Hanquinet et al. (2015)	[74]	Switzerland	Cholestatic infants	20	10	10	52.1 ± 29.2	NA	NA

BA—Biliary atresia; Non-BA—No Biliary atresia; NA—not available; [a] mean Age ± standard deviations, with ranges in parentheses; [b] median age, with interquartile range (IQR) in parentheses; [c] median age with range in parentheses; [R] Patients from retrospective study; [P] Patients from prospective study; [aR] mean age in the retrospective group; [aP] mean age in the prospective group; [T] Patients from the training cohort; [V] Patients from the validation cohort; [bT] median age training group; [bV] median age validation group.

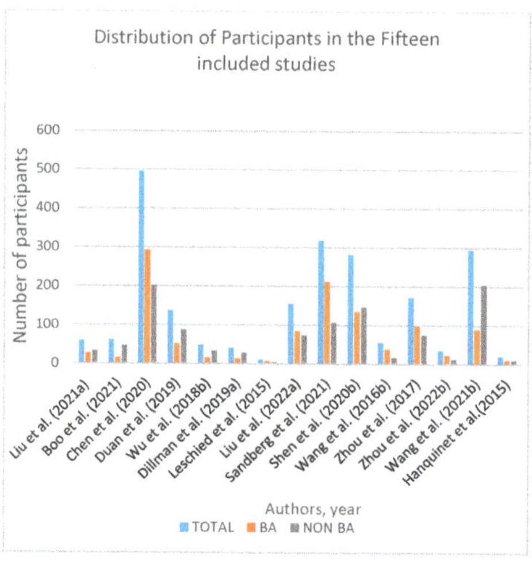

Figure 2. Frequency distribution of participants in the fifteen included studies [11,61–74].

Elastography ultrasound was the only advanced ultrasonography technique utilised in the included studies. The two indicators of liver stiffness measurements were shear wave velocity (SWV) (m/s) and the hepatic Young's modulus (SWE kPa). The detailed individual study characteristics are shown in Table 2.

Table 2. Main study characteristics of the included studies.

Author(s), Year.	Ref	Study Design	Type of Ultrasoumd Machine	Ultrasound Technique	Reference Standard	Ultrasound Parameter
Liu et al. (2021)	[61]	Prospective single center cohort	Siemens Acuson OXANA2 (Siemens Healthcare, Erlangen, Germany) with a 3–5.5 MHz 6C1 convex transducer probe and a 4–9 MHz 9L4 linear array probe.	VTQ and VTIQ	Surgical exploration	mean VTQ & VTIQ SWV
Boo et al. (2021)	[62]	prospective cohort study	TE (FibroScan 502 Touch; Echosens, Paris, France), S1 probe (5 MHz)	TE	IOC, surgical	Median TE kPa
Chen et al. (2020)	[11]	Prospective and retrospective analysis single center	Siemens Acuson S2000 (Siemens Medical Solutions) with a 4- to 9-MHz linear transducer.	VTQ	IOC and Intraoperative biopsy	median VTQ SWV
Duan et al. (2019)	[63]	Prospective, single center.	TUS-Aplio 500 scanner (Toshiba Medical Systems, Tokyo, Japan).14L5 linear array probe (10 MHz)	VTIQ	KPE and liver biopsy	Mean VTIQ kPa
Wu et al. (2018)	[64]	Prospective, single center	TE (Fibroscan 502 Touch; Echosens, Paris, France) S1 probe (5 MHz)	TE	IOC and liver biopsies	Median (kPa)
Dillman et al. (2019)	[65]	Prospective, multi-center study.	Acuson S2000 or S3000 (Siemens Healthcare, Erlangen, Germany); 9L4 linear transducer probe	VTIQ and VTQ	Not specified	Median VTQ and VTIQ SWV
Leschied et al. (2015)	[66]	Single-center retrospective	Acuson S3000 US system/ 9L4 transducer (Siemens Medical Solutions USA, Malvern, PA)	VTQ and VTIQ	liver biopsy andIOC	1. mean VTQ and VTIQ
Liu et al. (2022)	[72]	single-center retrospective study	Aixplorer ultrasound system (SuperSonic Imagine SA, Aix-en-Provence, France) with an L15-4 linear probe	VTIQ	IOC and Biopsy	
Sandberg et al. (2021)	[67]	prospective cohort	(Siemens), with C6 and L9 transducers,	VTQ & VTIQ 2 transducers & 2 ROI	biopsy	Median SWV
Shen et al. (2020)	[73]	retrospective	Aixplorer ultrasound system(SuperSonic Imagine SA, Aix-en-Provence, France), and L15–4 linear probe.	VTIQ	Kasai surgery	mean SWE kPa
Wang et al. (2016)	[68]	Single-center case control	Aixplorer ultrasound system (SuperSonic Imagine SA, Aix-en-Provence, France), an L15-4 linear probe.	VTIQ	Kasai surgery	mean SWE kPa
Zhou et al. (2017)	[69]	Single-center prospective cohort study	AixPlorer scanner (Supersonic Imagine, Paris, France) with a(1 to 6 MHz curvilinear transducer and 4 to 15 MHz linear array transducer 2.A linear array transducer (SL15-4)	VTIQ	surgical exploration, IOC and liver biopsy	Median kPA
Zhou et al. (2022)	[70]	Single-center prospective cohort study	Aixplorer scanner (SuperSonic Imagine, Aix-en-Provence, France), linear array transducer SL15-4 (5 to 14 MHz). Toshiba T-SWE used Aplio500 (Canon Medical System, Otawara, Tochigi, Japan), a linear array transducer 14-L5 (5 to 14 MHz)	S-SWE and T-SWE	surgical exploration, IOC and liver biopsy	mean SWE kPa
Wang et al. (2021)	[75]	Single-center prospective analysis	1. Aixplorer US system (SuperSonic Imagine, Aix-en-Provence, France), with linear probe. 2. HI VISION Ascendus (Hitachi Medical Systems, Japan) equipped with a 5–13 MHz linear-array transducer	VTIQ (2D SWE) training and validation groups	IOC	Mean SWEkPa
Hanquinet et al. (2015)	[74]	retrospective	Acuson® S2000 or S3000 US machine (Siemens Healthcare, Erlangen, Germany) a linear 9-MHz probe	VTQ	IOC & Liver biopsy	mean VTQ SWV

ROI—region of interest; IOC—Intraoperative cholangiography; VTQ—vital touch tissue quantification (point shear wave elastography); VTIQ—virtual touch tissue imaging quantification (2D-SWE); TE—transient elastography.

3.3. Diagnostic Performance of Shear Wave Elastography

The liver stiffness measurements (LSM) between BA and non-BA patients in the fifteen studies are shown in Table 3. A total of twenty-seven analyses were made and are depicted in Figure 3. Eight of the studies performed repeated analyses as they utilised different shear wave elastography modes, or categorised patients into different age groups. Among the twenty-seven analyses, fifteen were carried out in studies measuring the SWE kPa (Figure 4) whilst the remaining twelve analyses were performed for those studies in which the SWV was the outcome measure (Figure 5). The results from these analyses are presented below; first, for studies measuring the individual SWE parameters (SWE kPa and SWV) and, lastly, for all the studies to evaluate the diagnostic performance of the SWE ultrasonography technique.

Table 3. Liver stiffness measurements (LSM) values among patients with and without BA.

Author(s), Year	Ref	Elastography Technique	Hepatic Young's Modulus (kPA) BA	Hepatic Young's Modulus (kPA) Non BA	SWV(m/s) BA	SWV(m/s) Non BA	Main Finding
Liu et al. (2021)	[61]	VTIQ	NA	NA	[a] 2.43 ± 0.29	[a] 1.52 ± 0.29	VTQ and VTIQ can help distinguish BA from non-BA; VTIQ has higher sensitivity and specificity than VTQ
	[61]	VTQ	NA	NA	[a] 2.36 (0.36)	[a] 1.30 ± 0.28	
Boo et al. (2021)	[62]	(≤30) TE	[b] 8.4 (6.8–16.8) [ab] 10.1 (2.9)	[b] 4.2 (3.3–5.4) [ab] 4.3 (0.64)			Statistically significant difference between BA and non-BA TE values. A cutoff LSM > 7.7 kPa had high diagnostic accuracy for BA in all age groups, except for the group of 91–180 days of age.
	[62]	(31–60) TE	[b] 10 (5.5–13) [ab] 9.63 (2.15)	[b] 5.4 (3.8–6.2) [ab] 5.2 (0.72)			
	[62]	(61–90) TE	[b] 19.4 (19.1–19.7) [ab] 19.4 (0.27)	[b] 5.5 (4.5–6.1) [ab] 5.4 (0.51)			
	[62]	(91–180) TE	[b] 40.8 (26–55.5) [ab] 40.78 (8.52)	[b] 3.8 (3.2–8.8) [ab] 4.9 (1.65)			
Chen et al. (2020)	[11]	VTQ			[a] 1.77 (0.39)	[a] 1.30 (0.29)	Mean SWV is significantly higher in BA than in other causes of cholestasis, p< 0.001.
Duan et al. (2019)	[63]	T-SWE-VTQ	[a] 17.59 ± 5.65	[a] 9.84 ± 1.49			Both SWE and grayscale ultrasound have good performance in diagnosing BA. SWE increases the diagnostic specificity when combined with grayscale ultrasound.
	[63]	T-SWE VTIQ)	[a] 17.94 ± 6.44	[a] 9.91 ± 2.00			
Wu et al. (2018)	[64]	TE	[b] 10.50 (8.50–20.90) [ab] 12.6 (3.61)	[b] 4.60 (3.90–6.00) [ab] 4.78 (0.64)			LSM assessment during the workup of cholestatic infants may facilitate the diagnosis of BA.
Dillman et al. (2019)	[65]	2DSWE VTIQ			[b] 2.08 (1.90–2.50) [ab] 2.14 (0.27)	[b] 1.49 (1.34–1.80) [ab] 1.53 (0.24)	SWV were significantly different between BA and non-BA subjects, p = 0.0001 SWE showed better diagnostic performance for distinguishing BA from non-BA causes of neonatal cholestasis, p = 0.0014.
	[65]	Point SWE VTQ			[b] 1.95 (1.48–2.42) [ab] 1.95 (0.34)	[b] 1.21 (1.12–1.51) [ab] 1.26 (0.23)	
Leschied et al. (2015)	[66]	VTQ			[a] 2.08 ± 0.17 (1.90–2.30)	[a] 1.28 ± 0.13 (1.09–1.44)	A significant difference between the VTQ mean SWV of the BA and non-BA groups, p< 0.0001. The mean color pixel values were significantly different between BA and non-BA subjects, p < 0.0001.
	[66]	VTIQ			[a] 3.14 ± 0.73 (2.24–4.40)	[a] 1.61 ± 0.23 (1.34–1.87)	
Liu et al. (2022)	[72]	S-SWE	[b] 9.37 (7.30–11.45) [ab] 9.37 (1.22)	[b] 6.50 (5.95–7.65) [ab] 6.65 (0.53)			LSM measurement by SWE & Serum GGT level showed the best performances for differentiating BA fromNon BA LSM diagnostic value increased with age, and AUC = 0.91 in patients of (30–45) versus 0.74 in 1 (5–30) days old, p < 0.01.
Sandberg et al. (2021)	[67]	C6 VTQ 2.5			[b] 1.9 (1.6–2.3) [ab] 1.93 (0.29)	[b] 1.59 (1.3–1.7) [ab] 1.55 (0.23)	SWE had significantly better performance in differentiating BA from non-BA cases when compared to grayscale ultrasound.
	[67]	C6 VTQ 3.5			[b] 1.9 (1.6–2.3) [ab] 1.93 (0.29)	[b] 1.4 (1.3–1.7) [ab] 1.45 (0.2)	
	[67]	L9 VTQ			[b] 2.1 (1.7–2.4) [ab] 2.08 (0.29)	[b] 1.5 (1.3–1.9) [ab] 1.55 (0.27)	
	[67]	L9 VTIQ			[b] 2.2 (1.9–2.5) [ab] 2.2 (2.7)	[b] 1.8 (1.6–2.1) [ab] 1.83 (0.25)	
Shen et al. (2020)	[73]	2D S-SWE	[a] 12 (6.0)	[a] 8.1 (3.3)			Parallel testing of GGT and LSM in infants < 90 days decreases the rate of BA misdiagnosis, p < 0.001.
Wang et al. (2016)	[68]	2D S-SWE	[a] 20.46 ± 10.19	[a] 6.29 ± 0.99			Mean SWE values were significantly higher in BA than non-BA hepatitis syndrome and control groups, p< 0.01.
Zhou et al. (2017)	[66]	2D S-SWE	[b] 12.6 (10.6–18.8) [ab] 13.65 (2.39)	[b] 9.6 (7.5–11.7) [ab] 9.6 (1.23)			Diagnostic performance of LSM values in identifying BA was lower than that of grayscale ultrasound, p < 0.001. S-SWE was comparable to T-SWE (AUC 0.895 vs. 0.822, p = 0.071) in diagnosing BA. T-SWE had good performances in the diagnosis of BA and the assessment of liver fibrosis compared with S-SWE, p < 0.002.
Zhou et al. (2022)	[70]	2D S-SWE	[a] 14.0 (11.1–20.0)	[a] 8.2 (7.1–9.7)			
	[70]	2D T-SWE	[a] 11.0 (9.1–13.5)	[a] 8.5 (6.5–9.2)			
Wang et al. (2021)	[75]	2D S-SWE (TC)	[b] 9.9 (8.4–14.3) [ab] 10.63 (1.7)	[b] 6.6 (5.7–7.5) [ab] 6.6 (0.56)			Age (p = 0.009), gallbladder morphology (p = 0.001) and hepatic elasticity (p < 0.001) are independent predictive factors to differentiate between BA and other causes of cholestasis.
	[75]	2D S-SWE (VC)	[b] 11.1 (8.7–12.8) [ab] 10.93 (1.2)	[b] 6.3 (5.3–7.7) [ab] 6.4 (0.72)			

Table 3. *Cont.*

Author(s), Year	Ref	Elastography Technique	Hepatic Young's Modulus (kPA)		SWV(m/s)		Main Finding
			BA	Non BA	BA	Non BA	
Hanquinet et al. (2015)	[74]	VTQ			[a] 2.2 (0.4)	[a] 1.7 (0.6)	Significance difference between BA and non-BA SWV, *p* = 0.049

[a] mean values (SD); [b] median values (IQR); [ab] calculated mean from median values using formulae by Hozo et al. [24]; SWV—shear wave velocity; KPA—hepatic Young's modulus; 2D S-SWE—2 dimensional supersonic shearwave elastography; 2D T-SWE—2 dimensional Toshiba shearwave elastography; VTQ—vital touch tissue quantification (point shear wave elastography); VTIQ—virtual touch tissue imaging quantification (2D-SWE); TE—transient elastography; LSM—liver stiffness measurement; TC—Training cohort; VC—Validation cohort.

study name	Model	Std diff in	Standard error	Variance	Lower limit	Upper limit	Z-Value	p-Value	BA	NON BA	Weight (Random)	Relative weight
Liu et al. (2021) VTIQ		3.138	0.390	0.152	2.373	3.903	8.043	0.000	26	33	0.84	4.06
Liu et al. (2021) VTQ		3.338	0.404	0.163	2.546	4.129	8.263	0.000	26	33	0.83	4.02
Chen et al. (2020) VTQ		1.333	0.101	0.010	1.135	1.530	13.223	0.000	293	202	0.95	4.61
Dillman et al. (2019) VTIQ		2.444	0.431	0.185	1.600	3.288	5.674	0.000	13	28	0.82	3.95
Dillman et al. (2019) VTQ		2.568	0.439	0.193	1.707	3.429	5.845	0.000	13	28	0.81	3.93
Leschied et al. (2015) VTQ		5.211	1.265	1.601	2.731	7.691	4.118	0.000	6	5	0.38	1.83
Leschied et al. (2015) VTIQ		2.707	0.836	0.700	1.067	4.346	3.236	0.001	6	5	0.57	2.78
Sandberg et al. (2021) C6 VTQ 2.5		1.399	0.131	0.017	1.142	1.657	10.661	0.000	212	106	0.94	4.58
Sandberg et al. (2021) C6 VTQ 3.5		1.821	0.139	0.019	1.549	2.094	13.088	0.000	212	106	0.94	4.57
Sandberg et al. (2021) L9 VTQ		1.869	0.140	0.020	1.595	2.144	13.337	0.000	212	106	0.94	4.57
Sandberg et al. (2021) L9 VTIQ		0.167	0.119	0.014	-0.066	0.401	1.405	0.160	212	106	0.95	4.59
Hanquinet et al. (2015) VTQ		0.981	0.473	0.224	0.053	1.908	2.072	0.038	10	10	0.79	3.83
Boo et al. (2021) (<30) TE		3.622	0.640	0.409	2.369	4.876	5.662	0.000	8	20	0.69	3.34
Boo et al. (2021) (31-60) TE		4.544	0.938	0.881	2.705	6.383	4.843	0.000	3	18	0.52	2.52
Boo et al. (2021) (61-90) TE		29.669	7.973	63.576	14.042	45.297	3.721	0.000	2	5	0.02	0.07
Boo et al. (2021) (91-180) TE		7.035	2.405	5.783	2.322	11.748	2.926	0.003	2	3	0.15	0.71
Duan et al. (2019) T-SWE-F		1.824	0.303	0.092	1.230	2.417	6.025	0.000	33	29	0.88	4.28
Duan et al. (2019) T-SWE-M		2.261	0.326	0.106	1.622	2.901	6.931	0.000	18	58	0.87	4.22
Wu et al. (2018) TE		3.793	0.497	0.247	2.819	4.766	7.634	0.000	15	33	0.78	3.76
Liu et al. (2022) 2DS-SWE		2.830	0.227	0.051	2.385	3.274	12.480	0.000	83	73	0.92	4.44
Shen et al. (2020) 2D S-SWE		0.815	0.124	0.015	0.572	1.058	6.569	0.000	135	147	0.95	4.59
Wang et al. (2016) 2DS-SWE		1.661	0.332	0.110	1.010	2.312	5.003	0.000	38	17	0.87	4.21
Zhou et al. (2017) 2DS-SWE		2.055	0.190	0.036	1.684	2.426	10.843	0.000	97	75	0.93	4.50
Zhou et al. (2022) 2DS-SWE		3.184	0.517	0.267	2.171	4.197	6.160	0.000	22	13	0.76	3.70
Zhou et al. (2022) 2D T-SWE		2.581	0.466	0.218	1.667	3.495	5.534	0.000	22	13	0.79	3.85
Wang et al. (2021) 2D S-SWE-TC		3.943	0.291	0.084	3.373	4.512	13.570	0.000	43	107	0.89	4.31
Wang et al. (2021) 2D S-SWE-VC		5.032	0.346	0.120	4.353	5.710	14.534	0.000	46	98	0.86	4.17
	Random	2.516	0.220	0.048	2.084	2.947	11.429	0.000				

Model	Number Studies	Point estimate	Standard error	Variance	Lower limit	Upper limit	Z-value	P-value	Q-value	df (Q)	P-value	I-squared	Tau Squared	Standard Error	Variance	Tau
Fixed	27	1.596	0.043	0.002	1.511	1.680	36.991	0.000	528.373	26	0.000	95.079	1.041	0.488	0.238	1.020
Random	27	2.516	0.220	0.048	2.084	2.947	11.429	0.000								

Figure 3. A comparison of the liver stiffness value between the patients with and without BA for all the studies (KPa and SWV) [11,61–74].

Model	Study name	Statistics for each study						Sample size		Statistics for each study	Weight (Random)	Std diff in means and 95% CI
		Std diff in means	Standard error	Variance	Lower limit	Upper limit	Z-Value	Group-BA	Group-Non BA	p-Value	Relative weight	
	Boo et al. (2021) (?30) TE	3.622	0.640	0.409	2.369	4.876	5.662	8	20	0.000	6.76	
	Boo et al. (2021) (31-60) TE	4.544	0.938	0.881	2.705	6.383	4.843	3	18	0.000	5.58	
	Boo et al. (2021) (61-90) TE	29.669	7.973	63.576	14.042	45.297	3.721	2	5	0.000	0.23	
	Boo et al. (2021) (91-180) TE	7.035	2.405	5.783	2.322	11.748	2.926	2	3	0.003	1.98	
	Duan et al. (2019) T-SWE-F	1.824	0.303	0.092	1.230	2.417	6.025	33	29	0.000	7.88	
	Duan et al. (2019) T-SWE-M	2.261	0.326	0.106	1.622	2.901	6.931	18	58	0.000	7.82	
	Wu et al. (2018) TE	3.793	0.497	0.247	2.819	4.766	7.634	15	33	0.000	7.29	
	Liu et al. (2022) 2DS-SWE	2.830	0.227	0.051	2.385	3.274	12.480	83	73	0.000	8.05	
	Shen et al. (2020) 2D S-SWE	0.815	0.124	0.015	0.572	1.058	6.569	135	147	0.000	8.21	
	Wang et al. (2016) 2DS-SWE	1.661	0.332	0.110	1.010	2.312	5.003	38	17	0.000	7.80	
	Zhou et al. (2017) 2DS-SWE	2.055	0.190	0.036	1.684	2.426	10.843	97	75	0.000	8.12	
	Zhou et al. (2022) 2DS-SWE	3.184	0.517	0.267	2.171	4.197	6.160	22	13	0.000	7.22	
	Zhou et al. (2022) 2D T-SWE	2.581	0.466	0.218	1.667	3.495	5.534	22	13	0.000	7.39	
	Wang et al. (2021) 2D S-SWE-TC	3.943	0.291	0.084	3.373	4.512	13.570	43	107	0.000	7.91	
	Wang et al. (2021) 2D S-SWE-VC	5.032	0.346	0.120	4.353	5.710	14.534	46	98	0.000	7.77	
Random		3.018	0.388	0.151	2.256	3.779	7.769			0.000		

2D S-SWE-TC—two-dimensional supersonic shearwave elastography training cohort; 2D S-SWE-VC—two-dimensional supersonic shearwave elastography validation cohort, 2D S-SWE—two-dimensional supersonic shearwave elastography; T-SWE-F—two-dimensional Toshiba shearwave elastography female group; T-SWE-M—2 dimensional Toshiba shearwave elastography male group; VTQ—vital touch tissue quantification (point shear wave elastography); VTIQ—virtual touch tissue imaging quantification; TE—transient elastography.

Figure 4. A comparison of the liver stiffness parameter (kPa) between BA and non-BA patients [62,63,67–72].

Model	Study name	Statistics for each study							Statistics for	Sample size		Std diff in means and 95% CI	Weight (Random)	
		Std diff in means	Standard error	Variance	Lower limit	Upper limit	Z-Value	p-Value		BA	Non BA		Weight (Random)	Relative weight
	Liu et al. (2021) VTIQ	3.138	0.390	0.152	2.373	3.903	8.043	0.000		26	33		1.28	8.47
	Liu et al. (2021) VTQ	3.338	0.404	0.163	2.546	4.129	8.263	0.000		26	33		1.26	8.35
	Chen et al. (2020) VTQ	1.333	0.101	0.010	1.135	1.530	13.223	0.000		293	202		1.57	10.36
	Dillman et al. (2019) VTIQ	2.444	0.431	0.185	1.600	3.288	5.674	0.000		13	28		1.23	8.12
	Dillman et al. (2019) VTQ	2.568	0.439	0.193	1.707	3.429	5.845	0.000		13	28		1.22	8.05
	Leschied et al. (2015) VTQ	5.211	1.265	1.601	2.731	7.691	4.118	0.000		6	5		0.45	2.97
	Leschied et al. (2015) VTIQ	2.707	0.836	0.700	1.067	4.346	3.236	0.001		6	5		0.75	4.98
	Sandberg et al. (2021) C6 VTQ 2.5	1.399	0.131	0.017	1.142	1.657	10.661	0.000		212	106		1.55	10.24
	Sandberg et al. (2021) C6 VTQ 3.5	1.821	0.139	0.019	1.549	2.094	13.088	0.000		212	106		1.54	10.21
	Sandberg et al. (2021) L9 VTQ	1.869	0.140	0.020	1.595	2.144	13.337	0.000		212	106		1.54	10.20
	Sandberg et al. (2021) L9 VTIQ	0.167	0.119	0.014	-0.066	0.401	1.405	0.160		212	106		1.56	10.29
	Hanquinet et al. (2015) VTQ	0.981	0.473	0.224	0.053	1.908	2.072	0.038		10	10		1.17	7.76
Random		1.990	0.257	0.066	1.487	2.494	7.742	0.000						

Model		Effect size and 95% confidence interval						Test of null (2-Tail)		Heterogeneity				Tau-squared			
Model		Number Studies	Point estimate	Standard error	Variance	Lower limit	Upper limit	Z-value	P-value	Q-value	df (Q)	P-value	I-squared	Tau Squared	Standard Error	Variance	Tau
Fixed		12	1.371	0.053	0.003	1.267	1.474	25.982	0.000	195.660	11	0.000	94.378	0.628	0.414	0.172	0.793
Random		12	1.990	0.257	0.066	1.487	2.494	7.742	0.000								

Figure 5. A comparison of the liver stiffness parameter (SWV) between BA and non-BA patients [11,61,65–67,74].

3.3.1. Diagnostic Performance of the Hepatic Young Modulus (SWE KPa)

Nine of the included studies assessed the diagnostic efficacy of the liver stiffness indicator, the hepatic Young's modulus of elasticity (SWE kPa) in the assessment of cholestatic infants for the differential diagnosis of BA [62–64,68–73]. A total of four studies reported the liver stiffness measurements as mean SWE kPa [63,68,70,73], whilst five studies reported the SWE kPa median values [62,64,69,71,72] (Table 3). The difference in the median SWE kPa values between the BA and non-BA groups was statistically significant in all the studies utilizing the median SWE kPa values, with higher values observed in the BA group. Statistically significant findings ($p < 0.01$) were also observed between the mean SWE kPa values of BA and non-BA patients [63,68,73]. The cut-off point for the diagnosis of BA differed between the studies that used the mean SWE kPa values, and the reported cut-off values of the three studies were 12.35, 8.68, and 9.5 kPa, respectively [63,68,73]. The hepatic SWE kPa performance in the differential diagnosis of BA from cholestatic hepatic disease was reported to outperform that of conventional ultrasound parameters [63,75] with AUC values of 0.89 (95% CI: 0.829–0.935, $p < 0.001$ versus 0.748 (95% CI: 0.670–0.815, $p < 0.001$) in Wang et al. [75]. Contrary to these findings, one study observed that the diagnostic accuracy of SWE kPa does not surpass that of conventional grayscale ultrasound (AUC = 0.790 versus 0.893, respectively) [69]. The differentiating ability of SWE liver stiffness is reported to increase with the patient's age (days) at diagnosis [72,73]. Liu et al. [72], reported an AUC of 0.91 in the (30–45) versus an AUC of 0.74 in the (15–30), whereas Shen et al. [73] noted an AUC of 0.905 in the (91–120) versus AUC of 0.761 in the less than 60 days age group. Similarly, Zhou et al. [69] observed that the diagnostic performance of SWE kPa in patients of less than 60 days of age (AUC = 0.694, 95% CI: 0.579–0.793) was lower than that in patients of greater than 60 days of age (AUC = 0.779, 95% CI: 0.682–0.858). However, contrary to the above findings, only one study by Boo et al. [62] observed a lower diagnostic accuracy of 80% in older patients compared to the diagnostic accuracies of 92.9%, 95.2%, and 100% in the younger age groups (<30, 31–60 and 61–90) days, respectively. The results from the present meta-analysis showed statistically significant differences in liver stiffness SWE kPa values, with higher values observed in BA patients compared to the non-BA cholestatic patients.

The pooled statistics showed an overall effect size, indicated by the SMD, of 3.018 kPa with, 95% CI of 2.256–3.779 ($p < 0.0001$) (Figure 4). Shear wave elastography kPa demonstrated good discriminatory abilities between BA and non-BA patients. The observed pooled diagnostic performance was: sensitivity = 0.83 (95% CI: 0.80–0.86); specificity = 0.80 (95% CI: 0.77–0.82); AUC = 0.9066; DOR = 26.92 (95% CI: 13.34–54.34) (Figure 6a,b,c and d, respectively).

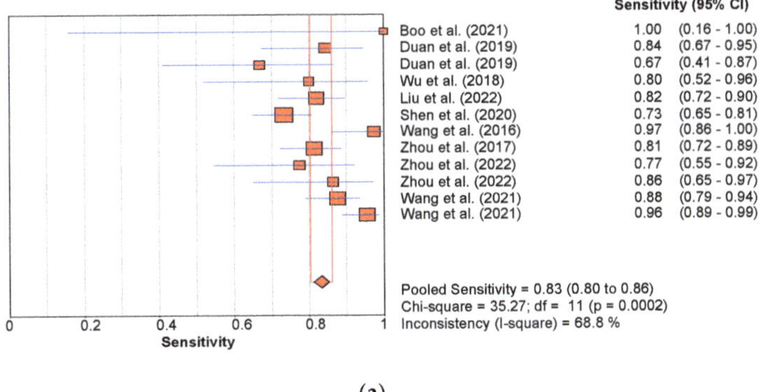

(**a**)

Figure 6. *Cont.*

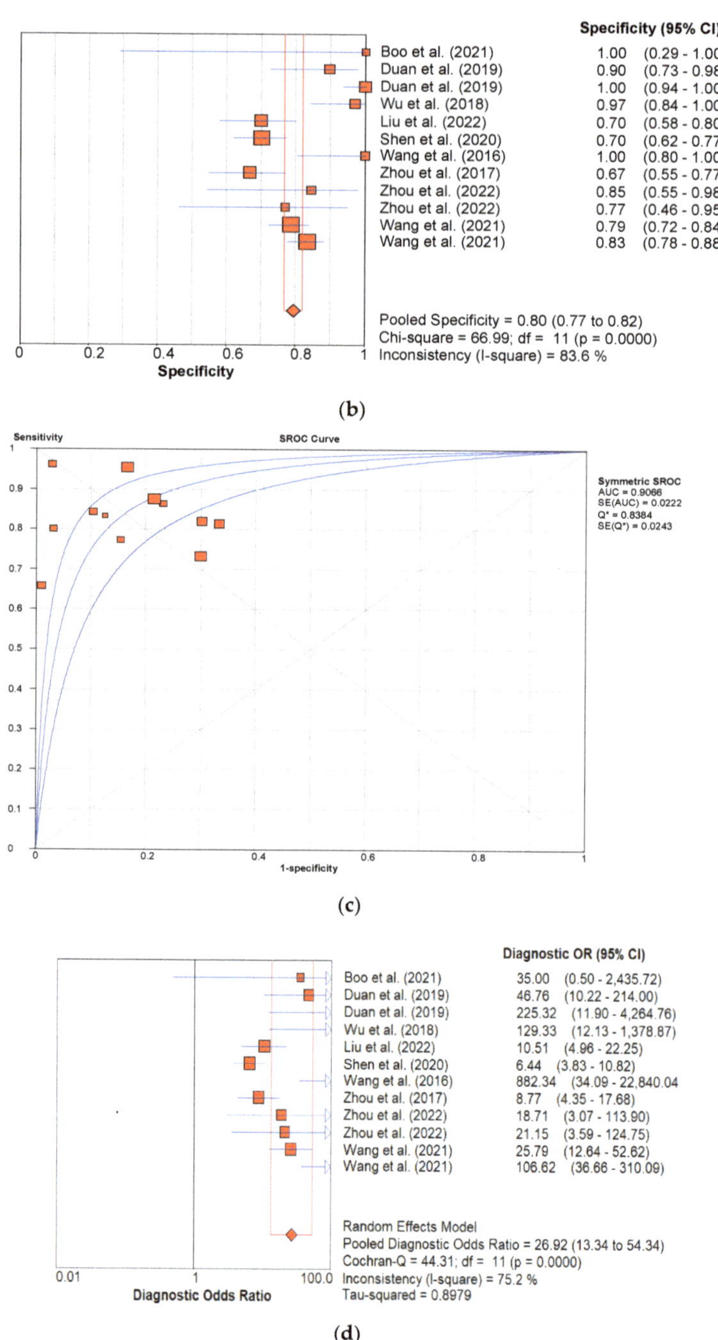

Figure 6. (**a**): Sensitivity forest plot for studies using SWE (kPa). (**b**): Specificity forest plot for studies using SWE (kPa). (**c**): Summary receiver operating characteristic curve for studies using SWE (kPa). (**d**): Forest plot showing overall diagnostic odds ratio for studies using SWE (kPa) [62–64,68–73].

3.3.2. Diagnostic Performance of Shear Wave Velocity (SWV in m/s)

Six studies demonstrated the clinical utility of shear wave velocity (SWV) in discriminating BA from other causes of infantile cholestasis [11,61,65–67,74]. Four of these studies [11,61,65,67] reported the sensitivity, specificity, and diagnostic accuracy (AUC) of the SWV elastography modes (VTQ and VTIQ), whereas two studies [66,74] reported only the *p*-values indicating statistically significant differences between the mean SWV of BA and non-BA patients, with no information on the other diagnostic performance measures. Contrary to the findings of Liu et al. [61], in which a higher diagnostic accuracy value of 0.918 (95% CI: 0.834–1), was observed in the mean SWV of the VTIQ modes (cut-off SWV = 1.92 m/s). Sandberg et al. [67] reported a moderate diagnostic accuracy value of 0.7 (95% CI: 0.7–0.8) at a median cut-off SWV of 2.0 m/s. A three-color risk stratification model was developed in which five variables, including an SWV greater than 1.35 m/s, had a high accuracy in discriminating BA infants from non-BA infants (AUC= 0.983, sensitivity = 98.7% and specificity = 91.4%) [11]. Regardless of whether the mean SWV [11,61,66,74] or median SWV values [65,67] was used, all six studies reported that the SWV of the liver in the BA group was significantly higher than that in the non-BA (Table 3).

Biliary atresia patients exhibited significantly higher liver stiffness values as indicated by the SWV compared to non-BA patients ($p < 0.0001$). The pooled effect size (SMD) and 95% confidence intervals were 1.99 and (95% CI:1.487 to 2.494), respectively (Figure 5). The studies however showed high inconsistencies, I^2 = 94.378. The pooled diagnostic performance for these studies was: sensitivity = 0.82 (95% CI: 0.80–0.84); specificity = 0.75 (95% CI: 0.72–0.78); AUC = 0.71; DOR = 18.22 (95% CI: 7.78–45.04) as shown in Figure 7a,b,c and d, respectively.

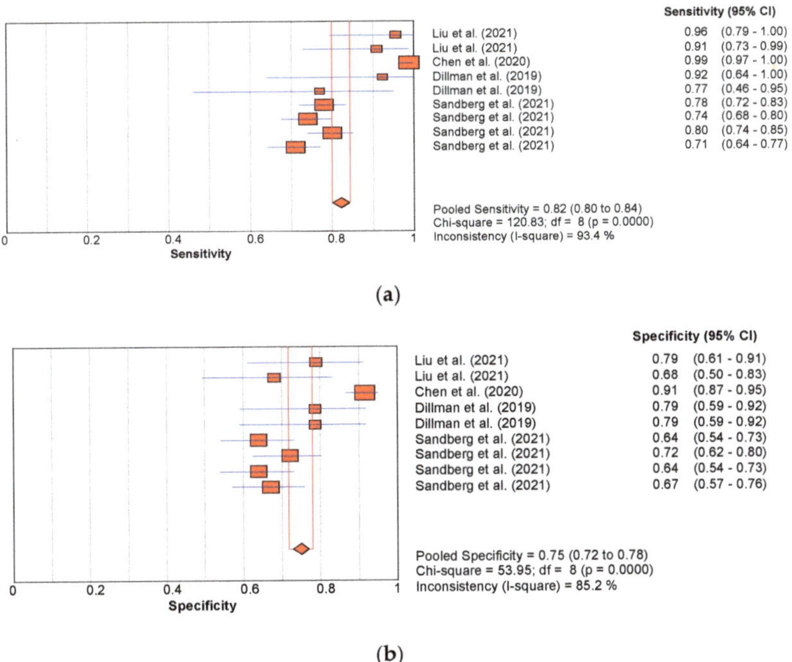

(a)

(b)

Figure 7. *Cont.*

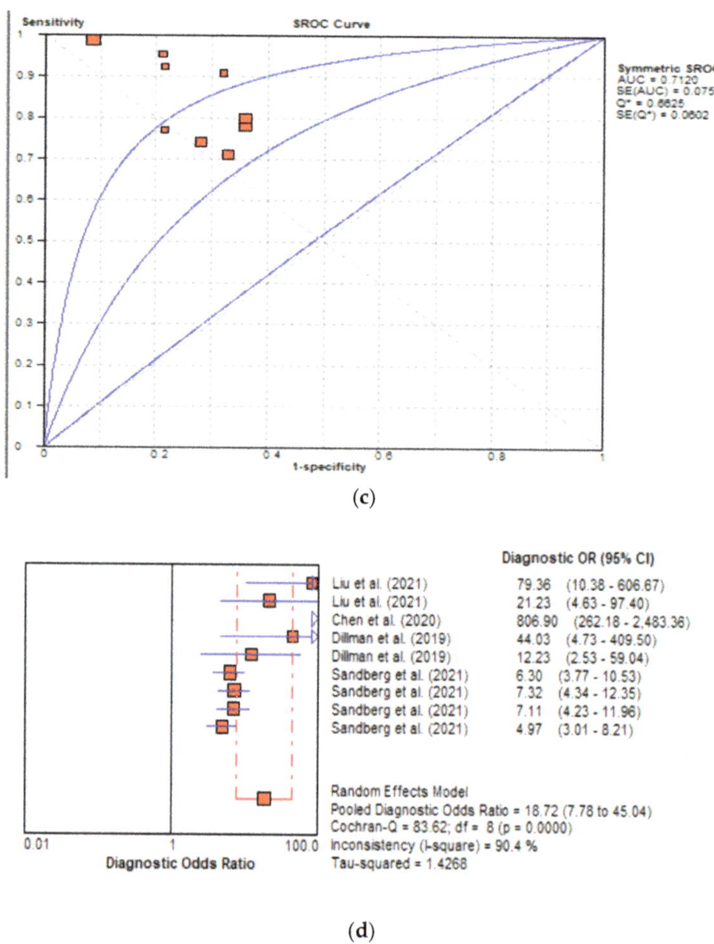

(c)

(d)

Figure 7. (**a**): Sensitivity forest plot for studies using shear wave velocity. (**b**): Specificity forest plot for studies using shear wave velocity. (**c**): Summary receiver-operating characteristic curve for studies using shear wave velocity. (**d**): Forest plot showing overall diagnostic odds ratio for studies using shear wave velocity. [11,61,65,67].

3.3.3. Diagnostic Performance of the Combined Studies

The statistical analysis of the combined studies showed that BA patients had higher liver stiffness values compared to non-BA patients. Shear-wave elastography showed high discriminative power in the diagnosis of BA. The overall SMD and 95% confidence intervals of all the studies evaluating the diagnostic performance of BA were 2.516 and (2.084 to 2.947), respectively, $p < 0.001$. The studies showed considerable heterogeneity, I^2 value of 95.079% (Figure 3). The pooled diagnostic performance was as follows: sensitivity = 0.83 (95% CI: 0.81–0.84); specificity = 0.77 (95% CI: 0.75–0.79); AUC = 0.896; DOR = 22.87 (95% CI: 13.16–39.75) as shown in Figure 8a, b, c and d, respectively.

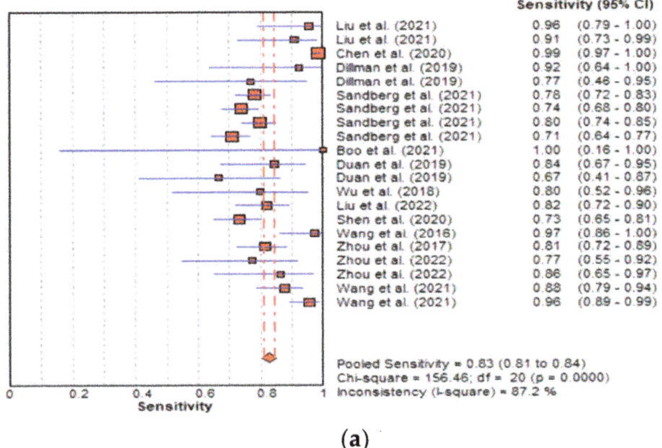

(**a**)

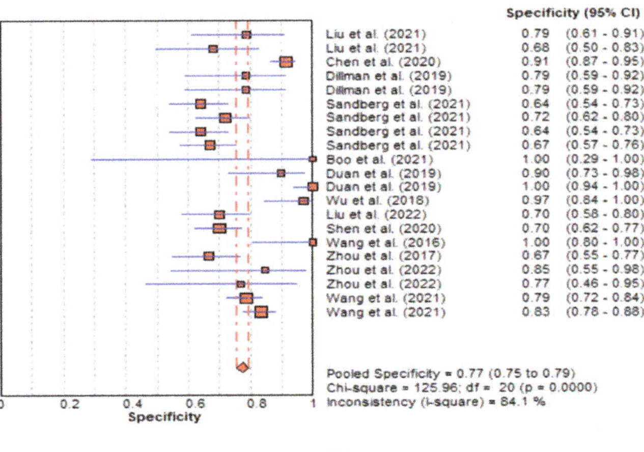

(**b**)

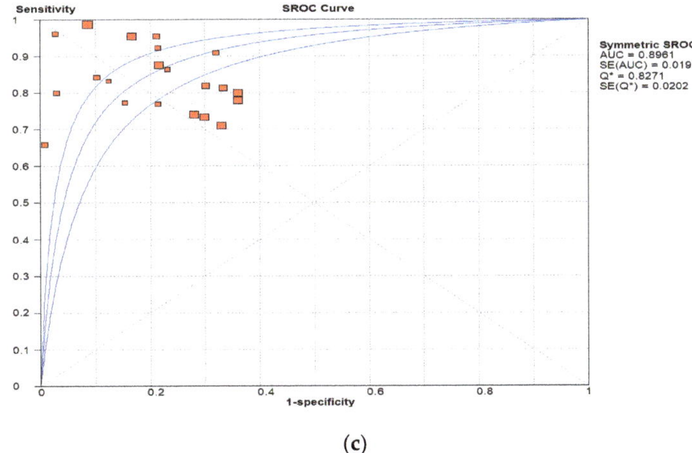

(**c**)

Figure 8. *Cont.*

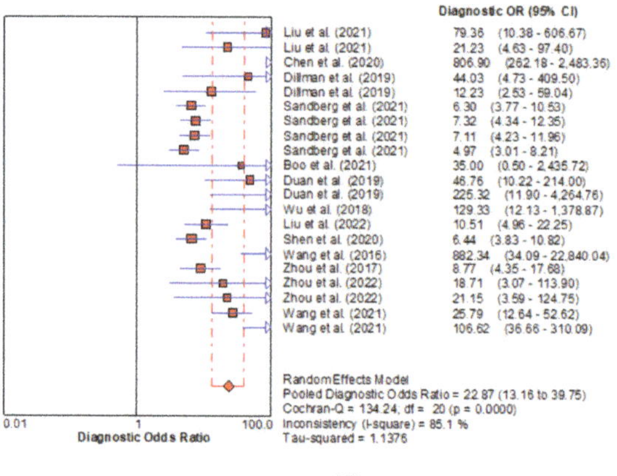

(d)

Figure 8. (**a**): Sensitivity forest plots for all included studies. (**b**): Specificity forest plots for all included studies. (**c**): Summary receiver operating characteristic curve for all included studies. (**d**): Forest plot showing overall diagnostic odds ratio for all included studies [11,61–65,67–73].

The pooled standardised mean difference of the six studies that evaluated the differentiating ability of SWV was 1.990 (95% CI: 1.487–2.494); however, considerable heterogeneity was observed in these studies, I^2 value of 94.378%, and, hence, a random effect model was adopted. A total of 11 out of the 12 analyses showed statistically significant differences between BA and non-BA patients' liver stiffness measures (SWV), whereas only one analysis from Sandberg et al. [67], utilising the L9 probe and the VTIQ mode, had an insignificant result (p = 0.160) and was seen to reach the line of no effect (Figures 3 and 5). The extracted data on the diagnostic performance indicators for the evaluated studies is shown in Table 4.

Table 4. Diagnostic performance indicators for each study.

Author (s)	Ref	Elastography Technique	Cutoff Value	Sen (%)	Spec (%)	PPV (%)	NPV (%)	AUC	DA	BA(n)	Non-BA(n)	TP	TN	FP	FN
Liu et al. (2021)	[61]	VTIQ	1.92	95.5	78.9	NA	NA	0.92	NA	26	33	24.83	26.04	6.96	1.17
	[61]	VTQ	1.77	90.9	68	NA	NA	0.89	NA	26	33	23.63	22.44	10.56	2.37
Chen et al. (2020)	[11]	VTQ	1.35	98.7	91.4	94	98.1	0.98	93.6	293	202	289.1	184.63	17.37	3.809
Dillman et al. (2019)	[65]	2DSWE VTIQ	1.84	92.3	78.6	66.7	95.7	0.89	NA	13	28	12	22.01	6	1.00
	[65]	Point SWE VTQ	1.53	76.9	78.6	62.5	88	0.81	NA	13	28	9.99	22.01	5.99	3.003
Leschied et al. (2015)	[66]	Mean SWV VTQ	NA	NA	NA	NA	NA	NA	NA	6	5	NA	NA	NA	NA
	[66]	Mean SWV VTIQ	NA	NA	NA	NA	NA	NA	NA	6	5	NA	NA	NA	NA
Sandberg et al. (2021)	[67]	C6 VTQ 2.5	1.5	78	64	NA	NA	0.8	NA	212	106	165.36	67.84	38.16	46.64
	[67]	C6 VTQ 3.5	1.6	74	72	NA	NA	0.8	NA	212	106	156.88	76.32	29.68	55.12
	[67]	L9 VTQ	1.6	80	64	NA	NA	0.8	NA	212	106	169.6	67.84	38.16	42.4
	[67]	L9 VTIQ	2	71	67	NA	NA	0.7	NA	212	106	150.52	71.02	34.98	61.48
Boo et al. (2021)	[62]	(91–180) TE	8.8	100	100	100	100	100	100	2	3	2	3	0	0
	[62]	(≤30) TE	7.7	NA	NA	100	90.9	NA	92.9	8	20	NA	NA	NA	NA
	[62]	(31–60) TE	7.7	NA	NA	100	94.7	NA	95.3	3	18	NA	NA	NA	NA
	[62]	(61–90) TE	7.7	NA	NA	100	100	NA	100	2	5	NA	NA	NA	NA
	[62]	(91–180) TE	7.7	NA	NA	66.7	100	NA	80	2	3	NA	NA	NA	NA
Duan et al. (2019)	[63]	T-SWE-VTQ-f	12.35	84.3	89.7	82.7	90.7	0.937	87.7	33	29	27.82	26.013	2.987	5.181
	[63]	T-SWE VTIQ-M	12.35	66.7	100	100	83.6	0.833	87.7	18	58	12.0	58	0	5.99

Table 4. *Cont.*

Author (s)	Ref	Elastography Technique	Cutoff Value	Sen (%)	Spec (%)	PPV (%)	NPV (%)	AUC	DA	BA(n)	Non-BA(n)	TP	TN	FP	FN
Wu et al. (2018)	[64]	TE	7.7	80	97	NA	NA	85.3	NA	15	33	12	32.01	0.99	3
Liu et al. (2022)	[72]	S-SWE	7.1	81.3	69.86	NA	NA	0.82	NA	83	73	68.00	50.9978	22.02	14.9981
Shen et al. (2020)	[73]	2D S-SWE	9.5	73.3	70.1	69.2	74.1	0.771	NA	135	147	98.96	103.047	43.95	36.045
Wang et al. (2016)	[68]	2DS-SWE	9.5	97.4	100	100	96.9	0.997	NA	38	17	37.01	17	0	0.988
Zhou et al. (2017)	[69]	2DS-SWE	10.2	81.4	66.7	76	73.5	0.79	NA	97	75	78.96	50.025	24.975	18.042
Zhou et al. (2022)	[70]	2DS-SWE	10.2	77.3	84.6	89.5	68.8	0.895	80	22	13	17.0	10.998	2.002	4.994
	[70]	2D T-SWE	8.7	86.4	76.9	86.4	76.9	0.822	82.9	22	13	19.0	9.997	3.003	2.992
Wang et al. (2021)	[75]	2D S-SWE-TV	7.81	87.6	78.5	63.9	93.6	0.888	81.3	89	205	77.964	160.925	44.075	11.036
	[75]	2D S-SWE-N	7.81	95.5	83.4	71.4	97.7	0.94	87.1	89	205	85	171	34.	4.00
Hanquinet et al. (2015)	[74]	VTQ	NA	NA	NA	NA	NA	NA	NA	10	10	NA	NA	NA	NA

NA—not available; Sen—sensitivity; Spec—specificity; PPV—positive predictive value; NPV—negative predictive value; DA—diagnostic accuracy AUC—area under receiver-operating curve; CI—confidence interval, 95% CI in parenthesis; mean values (TV—training + validation; N—normogram; TP—true positive; TN—true negative; FP—false positive; FN—false negative) were calculated based on the given data on sensitivity, specificity and the number of patients in each of the two groups (BA and non-BA groups) using Baratloo et al [76] formulae.

3.4. Studies Methodological Quality Assessment by the QUADAS Tool

The methodological quality of the studies was generally high, with the majority of studies exhibiting a low patient selection bias, as the consecutive selection of the participants was conducted in all studies except three [61,65,74] in which non-consecutive patient selection was used and unclear in each study, respectively (Table 5). In all the eligible studies, a case–control design was avoided. The inclusion–exclusion criteria were clear in all the studies, with low concerns of the selected patients not matching the review question that is focused on the diagnostic efficacy of advanced ultrasonography techniques for the diagnosis of biliary atresia among cholestatic infants. The reference tests were undertaken by different teams, who were blinded to the index test in all the studies; however, different reference standards were used, which could be a source of inhomogeneities. Despite the absence of an inter/intra-observer variability analysis among the two physicians who undertook the liver stiffness measurements for the index test in one study [73], the risk of bias in conducting the index test was deemed low, as the two physicians were reported to have more than five years of experience in abdominal ultrasonography. The reference standard was, however, not specified in one study [65]. The applicability concerns in the three domains of patient selection, index test, and reference standard were low in the majority of studies, except for two studies [69,70], in which three different reference standards (surgical exploration, intraoperative cholangiography under laparoscopy, or liver biopsy) were used to confirm the diagnosis of BA. The study flow timing in Liu et al. [72] was unclear; hence, it could have introduced bias as the time between the index test and reference test is not specified in the study.

The funnel plot in Figure 9, showed an asymmetrical distribution of the studies effects size, with the bottom of the plot showing a higher concentration of small studies only on one side of the mean effect size, demonstrating the small-study effects phenomena.

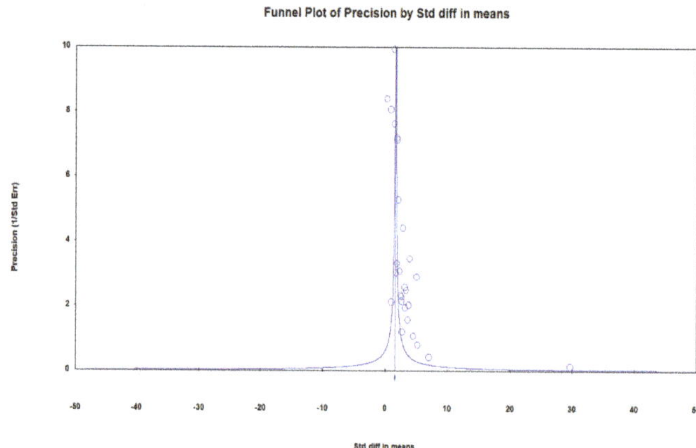

Figure 9. Funnel plot of precision (inverse standard error) by standardised difference in means assessing bias.

Table 5. QUADAS tool studies methodological quality assessment results (risk of bias and applicability concerns).

Aurthor(S), Year	Ref	Risk Of Bias				Applicability Concerns		
		Patient Selection	Index Test	Reference Standard	Flow and Timing	Patient Selection	Index Test	Reference Standard
Liu et al. (2021)	[61]	Unclear	Low	Low	Low	Low	Low	Low
Boo et al. (2021)	[62]	Low	Low	Low	Low	Low	Low	Low
Chen et al. (2020)	[11]	Low	Low	Low	Low	Low	Low	Low
Duan et al. (2019)	[63]	Low	Low	Low	Low	Low	Low	Low
Wu et al. (2018)	[64]	Low	Low	Low	Low	Low	Low	Low
Dillman et al. (2019)	[65]	High	Low	Unclear	Low	Low	Low	Unclear
Leschied et al. (2015)	[66]	Low	Low	Low	Low	Low	Low	Low
Liu et al. (2022)	[72]	Low	Low	Low	Unclear	Low	Low	Low
Sandberg et al. (2021)	[67]	Low	Low	Low	Low	Low	Low	Low
Shen et al. (2020)	[73]	Low	Low	Low	Low	Low	Low	Low
Wang et al. (2016)	[68]	Low	Low	Low	Low	Low	Low	Low
Zhou et al. (2017)	[69]	Low	Low	Low	Low	Low	Low	High
Zhou et al. (2022)	[70]	Low	Low	Low	Low	Low	Low	High
Wang et al. (2021)	[75]	Low	Low	Low	Low	Low	Low	Low
Hanquinet et al. (2015)	[74]	Unclear	Low	Low	Low	Low	Low	Low

Low = Low Risk; High = High Risk; Unclear = Unclear Risk.

3.5. Publication Bias Assessment

The possibility of publication bias was assessed using the funnel plot shown in Figure 9.

4. Discussion

The early and accurate diagnosis of BA, to rule out other causes of infantile cholestasis, is important for better prognostic outcomes. The current strategy for the differential diagnosis of BA from non-BA causes of infantile cholestasis involves invasive procedures such as intraoperative cholangiography [11]. The need for non-invasive accurate diagnostic tests, therefore, cannot be overemphasised. Ultrasonography is a non-invasive imaging technique and has seen several advances in its technology over recent years that have the potential to improve the differentiation of BA from non-BA causes of cholestasis in infants [16]. Systematic reviews of the diagnostic performance of conventional grayscale ultrasound techniques have been reported [36,42]. To the best of our knowledge, this is the first study to summarise the available evidence on the diagnostic performance of advanced ultrasonography techniques in the differential diagnosis of BA from other causes of infantile cholestasis.

The study results showed that only one advanced ultrasound imaging technique, shear wave elastography, was studied, to assess its diagnostic performance for the preoperative diagnosis of BA (Table 2). There are no studies assessing the diagnostic efficacy of other recent ultrasonography advances, such as microvascular imaging and contrast-enhanced ultrasound, that met the inclusion criteria. The two studies related to microvascular imaging technique in this review, however, were excluded from the analysis after a full article review, as they evaluated the clinical utility of MVI in a post-KPE procedure in BA patients and not for the preoperative diagnosis of BA [77]. The ability of MVI to detect capsular flows that conventional color Doppler could not among the BA group in the study by Lee et al. [77] is an indicator of its possible diagnostic utility among preoperative BA patients. It is, therefore, prudent to have studies assessing the diagnostic accuracy of MVI for the preoperative diagnosis of BA.

The significantly higher liver stiffness values observed in BA patients in comparison to non-BA patients; (overall SMD, 95% confidence intervals and p values) of (2.578, (2.136–3.02) and $p < 0.0001$), respectively (Figure 3), is an indicator that the shear wave elastography-based liver stiffness measurement can facilitate the differentiation of BA from other causes of infantile cholestasis. The technique involving an L9 probe in the VTIQ mode was assessed in only one study [67], and exhibited poor discriminatory ability ($p = 0.16$); hence, more studies are required to evaluate the clinical utility of this technique in discriminating BA from non BA cholestatic infants before concluding its relevance for clinical use. The effect size was higher in studies in which SWE (kPa) was the outcome measure, with an overall SMD of 3.08 in SWE kPa studies versus 2.078 for SWV studies.

The current study observed a good diagnostic performance of SWE with the pooled sensitivity of 0.83 (95% CI: 0.81–0.84), specificity of 0.77 (95% CI: 0.75–0.79), AUC of 0.896, and DOR of 22.87 (95% CI: 13.16–39.75) (Figure 8a–d). These findings are in agreement with those from a recent meta-analysis by Wagner et al. [40], which evaluated the diagnostic performance of SWE in which high diagnostic accuracy was reported (AUC = 0.91) versus the current study's AUC of 0.896. The results from the meta-analysis demonstrated that ultrasound-based liver stiffness assessment could be a valuable imaging marker for the diagnosis of infantile biliary atresia. It is, however, imperative to note that, despite the current study reporting SWE to have good diagnostic accuracy, the diagnostic performance of SWE does not exceed that of conventional grayscale ultrasound parameters, as reported from pooled studies in a meta-analysis by Yoon et al. [42], where the overall diagnostic accuracy (AUC = 0.97) for conventional grayscale parameters was higher than that for SWE reported in the current study (AUC = 0.896). The results from the systematic review showed that combining SWE and grayscale ultrasound yields a better diagnostic specificity [63], and similar findings were echoed by Wang et al. [71], who concluded that, despite the hepatic Young's modulus being an independent predictor of BA, the incorporation of the gallbladder structural features and age into a nomogram realized a better performance than the individual features. The subgroup analysis observed notable excellent diagnostic accuracy in studies utilising the hepatic Young's modulus compared to those reporting shear wave velocity: AUC was 0.906 versus 0.71, respectively. The systematic review demonstrated that the diagnostic performance of SWE increased with age and this can pose a potential clinical challenge in the utility of SWE for the early diagnosis of BA in young patients, which is key to obtaining good prognostic outcomes, as suggested by Napolitano [1].

It is imperative to note that the methodological approaches in the included studies were varied, as different machines, scanning protocols, reference index, and outcome measures were utilized (Table 2). Six of the studies used the Aixplorer ultrasound system (Super-Sonic Imagine SA, Aix-en-Provence, France) [69,70,72,73,75], five studies used the Acuson

S2000 or S3000 unit (Siemens Healthcare, Erlangen, Germany) [11,61,65–67], and two studies used the TUS-Aplio 500 scanner (Toshiba Medical Systems, Tokyo, Japan) [63,70]. The FibroScan 502 Touch (Echosens, Paris, France), in conjunction with a 5 MHz probe, was used in two studies [62,64]. Moreover, the measurement outcomes were reported differently in the studies, with some studies reporting mean values and others reporting median values (Table 3). These differences could account for the heterogeneities observed in the current study I^2 = 87.2%, chi square = 156.46%, p < 0.0001 (Figure 8a). In one of the studies, different diagnostic performances were reported across different SWE modes (VTIQ and VTQ), probes, and scanning regions of interest (ROI) [67]. The liver stiffness measures were also not uniformly reported, as these were reported either as mean or median values. Hence, to facilitate the meta-analysis, the median values were converted to the mean values using established formula [24]. The current study findings point toward the need for future standardization of SWE protocols for the diagnosis of BA, which will allow for an accurate pooling of the studies of diagnostic performance.

The bias assessment is represented by the funnel plot in Figure 9. The concentration of low-precision studies shown at the base of the plot is an indicator that there are more small studies reported in comparison to large-sample-size studies. The observed funnel plot asymmetry is indicative of the small-study effect phenomena, in which all of the evaluated low-precision studies are observed to concentrate only on the positive side of the mean effect size. These findings could suggest the presence of publication bias, although they do not rightly imply that publication bias was present [78–80] as funnel plot asymmetry may be due to other causes, including but not limited to, between-study heterogeneity and chance [80].

5. Limitations of the Study

The study, however, is limited, as only a few studies with a small number of patients met the inclusion criteria, which could restrict the generalizability of the study results. It should be noted that the included studies were mainly limited to the Asian and American population, further limiting the external validity of the results to other populations. The possibility of publication bias is another limitation of this study, as this could lead to an overestimated observed mean effect size. The evaluated studies utilised different reference standards and there were inconsistencies in outcome reporting, with some studies reporting mean values, whereas others reported median values, which could be a source of inhomogeneities.

6. Conclusions

The results from the current systematic review and meta-analysis have demonstrated that shear wave elastography has a good diagnostic performance and could, therefore, be a useful complementary tool to other diagnostic methods in differentiating BA from non-BA causes of infantile cholestasis. Liver stiffness indicators were significantly higher in BA patients compared to non-BA patients. Future studies assessing the utility of other advanced ultrasonography techniques are recommended.

Supplementary Materials: The following supporting information can be downloaded at: https://www.mdpi.com/article/10.3390/children9111676/s1, Table S1: Database search strings.

Author Contributions: Conceptualization, S.T.G., M.T.-c.Y. and N.C.; methodology, S.T.G., M.T.-c.Y. and N.C.; validation, S.T.G., M.T.-c.Y., N.C., X.F.C. and M.Y.C.P.; formal analysis, S.T.G. and M.T.-c.Y.; investigation, S.T.G., M.T.-c.Y. and N.C.; data curation, S.T.G., M.T.-c.Y., X.F.C., N.C. and M.Y.C.P.; writing-original draft preparation, S.T.G.; writing-review and editing, S.T.G., M.T.-c.Y., X.F.C., M.Y.C.P. and N.C.; visualization, S.T.G., M.T.-c.Y., N.C., X.F.C. and M.Y.C.P.; supervision, M.T.-c.Y., X.F.C. and M.Y.C.P.; project administration, S.T.G. and M.T.-c.Y.; funding acquisition, M.T.-c.Y. All authors have read and agreed to the published version of the manuscript.

Funding: This research was supported by a research studentship grant (R006) of The Hong Kong Polytechnic University, Hung Hom, Kowloon, Hong Kong, SAR, China.

Institutional Review Board Statement: Not applicable.

Informed Consent Statement: Not applicable.

Data Availability Statement: Not applicable.

Conflicts of Interest: The authors declare no conflict of interest.

References

1. Napolitano, M. Imaging in biliary atresia. *Pediatr. Radiol.* **2019**, *49*, S297. [CrossRef]
2. Lendahl, U.; Lui, V.C.H.; Chung, P.H.Y.; Tam, P.K.H. Biliary Atresia—emerging diagnostic and therapy opportunities. *eBioMedicine* **2021**, *74*, 103689. [CrossRef] [PubMed]
3. Dike, P.; Mahmood, N.; Harpavat, S. Recent advances in the use of ultrasound and related techniques in diagnosing and predicting outcomes in biliary atresia. *Curr. Opin. Pediatr.* **2021**, *33*, 515–520. [CrossRef]
4. Fanna, M.; Masson, G.; Capito, C.; Girard, M.; Guerin, F.; Hermeziu, B.; Lachaux, A.; Roquelaure, B.; Gottrand, F.; Broue, P.; et al. Management of Biliary Atresia in France 1986 to 2015: Long-term Results. *J. Pediatr. Gastroenterol. Nutr.* **2019**, *69*, 416–424. [CrossRef] [PubMed]
5. Lakshminarayanan, B.; Davenport, M. Biliary atresia: A comprehensive review. *J. Autoimmun.* **2016**, *73*, 1–9. [CrossRef] [PubMed]
6. Chiu, C.-Y.; Chen, P.-H.; Chan, C.-F.; Chang, M.-H.; Wu, T.-C. Biliary Atresia in Preterm Infants in Taiwan: A Nationwide Survey. *J. Pediatr.* **2013**, *163*, 100–103.e101. [CrossRef]
7. Chardot, C.; Buet, C.; Serinet, M.-O.; Golmard, J.-L.; Lachaux, A.; Roquelaure, B.; Gottrand, F.; Broué, P.; Dabadie, A.; Gauthier, F.; et al. Improving outcomes of biliary atresia: French national series 1986–2009. *J. Hepatol.* **2013**, *58*, 1209–1217. [CrossRef]
8. Chung, P.H.Y.; Zheng, S.; Tam, P.K.H. Biliary atresia: East versus west. *Semin. Pediatr. Surg.* **2020**, *29*, 150950. [CrossRef]
9. Nio, M.; Sasaki, H.; Wada, M.; Kazama, T.; Nishi, K.; Tanaka, H. Impact of age at Kasai operation on short- and long-term outcomes of type III biliary atresia at a single institution. *J. Pediatr. Surg.* **2010**, *45*, 2361–2363. [CrossRef]
10. Pakarinen, M.P.; Johansen, L.S.; Svensson, J.F.; Bjørnland, K.; Gatzinsky, V.; Stenström, P.; Koivusalo, A.; Kvist, N.; Almström, M.; Emblem, R.; et al. Outcomes of biliary atresia in the Nordic countries—A multicenter study of 158 patients during 2005–2016. *J. Pediatr. Surg.* **2018**, *53*, 1509–1515. [CrossRef]
11. Chen, Y.; Zhao, D.; Gu, S.; Li, Y.; Pan, W.; Zhang, Y. Three-color risk stratification for improving the diagnostic accuracy for biliary atresia. *Eur. Radiol.* **2020**, *30*, 3852–3861. [CrossRef] [PubMed]
12. Choi, H.-Y. Carotid duplex ultrasound: Interpretations and clinical applications. *Ann. Clin. Neurophysiol.* **2021**, *23*, 82–91. [CrossRef]
13. Di Serafino, M.; Gioioso, M.; Severino, R.; Esposito, F.; Vezzali, N.; Ferro, F.; Pelliccia, P.; Caprio, M.G.; Iorio, R.; Vallone, G. Ultrasound findings in paediatric cholestasis: How to image the patient and what to look for. *J. Ultrasound* **2020**, *23*, 1–12. [CrossRef] [PubMed]
14. Zhou, W.; Chen, D.; Jiang, H.; Shan, Q.; Zhang, X.; Xie, X.; Zhou, L. Ultrasound Evaluation of Biliary Atresia Based on Gallbladder Classification: Is 4 Hours of Fasting Necessary? *J. Ultrasound Med.* **2019**, *38*, 2447–2455. [CrossRef] [PubMed]
15. Ho, A.; Sacks, M.A.; Sapra, A.; Khan, F.A. The Utility of Gallbladder Absence on Ultrasound for Children With Biliary Atresia. *Front. Pediatr.* **2021**, *9*, 685268. [CrossRef]
16. Hwang, M.; Piskunowicz, M.; Darge, K. Advanced Ultrasound Techniques for Pediatric Imaging. *Pediatrics* **2019**, *143*, e20182609. [CrossRef] [PubMed]
17. Riccabona, M.; Fritz, G.A.; Schöllnast, H.; Schwarz, T.; Deutschmann, M.J.; Mache, C.J. Hydronephrotic Kidney: Pediatric Three-dimensional US for Relative Renal Size Assessment—Initial Experience. *Radiology* **2005**, *236*, 276–283. [CrossRef]
18. Haratz, K.; Nardozza, L.; Oliveira, P.; Rolo, L.; Milani, H.; Sá Barreto, E.; Araujo Júnior, E.; Ajzen, S.; Moron, A. Morphological evaluation of lateral ventricles of fetuses with ventriculomegaly by three-dimensional ultrasonography and magnetic resonance imaging: Correlation with etiology. *Arch. Gynecol. Obstet.* **2010**, *284*, 331–336. [CrossRef]
19. Riccabona, M. Editorial review: Pediatric 3D ultrasound. *J. Ultrason* **2014**, *14*, 5–20. [CrossRef]
20. Csutak, R.; Unterassinger, L.; Rohrmeister, C.; Weninger, M.; Vergesslich, K.A. Three-dimensional volume measurement of the lateral ventricles in preterm and term infants: Evaluation of a standardised computer-assisted method in vivo. *Pediatr. Radiol.* **2003**, *33*, 104–109. [CrossRef]
21. Hwang, M.; Riggs, B.J.; Katz, J.; Seyfert, D.; Northington, F.; Shenandoah, R.; Burd, I.; McArthur, J.; Darge, K.; Thimm, M.A.; et al. Advanced Pediatric Neurosonography Techniques: Contrast-Enhanced Ultrasonography, Elastography, and Beyond. *J. Neuroimaging* **2018**, *28*, 150–157. [CrossRef] [PubMed]
22. Page, M.J.; McKenzie, J.E.; Bossuyt, P.M.; Boutron, I.; Hoffmann, T.C.; Mulrow, C.D.; Shamseer, L.; Tetzlaff, J.M.; Akl, E.A.; Brennan, S.E.; et al. The PRISMA 2020 statement: An updated guideline for reporting systematic reviews. *Syst. Rev.* **2021**, *10*, 89. [CrossRef] [PubMed]
23. Šimundić, A.-M. Measures of Diagnostic Accuracy: Basic Definitions. *EJIFCC* **2009**, *19*, 203–211. [PubMed]
24. Hozo, S.P.; Djulbegovic, B.; Hozo, I. Estimating the mean and variance from the median, range, and the size of a sample. *BMC Med. Res. Methodol.* **2005**, *5*, 13. [CrossRef] [PubMed]

25. Urakami, Y.; Seki, H.; Kishi, S. Endoscopic retrograde cholangiopancreatography (ERCP) performed in children. *Endoscopy* **1977**, *9*, 86–91. [CrossRef] [PubMed]
26. Saito, T.; Terui, K.; Mitsunaga, T.; Nakata, M.; Kuriyama, Y.; Higashimoto, Y.; Kouchi, K.; Onuma, N.; Takahashi, H.; Yoshida, H. Role of pediatric endoscopic retrograde cholangiopancreatography in an era stressing less-invasive imaging modalities. *J Pediatr. Gastroenterol. Nutr.* **2014**, *59*, 204–209. [CrossRef]
27. Petersen, C.; Meier, P.N.; Schneider, A.; Turowski, C.; Pfister, E.D.; Manns, M.P.; Ure, B.M.; Wedemeyer, J. Endoscopic retrograde cholangiopancreaticography prior to explorative laparotomy avoids unnecessary surgery in patients suspected for biliary atresia. *J. Hepatol.* **2009**, *51*, 1055–1060. [CrossRef]
28. Larrosa–Haro, A.; Caro–López, A.M.; Coello–Ramírez, P.; Zavala–Ocampo, J.; Vázquez–Camacho, G. Duodenal Tube Test in the Diagnosis of Biliary Atresia. *J. Pediatr. Gastroenterol. Nutr.* **2001**, *32*, 311–315. [CrossRef]
29. Yoshii, D.; Inomata, Y.; Yamamoto, H.; Irie, T.; Kadohisa, M.; Okumura, K.; Isono, K.; Honda, M.; Hayashida, S.; Oya, Y.; et al. The duodenal tube test is more specific than hepatobiliary scintigraphy for identifying bile excretion in the differential diagnosis of biliary atresia. *Surg. Today* **2020**, *50*, 1232–1239. [CrossRef]
30. Rafeey, M.; Saboktakin, L.; Hasani, J.S.; Naghashi, S. Diagnostic value of anti-smooth muscle antibodies and liver enzymes in differentiation of extrahepatic biliary atresia and idiopathic neonatal hepatitis. *Afr. J. Paediatr. Surg.* **2016**, *13*, 63–68. [CrossRef]
31. Rafeey, M.; Saboktakin, L.; Shoa Hassani, J.; Farahmand, F.; Aslanabadi, S.; Ghorbani-Haghjou, A.; Poorebrahim, S. Diagnostic value of procalcitonin and apo-e in extrahepatic biliary atresia. *Iran J. Pediatr.* **2014**, *24*, 623–629. [PubMed]
32. Guo, Y.; Parthasarathy, S.; Goyal, P.; McCarthy, R.J.; Larson, A.C.; Miller, F.H. Magnetic resonance elastography and acoustic radiation force impulse for staging hepatic fibrosis: A meta-analysis. *Abdom. Imaging* **2015**, *40*, 818–834. [CrossRef] [PubMed]
33. He, J.-P.; Hao, Y.; Wang, X.-L.; Yang, X.-J.; Shao, J.-F.; Feng, J.-X. Comparison of different noninvasive diagnostic methods for biliary atresia: A meta-analysis. *World J. Pediatr.* **2016**, *12*, 35–43. [CrossRef]
34. Wang, L.; Yang, Y.; Chen, Y.; Zhan, J. Early differential diagnosis methods of biliary atresia: A meta-analysis. *Pediatr. Surg. Int.* **2018**, *34*, 363–380. [CrossRef]
35. Zhou, L.; Shan, Q.; Tian, W.; Wang, Z.; Liang, J.; Xie, X. Ultrasound for the Diagnosis of Biliary Atresia: A Meta-Analysis. *Am. J. Roentgenol.* **2016**, *206*, W73–W82. [CrossRef] [PubMed]
36. Sun, C.; Wu, B.; Pan, J.; Chen, L.; Zhi, W.; Tang, R.; Zhao, D.; Guo, W.; Wang, J.; Huang, S. Hepatic Subcapsular Flow as a Significant Diagnostic Marker for Biliary Atresia: A Meta-Analysis. *Dis. Mrk.* **2020**, *2020*, 5262565. [CrossRef]
37. He, L.; Ip, D.K.M.; Tam, G.; Lui, V.C.H.; Tam, P.K.H.; Chung, P.H.Y. Biomarkers for the diagnosis and post-Kasai portoenterostomy prognosis of biliary atresia: A systematic review and meta-analysis. *Sci. Rep.* **2021**, *11*, 11692. [CrossRef]
38. Kim, D.W.; Park, C.; Yoon, H.M.; Jung, A.Y.; Lee, J.S.; Jung, S.C.; Cho, Y.A. Technical performance of shear wave elastography for measuring liver stiffness in pediatric and adolescent patients: A systematic review and meta-analysis. *Eur. Radiol.* **2019**, *29*, 2560–2572. [CrossRef]
39. Liu, Y.; Tan, H.-Y.; Zhang, X.-G.; Zhen, Y.-H.; Gao, F.; Lu, X.-F. Prediction of high-risk esophageal varices in patients with chronic liver disease with point and 2D shear wave elastography: A systematic review and meta-analysis. *Eur. Radiol.* **2022**, *32*, 4616–4627. [CrossRef]
40. Wagner, E.S.; Abdelgawad, H.A.H.; Landry, M.; Asfour, B.; Slidell, M.B.; Azzam, R. Use of shear wave elastography for the diagnosis and follow-up of biliary atresia: A meta-analysis. *World J. Gastroenterol.* **2022**, *28*, 4726–4740. [CrossRef]
41. Yan, H.; Du, L.; Zhou, J.; Li, Y.; Lei, J.; Liu, J.; Luo, Y. Diagnostic performance and prognostic value of elastography in patients with biliary atresia and after hepatic portoenterostomy: Protocol for a systematic review and meta-analysis. *BMJ Open* **2021**, *11*, e042129. [CrossRef] [PubMed]
42. Yoon, H.M.; Suh, C.H.; Kim, J.R.; Lee, J.S.; Jung, A.Y.; Cho, Y.A. Diagnostic Performance of Sonographic Features in Patients With Biliary Atresia: A Systematic Review and Meta-analysis. *J. Ultrasound Med.* **2017**, *36*, 2027–2038. [CrossRef] [PubMed]
43. Kianifar, H.R.; Tehranian, S.; Shojaei, P.; Adinehpoor, Z.; Sadeghi, R.; Kakhki, V.R.D.; Keshtgar, A.S. Accuracy of hepatobiliary scintigraphy for differentiation of neonatal hepatitis from biliary atresia: Systematic review and meta-analysis of the literature. *Pediatr. Radiol.* **2013**, *43*, 905–919. [CrossRef] [PubMed]
44. Zhang, X.; Chen, C.; Yan, C.; Song, T. Accuracy of 2D and point shear wave elastography-based measurements for diagnosis of esophageal varices: A systematic review and meta-analysis. *Diagn. Interv. Radiol.* **2022**, *28*, 138–148. [CrossRef]
45. Sandberg, J.; Sun, Y.; Ju, Z.; Liu, S.; Jiang, J.; Koci, M.; Willemink, M.; Rosenberg, J.; Rubesova, E.; Barth, R. Biliary atresia versus other causes of neonatal jaundice: What is the value of shear wave elastography complementing grayscale findings? *Pediatr. Radiol.* **2019**, *49*, S134–S135. [CrossRef]
46. Dabadie, A.; Pariente, D.; Guerin, F.; Hermeziu, B.; Gonzales, E.; Adamsbaum, C.; Franchi-Abella, S. Can liver and spleen stiffness measurements help to differentiate biliary atresia from other neonatal cholestasis? *Pediatr. Radiol.* **2018**, *48*, S408. [CrossRef]
47. Chen, H.; Zhou, L.; Liao, B.; Cao, Q.; Jiang, H.; Zhou, W.; Wang, G.; Xie, X. Two-Dimensional Shear Wave Elastography Predicts Liver Fibrosis in Jaundiced Infants with Suspected Biliary Atresia: A Prospective Study. *Korean J. Radiol.* **2021**, *22*, 959. [CrossRef]
48. Dillman, J.R.; Heider, A.; Bilhartz, J.L.; Smith, E.A.; Keshavarzi, N.; Rubin, J.M.; Lopez, M.J. Ultrasound shear wave speed measurements correlate with liver fibrosis in children. *Pediatr. Radiol.* **2015**, *45*, 1480–1488. [CrossRef]
49. Farmakis, S.G.; Buchanan, P.M.; Guzman, M.A.; Hardy, A.K.; Jain, A.K.; Teckman, J.H. Shear wave elastography correlates with liver fibrosis scores in pediatric patients with liver disease. *Pediatr. Radiol.* **2019**, *49*, 1742–1753. [CrossRef]

50. Galina, P.; Alexopoulou, E.; Mentessidou, A.; Mirilas, P.; Zellos, A.; Lykopoulou, L.; Patereli, A.; Salpasaranis, K.; Kelekis, N.L.; Zarifi, M. Diagnostic accuracy of two-dimensional shear wave elastography in detecting hepatic fibrosis in children with autoimmune hepatitis, biliary atresia and other chronic liver diseases. *Pediatr. Radiol.* **2021**, *51*, 1358–1368. [CrossRef]

51. Gao, F.; Chen, Y.Q.; Fang, J.; Gu, S.L.; Li, L.; Wang, X.Y. Acoustic Radiation Force Impulse Imaging for Assessing Liver Fibrosis Preoperatively in Infants With Biliary Atresia: Comparison With Liver Fibrosis Biopsy Pathology. *J. Ultrasound Med. Off. J. Am. Inst. Ultrasound Med.* **2017**, *36*, 1571–1578. [CrossRef] [PubMed]

52. Hanquinet, S.; Rougemont, A.-L.; Courvoisier, D.; Rubbia-Brandt, L.; McLin, V.; Tempia, M.; Anooshiravani, M. Acoustic radiation force impulse (ARFI) elastography for the noninvasive diagnosis of liver fibrosis in children. *Pediatr. Radiol.* **2013**, *43*, 545–551. [CrossRef] [PubMed]

53. Shen, Q.L.; Chen, Y.J.; Wang, Z.M.; Zhang, T.C.; Pang, W.B.; Shu, J.; Peng, C.H. Assessment of liver fibrosis by Fibroscan as compared to liver biopsy in biliary atresia. *World J. Gastroenterol.* **2015**, *21*, 6931–6936. [CrossRef] [PubMed]

54. Teufel-Schäfer, U.; Flechtenmacher, C.; Fichtner, A.; Hoffmann, G.F.; Schenk, J.P.; Engelmann, G. Transient elastography correlated to four different histological fibrosis scores in children with liver disease. *Eur. J. Pediatr.* **2021**, *180*, 2237–2244. [CrossRef]

55. Ding, C.; Wang, Z.; Peng, C.; Pang, W.; Tan, S.S.; Chen, Y. Diagnosis of liver cirrhosis with two-dimensional shear wave elastography in biliary atresia before Kasai portoenterostomy. *Pediatr. Surg. Int.* **2022**, *38*, 209–215. [CrossRef]

56. Uchikawa, S.; Kawaoka, T.; Fujino, H.; Ono, A.; Nakahara, T.; Murakami, E.; Yamauchi, M.; Miki, D.; Imamura, M.; Aikata, H. The effect of the skin-liver capsule distance on the accuracy of ultrasound diagnosis for liver steatosis and fibrosis. *J. Med. Ultrason. 2001* **2022**, *49*, 443–450. [CrossRef]

57. Voutilainen, S.; Kivisaari, R.; Lohi, J.; Jalanko, H.; Pakarinen, M.P. A Prospective Comparison of Noninvasive Methods in the Assessment of Liver Fibrosis and Esophageal Varices in Pediatric Chronic Liver Diseases. *J. Clin. Gastroenterol.* **2016**, *50*, 658–663. [CrossRef]

58. Zhou, W.; Yang, Y.; Yu, C.; Liu, J.; Duan, X.; Weng, Z.; Chen, D.; Liang, Q.; Fang, Q.; Zhou, J.; et al. Ensembled deep learning model outperforms human experts in diagnosing biliary atresia from sonographic gallbladder images. *Nat. Commun.* **2021**, *12*, 1259. [CrossRef]

59. Zhou, L.; Xie, J.; Gao, P.; Chen, H.; Chen, S.; Wang, G.; Zhou, W.; Xie, X. Percutaneous ultrasound-guided cholecystocholangiography with microbubbles combined with liver biopsy for the assessment of suspected biliary atresia. *Pediatr. Radiol.* **2022**, *52*, 1075–1085. [CrossRef]

60. Zhou, L.-Y.; Chen, S.-L.; Chen, H.-D.; Huang, Y.; Qiu, Y.-X.; Zhong, W.; Xie, X.-Y. Percutaneous US-guided Cholecystocholangiography with Microbubbles for Assessment of Infants with US Findings Equivocal for Biliary Atresia and Gallbladder Longer than 1.5 cm: A Pilot Study. *Radiology* **2018**, *286*, 1033–1039. [CrossRef]

61. Liu, Y.F.; Ni, X.W.; Pan, Y.; Luo, H.X. Comparison of the diagnostic value of virtual touch tissue quantification and virtual touch tissue imaging quantification in infants with biliary atresia. *Int. J. Clin. Pract.* **2021**, *75*, e13860. [CrossRef] [PubMed]

62. Boo, Y.A.; Chang, M.H.; Jeng, Y.M.; Peng, S.F.; Hsu, W.M.; Lin, W.H.; Chen, H.L.; Ni, Y.H.; Hsu, H.Y.; Wu, J.F. Diagnostic Performance of Transient Elastography in Biliary Atresia Among Infants With Cholestasis. *Hepatol. Commun.* **2021**, *5*, 882–890. [CrossRef]

63. Duan, X.; Peng, Y.; Liu, W.; Yang, L.; Zhang, J. Does Supersonic Shear Wave Elastography Help Differentiate Biliary Atresia from Other Causes of Cholestatic Hepatitis in Infants Less than 90 Days Old? Compared with Grey-Scale US. *BioMed. Res. Int.* **2019**, *2019*, 9036362. [CrossRef] [PubMed]

64. Wu, J.-F.; Lee, C.-S.; Lin, W.-H.; Jeng, Y.-M.; Chen, H.-L.; Ni, Y.-H.; Hsu, H.-Y.; Chang, M.-H. Transient elastography is useful in diagnosing biliary atresia and predicting prognosis after hepatoportoenterostomy. *Hepatology* **2018**, *68*, 616–624. [CrossRef] [PubMed]

65. Dillman, J.R.; DiPaola, F.W.; Smith, S.J.; Barth, R.A.; Asai, A.; Lam, S.; Campbell, K.M.; Bezerra, J.A.; Tiao, G.M.; Trout, A.T. Prospective Assessment of Ultrasound Shear Wave Elastography for Discriminating Biliary Atresia from other Causes of Neonatal Cholestasis. *J. Pediatr.* **2019**, *212*, 60–65. [CrossRef] [PubMed]

66. Leschied, J.R.; Dillman, J.R.; Bilhartz, J.; Heider, A.; Smith, E.A.; Lopez, M.J. Shear wave elastography helps differentiate biliary atresia from other neonatal/infantile liver diseases. *Pediatr Radiol* **2015**, *45*, 366–375. [CrossRef]

67. Sandberg, J.K.; Sun, Y.; Ju, Z.; Liu, S.; Jiang, J.; Koci, M.; Rosenberg, J.; Rubesova, E.; Barth, R.A. Ultrasound shear wave elastography: Does it add value to gray-scale ultrasound imaging in differentiating biliary atresia from other causes of neonatal jaundice? *Pediatr. Radiol.* **2021**, *51*, 1654–1666. [CrossRef]

68. Wang, X.; Qian, L.; Jia, L.; Bellah, R.; Wang, N.; Xin, Y.; Liu, Q. Utility of Shear Wave Elastography for Differentiating Biliary Atresia From Infantile Hepatitis Syndrome. *J. Ultrasound Med.* **2016**, *35*, 1475–1479. [CrossRef]

69. Zhou, L.Y.; Jiang, H.; Shan, Q.Y.; Chen, D.; Lin, X.N.; Liu, B.X.; Xie, X.Y. Liver stiffness measurements with supersonic shear wave elastography in the diagnosis of biliary atresia: A comparative study with grey-scale US. *Eur. Radiol.* **2017**, *27*, 3474–3484. [CrossRef]

70. Zhou, W.; Liang, J.; Shan, Q.; Chen, H.; Gao, P.; Cao, Q.; Wang, G.; Xie, X.; Zhou, L. Comparison of Two Kinds of Two-Dimensional Shear Wave Elastography Techniques in the Evaluation of Jaundiced Infants Suspected of Biliary Atresia. *Diagnostics* **2022**, *12*, 1092. [CrossRef]

71. Wang, Y.; Jia, L.Q.; Hu, Y.X.; Xin, Y.; Yang, X.; Wang, X.M. Development and Validation of a Nomogram Incorporating Ultrasonic and Elastic Findings for the Preoperative Diagnosis of Biliary Atresia. *Acad. Radiol.* **2021**, *28* (Suppl. S1), S55–S63. [CrossRef] [PubMed]

72. Liu, Y.; Peng, C.; Wang, K.; Wu, D.; Yan, J.; Tu, W.; Chen, Y. The utility of shear wave elastography and serum biomarkers for diagnosing biliary atresia and predicting clinical outcomes. *Eur. J. Pediatr.* **2022**, *181*, 73–82. [CrossRef] [PubMed]

73. Shen, Q.; Tan, S.S.; Wang, Z.; Cai, S.; Pang, W.; Peng, C.; Chen, Y. Combination of gamma-glutamyl transferase and liver stiffness measurement for biliary atresia screening at different ages: A retrospective analysis of 282 infants. *BMC Pediatr.* **2020**, *20*, 276. [CrossRef] [PubMed]

74. Hanquinet, S.; Courvoisier, D.S.; Rougemont, A.-L.; Dhouib, A.; Rubbia-Brandt, L.; Wildhaber, B.E.; Merlini, L.; McLin, V.A.; Anooshiravani, M. Contribution of acoustic radiation force impulse (ARFI) elastography to the ultrasound diagnosis of biliary atresia. *Pediatr. Radiol.* **2015**, *45*, 1489–1495. [CrossRef]

75. Wang, G.; Zhang, N.; Zhang, X.; Zhou, W.; Xie, X.; Zhou, L. Ultrasound characteristics combined with gamma-glutamyl transpeptidase for diagnosis of biliary atresia in infants less than 30 days. *Pediatr. Surg. Int.* **2021**, *37*, 1175–1182. [CrossRef]

76. Baratloo, A.; Hosseini, M.; Negida, A.; El Ashal, G. Part 1: Simple Definition and Calculation of Accuracy, Sensitivity and Specificity. *Emergency* **2015**, *3*, 48–49.

77. Lee, S.; Kim, M.-J.; Lee, M.-J.; Yoon, H.; Han, K.; Han, S.J.; Koh, H.; Kim, S.; Shin, H.J. Hepatic subcapsular or capsular flow in biliary atresia: Is it useful imaging feature after the Kasai operation? *Eur. Radiol.* **2020**, *30*, 3161–3167. [CrossRef]

78. Sterne, J.A.C.; Sutton, A.J.; Ioannidis, J.P.A.; Terrin, N.; Jones, D.R.; Lau, J.; Carpenter, J.; Rucker, G.; Harbord, R.M.; Schmid, C.H.; et al. Recommendations for examining and interpreting funnel plot asymmetry in meta-analyses of randomised controlled trials. *BMJ* **2011**, *343*, d4002. [CrossRef]

79. Egger, M.; Smith, G.D.; Schneider, M.; Minder, C. Bias in meta-analysis detected by a simple, graphical test. *BMJ* **1997**, *315*, 629–634. [CrossRef]

80. Page, M.J.; Sterne, J.A.C.; Higgins, J.P.T.; Egger, M. Investigating and dealing with publication bias and other reporting biases in meta-analyses of health research: A review. *Res. Synth. Methods* **2021**, *12*, 248–259. [CrossRef]

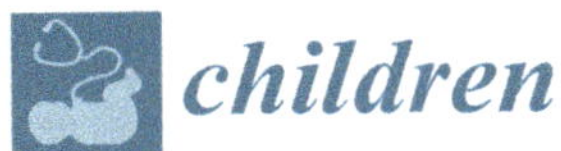

Systematic Review

Cumulative Radiation Dose from Medical Imaging in Children with Congenital Heart Disease: A Systematic Review

Emer Shelly [1], Michael G. Waldron [2,*], Erica Field [1], Niamh Moore [1], Rena Young [1], Andy Scally [1], Andrew England [1], Michael Maher [2,3] and Mark F. McEntee [1]

1   Discipline of Medical Imaging & Radiation Therapy, University College Cork, T12AK54 Cork, Ireland
2   Department of Radiology, Cork University Hospital, T12 DC4A Cork, Ireland
3   Department of Medicine, University College Cork, T12 AK54 Cork, Ireland
*   Correspondence: mwaldron@ucc.ie

Abstract: Children with congenital heart disease are exposed to repeated medical imaging throughout their lifetime. Although the imaging contributes to their care and treatment, exposure to ionising radiation is known to increase one's lifetime attributable risk of malignancy. A systematic search of multiple databases was performed. Inclusion and exclusion criteria were applied to all relevant papers and seven were deemed acceptable for quality assessment and risk of bias assessment. The cumulative effective dose (CED) varied widely across the patient cohorts, ranging from 0.96 mSv to 53.5 mSv. However, it was evident across many of the included studies that a significant number of patients were exposed to a CED >20 mSv, the current annual occupational exposure limit. Many factors affected the dose which patients received, including age and clinical demographics. The imaging modality which contributed the most radiation dose to patients was cardiology interventional procedures. Paediatric patients with congenital heart disease are at an increased risk of receiving an elevated cumulative radiation dose across their lifetime. Further research should focus on identifying risk factors for receiving higher radiation doses, keeping track of doses, and dose optimisation where possible.

Keywords: cumulative; radiation dose; medical imaging; congenital heart disease

Citation: Shelly, E.; Waldron, M.G.; Field, E.; Moore, N.; Young, R.; Scally, A.; England, A.; Maher, M.; McEntee, M.F. Cumulative Radiation Dose from Medical Imaging in Children with Congenital Heart Disease: A Systematic Review. *Children* **2023**, *10*, 645. https://doi.org/10.3390/children10040645

Academic Editor: Curtise Ng

Received: 7 March 2023
Revised: 18 March 2023
Accepted: 27 March 2023
Published: 30 March 2023

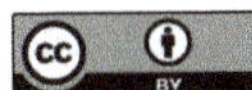

1. Introduction

Congenital heart disease is a defect in the structure of the heart or the great vessels, which is present at birth and occurs in approximately 1% of births per year in the United States [1]. Many of the diagnostic and interventional tools used to investigate and treat congenital heart disease involve the use of medical ionising radiation. The main concern with these procedures is the potential increase in the lifetime attributable risk of radiation-induced malignancy [2]. Patients with congenital heart disease are often exposed to relatively high doses of ionising radiation from medical sources from a very young age, often even from birth [3]. Malignancy due to ionising radiation poses a particular risk to children due to their rapidly dividing cells and longer life span in which the radiation can potentially cause damage [4]. Awareness of radiation safety and its possible long-term effects is suboptimal among many doctors, including paediatricians [5,6].

Lifetime cumulative radiation dose and the associated risk of developing cancer is a poorly understood subject. Much of our current understanding of the effects of radiation is based on atomic bomb survivors [2] or studies based on large single doses of radiation of >100 mSv [7]. Recent evidence would suggest that a high cumulative dose does carry an increased risk of developing cancer [8]. However, it remains unclear if this risk is the same as receiving the equivalent amount of radiation in one dose. Notably, according to the linear no-threshold (LNT) hypothesis, any dose, irrelevant of size, carries an inherent risk [9,10]. Therefore, the cumulative exposure burden to children with congenital heart disease calls for better understanding and awareness so that those involved in their care can make more informed decisions and, where possible, use a dose as low as reasonably acceptable.

The importance of understanding the risks associated with repeated exposure to ionising radiation, particularly in childhood, is emphasised by epidemiological studies. Researchers analysed the data of 11 million Australians to assess the malignancy risk in children and adolescents by analysing cancer incidence rates in those who had a CT more than one year before diagnosis compared to a group unexposed to CT imaging prior to malignancy diagnosis. They highlighted an elevated risk with an absolute excess incidence of 9.38 per 100,000 person-years at risk [11]. It must, however, be recognised that many of these types of studies have limitations, such as the dose estimation methods (which may over/underestimate risks), and the eventual lifetime risk of cancer is difficult to estimate due to the time limits of the studies (which may minimise risks).

The Alliance for Radiation in Paediatric Imaging has recognised the importance of monitoring low-dose ionising radiation in the "Image Gently" campaign to improve safe and effective imaging care for children worldwide. Image Gently advocates methods to reduce unnecessary ionising radiation by sharing best practices of imaging protocols for children and using alternative imaging that avoids ionising radiation. They have also created informational and advocacy information for each ionising radiation modality [12]. More recently, in 2017, a document from the Image Gently Alliance highlighted the relatively high cumulative lifetime burden of ionising radiation in children with complex congenital and acquired heart disease (CAHD) from the multiple imaging studies and procedures over their lifetime [3]. In this document, they emphasised the need to achieve high-quality studies with the lowest achievable radiation dose and to standardise dose metrics across imaging modalities to encourage comparative effectiveness studies across the spectrum of CAHD in children.

Many efforts have been made so far to reduce the radiation dose to CHD patients [13–15], including an interesting study by Patel et al. [16], which implemented several system-based interventions in the congenital cardiac catheterisation lab to reduce radiation exposure to paediatric CHD patients, including the utilisation of lower fluoroscopy and digital angiography doses, increasing staff and physician awareness, focusing on tighter collimation, and changing the default fluoroscopy and DA doses to lower settings [17]. Studies like these demonstrate the potential change that is possible on a broader scale to reduce radiation dose, ultimately lowering the cumulative radiation burden that CHD patients are exposed to.

The concepts of justification and the 'As Low as Reasonably Achievable' (ALARA) principle are imperative in medical imaging, especially regarding patients repeatedly exposed to radiation. A study assessing the rate of patients receiving high cumulative doses over 100 mSv highlighted an incidence of 0.21% over five years across 35 countries [18]. An up-to-date systematic review must be undertaken to establish the CED that this cohort of patients is receiving in a wide variety of settings, in addition to the modalities utilised and conditions that put these patients at a higher risk of receiving a higher cumulative radiation dose. This study aims to systematically review published data regarding the cumulative exposure from medical sources of ionising radiation in paediatric patients with CHD. We aim to provide the medical imaging community with a better understanding of dose estimation, cumulative dose, and risk factors for CHD patients who may be exposed to higher/repeated radiation. This will allow future practice to be improved and further work to be done surrounding the monitoring and reducing the cumulative dose of these patients.

2. Materials and Methods

The systematic review was performed in accordance with the pre-specified protocol, which was registered on PROSPERO, the prospective international register of systematic reviews.

2.1. Search Strategy

A comprehensive search of the current literature was performed in accordance with the Preferred Reporting Items for Systematic Reviews and Meta-Analyses (PRISMA) guidelines [19]. PubMed, Science Direct, Scopus, and Embase were searched. The 'year published' filter was applied for each database to only capture studies published between 1 January 2010 and 1 March 2023. Several pre-determined keywords were pooled for the systematic search and subsequent MeSH terms were generated. The MeSH terms used were "cumulative effective dose", "cumulative dose", "cumulative exposure", "cumulative radiation dose", "cumulative medical radiation exposure", "CHD", "congenital heart disease", "pediatric", "paediatric", "child", and "children". The MeSH terms were then combined according to the specifications of each database using link words such as "AND", "OR", and "NOT".

2.2. Data Synthesis

An initial screen of the literature was performed using the titles and abstracts of all articles that had been identified. Only articles that contained data from cumulative radiation dose in a follow-up period of one year minimum for children aged ≤ 18 years were included for a full-text review. Meta-analysis and review articles were excluded. For each study, reviewers applied inclusion/exclusion criteria as outlined below:

Clinical trials and observational studies were published between 2010 and 2020 in the English language.

(1)   Only studies involving a minimum of 20 paediatric patients.
(2)   Only studies involving the monitoring of cumulative radiation dose over at least one year.
(3)   Only studies involving the monitoring of cumulative radiation dose from medical sources (both interventional and diagnostic) as opposed to other sources.
(4)   Only studies where the patients had some form of congenital heart disease and/or had several cardiac interventional/diagnostic procedures carried out.
(5)   Only studies where the outcome measures included the cumulative radiation dose of included patients.
(6)   Only original cross-sectional studies, case-control studies, cohort studies, or randomised control trials.

Quality assessment was carried out using the STROBE quality assessment tool [20], and a risk of bias was applied to all included studies [21].

3. Results

3.1. Study Selection and Quality Assessment

The systematic search revealed 296 papers from PubMed/Science Direct, 66 from SCOPUS, and 61 from EMBASE. Hand-searching reference lists also found six further studies from other papers. After removing the duplicates, 337 titles and/or abstracts were assessed for relevance, and this resulted in 26 papers which were relevant to this review question. The full text of these 20 articles was reviewed, and inclusion/exclusion criteria were applied. Two reviewers (ES and EF) carried out this step to reduce bias. Any discrepancies at this stage were discussed, and updates were made where necessary. Seven of these 20 papers were agreed upon to be eligible for inclusion in this systematic review (Figure 1) (Supplementary Table S1).

Qualitative analysis was applied to these seven papers using the STROBE quality assessment tool by two independent reviewers (ES and EF). According to STROBE, all seven studies reached an acceptable level of quality. Certain limitations were identified outside of STROBE that included potential unrecorded radiation doses for investigations performed outside the facility of the study. The sample size for each paper was spread across an extensive range. Some papers had a low sample size (McDonnel et al. sampled 31 patients), with some cohorts followed for a relatively short time (Ait-Ali et al. [22] followed patients for one year). These factors need to be taken into consideration when interpreting the results. The level of homogeneity across these studies also proved to be a challenge, with several papers presenting their outcomes differently. Also, we assessed papers performed across a range of modalities that these papers collected data, which allowed us to understand the overall picture of the cumulative radiation dose of CHD patients from all their medical imaging.

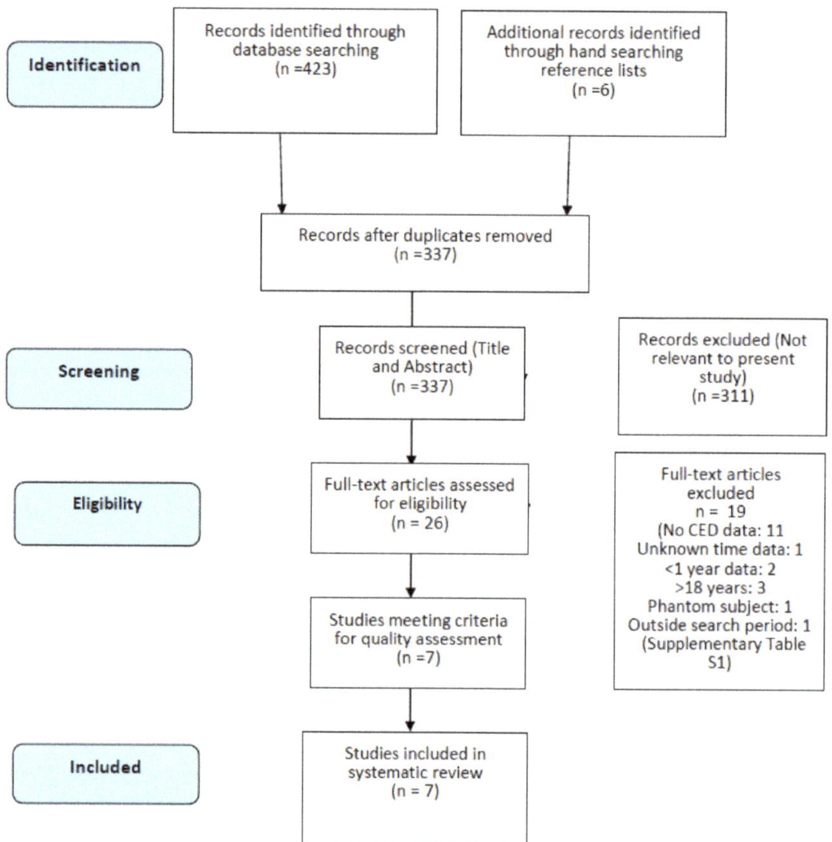

Figure 1. PRISMA flow diagram.

3.2. Data Extraction

A risk of bias assessment (Figure 2) was performed using questions designed to review cohort studies developed by the Clarity Group at McMaster University [21]. The overall risk of bias across all seven studies was relatively low. Due to the nature of the assessment of exposure and the variation of estimation techniques across the studies, there was likely a degree of information bias across all seven studies. It is also important to note that the exposure assessment may represent some bias since the patients were only followed in a single centre except for Ait-Ali et al. [22]. Assessment of confidence in the outcome was high across all papers but may be slightly lower in Ait-Ali et al., since the lifetime radiological exposure was derived from patient records. This may cause an underestimation in the calculation of the cumulative radiation dose.

Table 1 summarises the cumulative radiation exposure of included studies, the study type, the number of patients, the x-ray procedures recorded, and the effective dose estimation method. The contribution of different imaging modalities to the cumulative recorded radiation dose is recorded (Supplementary Table S2).

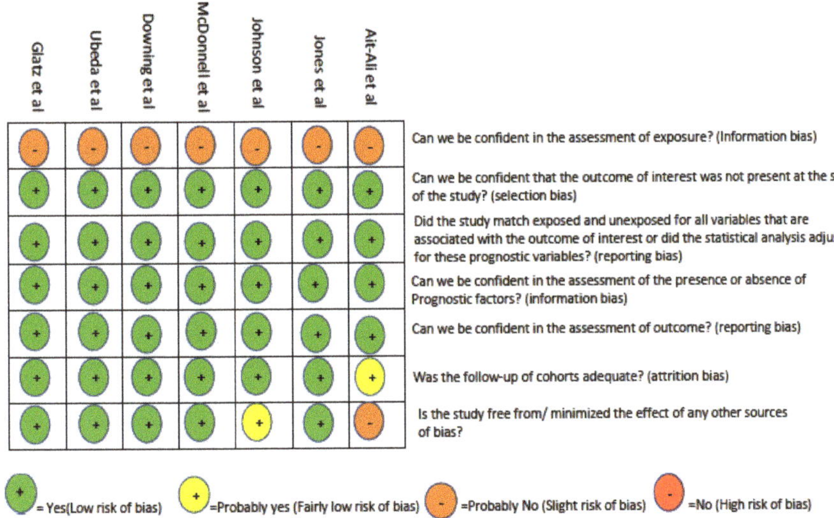

Figure 2. Risk of bias [22–28].

Table 1. Summary of included studies and cumulative effective radiation.

Author (Year)	Study Type	Number of Participants	Age of Participants, Years	Radiation Source	Overall Cumulative Effective Dose (mSv)	[1] Participants Cumulative Effective Dose >20 mSv
Ait-Ali (2010) [22]	Prospective cohort	59	2.8 (mean)	All ionising radiation	7.7 (median)	0/59
Jones (2017) [23]	Retrospective cohort	117	0–17 (range)	Interventional procedures	16.5 (median)	14/117
Ubeda (2019) [24]	Prospective/ retrospective cohort	1521	2–8 (range)	Interventional procedures	8.7 (>four procedures) (mean)	0/1521
McDonnell (2014) [25]	Retrospective cohort	31	13.6 (median at heart transplant)	All ionising radiation	53.5 (mean)	Unknown
Glatz (2014) [26]	Retrospective cohort	4132	0.3 (mean)	All ionising radiation	0.96 (median)	218/4132
Downing (2015) [27]	Retrospective cohort	38	[2] Birth-Fontan closure	All ionising radiation	25.7 (mean)	2.9
Johnson (2014) [28]	Retrospective cohort	337	0.24 (median at heart transplant)	All ionising radiation	2.67 (median)	94/337

[1] 20 mSv used as it is the current limit on effective dose for occupational exposure. [2] Fontan completion is a procedure to re-route the systemic deoxygenated blood from the venous circulation into the pulmonary vasculature.

4. Discussion

The seven included papers [22–28] utilised CED to measure ionising radiation exposure. CED is the total dose resulting from repeated exposures to ionising radiation from all radiologic studies [29]. Translating the relatively low levels of medical ionising radiation these patients receive into mutagenic effects is difficult due to sparse data, as most of our understanding of cancer risks stems from data on atomic bomb survivors [8]. Although the elevated risk associated with a single large radiation dose is known, the effects of recurrent smaller exposures are not well defined. However, the linear no-threshold model (whereby the risk of cancer increases linearly with the increase in radiation dose with no lower radiation dose limit) is widely accepted and provides the best description of the relationship between ionising radiation dose received and the risk of stochastic effects. Over 85% of infants born with modern or complex heart disease live to adulthood, with medical imaging involving ionising radiation playing a significant role in their diagnosis, treatment, and survival [30]. A large population-based study by Mathews et al. [11] suggested that each sievert of effective dose from CT scans can be attributed to 0.125 excess cancers in an average follow-up of 9.5 years. Therefore, it is more imperative than ever to assess and manage the doses being administered to these patients, following ALARA principles.

Unsurprisingly, diagnostic and interventional cardiac catheterisation represented the most significant percentage of cumulative effective dose across all seven included studies. In a previous study, the median exposure was reduced by 30% for all cases by employing institution-specific quality improvement intervention techniques [31]. Conversely, radiographs represented the lowest contribution to cumulative exposure across all studies where it was recorded. Although CT was only recorded in two papers, it represented a small percentage of examinations in both cases whilst contributing a large proportion of the overall radiation dose. CT is frequently used in diagnosing and treating CHD [32] and is a significant contributor to CED. Therefore, further studies should focus on reducing CED in CHD patients. Substantial efforts have been made to manage the radiation dose for paediatric cardiac CT via the Image Gently 'Have-a-Heart' campaign [33]. They found that understanding CT technical parameters and how to apply them to children of various sizes and heart rates is necessary to optimise image quality at the lowest possible radiation dose. A CT dose management program should be implemented to ensure regulatory compliance and to optimise ionising radiation use in patients exposed to long-term cumulative radiation due to their high risk of repeated and elevated exposure. Currently, the limit on effective dose for occupational exposure is 20 mSv, according to the 'Radiological Protection Act 1991- Ionising Radiation Regulation S.I No. 30 2019' [34]. It is, therefore, even more crucial that we consistently monitor and assess every single dose of ionising radiation and whether it can be reduced or avoided altogether.

There are many ways in which dose reduction can be achieved. These are generally classified as justification, optimisation, and dose limitation. iRefer guidelines [35] and the European Society of Radiology iGuide [36] tools can aid clinician decision-making for the justification of the use of medical imaging with suggestions for decisions including information related to radiation reduction and cost efficiency. Appropriate use of ionising radiation is essential in minimising the cumulative radiation dose to CHD paediatric patients. Optimisation strategies across different imaging modalities are possible. For example, in cardiac CT, the lowest practical radiation dose which can achieve acceptable image quality should be used. The use of ECG-gated tube current modulation for functional imaging, can greatly reduce dose [3]. In nuclear cardiology, using advanced hardware (e.g., PET, CZT) or software technology to reduce administered activity can also aid in dose optimisation [3]. The introduction of iterative algorithms in CT reconstruction offers promise of further reduction in the radiation dose to CHD patients. The second way of reducing dose can be by using alternative modalities which do not use ionising radiation, such as ultrasound or magnetic resonance imaging. Echocardiography is the first-line imaging technique used for CHD, as it is capable of providing excellent depiction of intracardiac and valvular anatomy, cardiac function, and hemodynamic [29]. Dose reduction can also be implemented with the help of diagnostic reference levels (DRLs). There is currently limited data in Ireland for DRLs for paediatric catheterisation. However, Eurosafe Imaging has provided a document on European DRLs for paediatric imaging that can assist dose optimisation [37].

A limitation of this review is that all studies assessing CED in CHD were included (both diagnostic and therapeutic). Some studies derived the cumulative effective dose from solely cardiac procedures as opposed to from all imaging modalities [27,28], which may represent an underestimation. This increased the heterogenicity between the studies, as such a meta-analysis could not be performed and increased difficulties in comparing the studies. A multi-centre study is required to gain a more accurate estimation of CED, with a separate investigation of radiation from diagnostic and interventional procedures (and overall CED), which should be aided by a state-wide dose estimation programme. A strength of this study was that the risk of bias within the review was kept as low as possible with two reviewers carrying out the search strategy, quality assessment, data extraction, and risk of bias assessment.

For patients with chronic conditions like CHD, it is evident that further multi-centre studies, involving larger patient cohorts and longer follow-up, are required to better understand the true estimate of CED accrued across their lifetime. Implementation of dose reduction measures should be applied more rigorously by those involved in their care to reduce unnecessary radiation and ultimately reduce their chance of developing a radiation-induced cancer.

5. Conclusions

It has long been accepted that children are at a higher risk than adults for radiation-induced cancer. This review has demonstrated that the radiation burden from medical imaging is elevated in paediatric patients with congenital heart disease, with radiation from diagnostic and interventional cardiac catheterisation representing the greatest cumulative dose. Overall, the importance of following ALARA principles is vital. Efforts on dose optimisation, limiting radiation exposure, and the use of alternative modalities without ionising radiation where possible are crucial to minimise lifetime CED in this cohort.

Supplementary Materials: The following supporting information can be downloaded at: https://www.mdpi.com/article/10.3390/children10040645/s1, Table S1: Excluded studies after full-text review [38–51]; Table S2: Contribution of total radiation exposure from various imaging modalities.

Author Contributions: E.S. and M.F.M. were responsible for conceptualisation and methodology. E.S. and E.F. were responsible for data collection and data interpretation. E.S. was responsible for writing the report. A.E., A.S., M.G.W., M.M., M.F.M., N.M. and R.Y. were responsible for the critical review of the final report. All authors have read and agreed to the published version of the manuscript.

Funding: This research received no external funding.

Institutional Review Board Statement: Not applicable.

Informed Consent Statement: Not applicable.

Data Availability Statement: Not applicable.

Acknowledgments: The corresponding author certifies that no other persons have made substantial contributions to the research and/or manuscript.

Conflicts of Interest: The authors declare no conflict of interest.

Abbreviations

ALARA—As low as reasonably achievable; CAHD—congenital and acquired heart disease; CED—cumulative effective dose; CHD—congenital heart disease; CT—computed tomogram; DRL—diagnostic reference level.

References

1. Reller, M.D.; Strickland, M.J.; Riehle-Colarusso, T.; Mahle, W.T.; Correa, A. Prevalence of congenital heart defects in metropolitan Atlanta, 1998–2005. *J. Pediatr.* **2008**, *153*, 807–813. [CrossRef] [PubMed]
2. National Research Council. *Health Risks from Exposure to Low Levels of Ionizing Radiation: BEIR VII Phase 2*; The National Academies Press: Washington, DC, USA, 2006.
3. Hill, K.D.; Frush, D.P.; Han, B.K.; Abbott, B.G.; Armstrong, A.K.; DeKemp, R.A.; Glatz, A.C.; Greenberg, S.B.; Herbert, A.S.; Justino, H.; et al. Radiation Safety in Children with Congenital and Acquired Heart Disease: A Scientific Position Statement

on Multimodality Dose Optimization from the Image Gently Alliance. *JACC Cardiovasc. Imaging* **2017**, *10*, 797–818. [CrossRef] [PubMed]

4. Meinert, R.; Kaletsch, U.; Kaatsch, P.; Schüz, J.; Michaelis, J. Associations between childhood cancer and ionising radiation: Results of a population-based case-control study in Germany. *Cancer Epidemiol. Biomark. Prev.* **1999**, *8*, 793–799.

5. Han, B.K.; Grant, K.L.R.; Garberich, R.; Sedlmair, M.; Lindberg, J.; Lesser, J.R. Assessment of an iterative reconstruction algorithm [SAFIRE] on image quality in pediatric cardiac CT datasets. *J. Cardiovasc. Comput. Tomogr.* **2012**, *6*, 200–204. [CrossRef] [PubMed]

6. Thomas, K.E.; Parnell-Parmley, J.E.; Haidar, S.; Moineddin, R.; Charkot, E.; BenDavid, G.; Krajewski, C. Assessment of radiation dose awareness among pediatricians. *Pediatr. Radiol.* **2006**, *36*, 823–832. [CrossRef]

7. Einstein, A.J.; Henzlova, M.J.; Rajagopalan, S. Estimating risk of cancer associated with radiation exposure from 64-slice computed tomography coronary angiography. *JAMA* **2007**, *298*, 317–323. [CrossRef]

8. Einstein, A.J. Beyond the bombs: Cancer risks of low-dose medical radiation. *Lancet* **2012**, *380*, 455–457. [CrossRef]

9. UNSCEAR. *Effects of Ionizing Radiation Volume 1*; United Nations Scientific Committee: Vienna, Austria, 2006.

10. Cohen, B.L. Cancer Risk from Low-Level Radiation. *Am. J. Roentgenol.* **2002**, *179*, 1137–1143. [CrossRef]

11. Mathews, J.D.; Forsythe, A.V.; Brady, Z.; Butler, M.W.; Goergen, S.K.; Byrnes, G.B.; Giles, G.G.; Wallace, A.B.; Anderson, P.R.; Guiver, T.A.; et al. Cancer risk in 680 000 people exposed to computed tomography scans in childhood or adolescence: Data linkage study of 11 million Australians. *BMJ Br. Med. J.* **2013**, *346*, f2360. [CrossRef]

12. Applegate, K.E.; Cost, N.G. Image Gently: A campaign to reduce children's and adolescents' risk for cancer during adulthood. *J. Adolesc. Heal.* **2013**, *52* (Suppl. S5), S93–S97. [CrossRef]

13. Ghelani, S.J.; Glatz, A.C.; David, S.; Leahy, R.; Hirsch, R.; Armsby, L.B.; Trucco, S.M.; Holzer, R.J.; Bergersen, L. Radiation Dose Benchmarks During Cardiac Catheterization for Congenital Heart Disease in the United States. *JACC Cardiovasc. Interv.* **2014**, *7*, 1060–1069. [CrossRef] [PubMed]

14. Haas, N.A.; Happel, C.M.; Mauti, M.; Sahyoun, C.; Tebart, L.Z.; Kececioglu, D.; Laser, K.T. Substantial radiation reduction in pediatric and adult congenital heart disease interventions with a novel X-ray imaging technology. *IJC Hear. Vasc.* **2015**, *6*, 101–109. [CrossRef] [PubMed]

15. Partington, S.L.; Valente, A.M.; Bruyere, J.; Rosica, D.; Shafer, K.M.; Landzberg, M.J.; Taqueti, V.R.; Blankstein, R.; Skali, H.; Kwatra, N.; et al. Reducing radiation dose from myocardial perfusion imaging in subjects with complex congenital heart disease. *J. Nucl. Cardiol.* **2019**, *28*, 1395–1408. [CrossRef] [PubMed]

16. Patel, C.; Grossman, M.; Shabanova, V.; Asnes, J. Reducing Radiation Exposure in Cardiac Catheterizations for Congenital Heart Disease. *Pediatr. Cardiol.* **2019**, *40*, 638–649. [CrossRef]

17. Rehani, M.M.; Hauptmann, M. Estimates of the number of patients with high cumulative doses through recurrent CT exams in 35 OECD countries. *Phys. Med.* **2020**, *76*, 173–176. [CrossRef]

18. Brambilla, M.; De Mauri, A.; Lizio, D.; Leva, L.; Carriero, A.; Carpeggiani, C.; Picano, E. Cumulative radiation dose estimates from medical imaging in paediatric patients with non-oncologic chronic illnesses. A systematic review. *Phys. Med.* **2014**, *30*, 403–412. [CrossRef]

19. Page, M.J.; McKenzie, J.E.; Bossuyt, P.M.; Boutron, I.; Hoffmann, T.C.; Mulrow, C.D.; Shamseer, L.; Tetzlaff, J.M.; Akl, E.A.; Brennan, S.E.; et al. The PRISMA 2020 statement: An updated guideline for reporting systematic reviews. *BMJ* **2021**, *88*, 372.

20. STROBE. Strengthening the Reporting of Observational Studies in Epidemiology. 2007. Available online: https://www.strobe-statement.org/index.php?id=available-checklists (accessed on 1 February 2023).

21. Clarity Group at McMaster University. Tool to Assess Risk of Bias in Cohort Studies. 2011. Available online: https://methods.cochrane.org/bias/sites/methods.cochrane.org.bias/files/public/uploads/TooltoAssessRiskofBiasinCohortStudies.pdf (accessed on 1 February 2023).

22. Ait-Ali, L.; Andreassi, M.G.; Foffa, I.; Spadoni, I.; Vano, E.; Picano, E. Cumulative patient effective dose and acute radiation-induced chromosomal DNA damage in children with congenital heart disease. *Heart* **2010**, *96*, 269–274. [CrossRef]

23. Jones, T.P.; Brennan, P.C.; Ryan, E. Cumulative Effective and Individual Organ Dose Levels in Paediatric Patients Undergoing Multiple Catheterisations for Congenital Heart Disease. *Radiat. Prot. Dosim.* **2017**, *176*, 252–257. [CrossRef]

24. Ubeda, C.; Vano, E.; Miranda, P.; Figueroa, X. Organ and effective doses detriment to paediatric patients undergoing multiple interventional cardiology procedures. *Phys. Med.* **2019**, *60*, 182–187. [CrossRef]

25. McDonnell, A.; Downing, T.E.; Zhu, X.; Ryan, R.; Rossano, J.W.; Glatz, A.C. Cumulative exposure to medical sources of ionising radiation in the first year after pediatric heart transplantation. *J. Hear. Lung Transpl.* **2014**, *33*, 1126–1132. [CrossRef] [PubMed]

26. Glatz, A.C.; Purrington, K.S.; Klinger, A.; King, A.R.; Hellinger, J.; Zhu, X.; Gruber, S.B.; Gruber, P.J. Cumulative exposure to medical radiation for children requiring surgery for congenital heart disease. *J. Pediatr.* **2014**, *164*, 789–794.e10. [CrossRef] [PubMed]

27. Downing, T.E.; McDonnell, A.; Zhu, X.; Dori, Y.; Gillespie, M.J.; Rome, J.J.; Glatz, A.C. Cumulative medical radiation exposure throughout staged palliation of single ventricle congenital heart disease. *Pediatr. Cardiol.* **2015**, *36*, 190–195. [CrossRef] [PubMed]

28. Johnson, J.N.; Hornik, C.P.; Li, J.S.; Benjamin, D.K., Jr.; Yoshizumi, T.T.; Reiman, R.E.; Frush, D.P.; Hill, K.D. Cumulative radiation exposure and cancer risk estimation in children with heart disease. *Circulation* **2014**, *130*, 161–167. [CrossRef] [PubMed]

29. Kim, P.K.; Gracias, V.H.; Maidment, A.D.; O'Shea, M.; Reilly, P.M.; Schwab, C.W. Cumulative radiation dose caused by radiologic studies in critically ill trauma patients. *J. Trauma* **2004**, *57*, 510–514. [CrossRef]

30. Moodie, D. Adult congenital heart disease: Past, present, and future. *Tex. Hear. Inst. J.* **2011**, *38*, 705–706.

31. Quinn, B.P. Longitudinal Improvements in Radiation Exposure in Cardiac Catheterisation for Congenital Heart Disease: A Prospective Multicenter C3P0-QI Study. *Circ. Cardiovasc. Interv.* **2020**, *13*, e008172. [CrossRef]
32. Puranik, R.; Muthurangu, V.; Celermajer, D.S.; Taylor, A.M. Congenital heart disease and multi-modality imaging. *Heart Lung Circ.* **2010**, *19*, 133–144. [CrossRef]
33. Rigsby, C.K.; McKenney, S.E.; Hill, K.D.; Chelliah, A.; Einstein, A.J.; Han, B.K.; Robinson, J.D.; Sammet, C.L.; Slesnick, T.C.; Frush, D.P. Radiation dose management for pediatric cardiac computed tomography: A report from the Image Gently "Have-A-Heart" campaign. *Pediatr. Radiol.* **2018**, *48*, 5–20. [CrossRef]
34. Radiological Protection Act 1991 [Ionising Radiation] Regulations S.I No.30. 2019. Available online: http://www.irishstatutebook.ie/eli/2019/si/30/made/en/pdf (accessed on 1 February 2023).
35. Royal College of Radiologists. iRefer Guidelines. Available online: https://www.irefer.org.uk/guidelines (accessed on 1 February 2023).
36. Gabelloni, M.; Di Nasso, M.; Morganti, R.; Faggioni, L.; Masi, G.; Falcone, A.; Neri, E. Application of the ESR iGuide clinical decision support system to the imaging pathway of patients with hepatocellular carcinoma and cholangiocarcinoma: Preliminary findings. *Radiol. Med.* **2020**, *125*, 531–537. [CrossRef]
37. European Diagnostic Reference Levels for Paediatric Imaging. Eurosafe Imaging. Available online: http://www.eurosafeimaging.org/wp/wp-content/uploads/2018/09/rp_185.pdf (accessed on 1 February 2023).
38. El Sayed, M.H.; Roushdy, A.M.; El Farghaly, H.; El Sherbini, A. Radiation exposure in children during the current era of pediatric cardiac intervention. *Pediatr. Cardiol.* **2012**, *33*, 27–35. [CrossRef] [PubMed]
39. Glatz, A.C.; Patel, A.; Zhu, X.; Dori, Y.; Hanna, B.D.; Gillespie, M.J.; Rome, J.J. Patient Radiation Exposure in a Modern, Large-Volume, Pediatric Cardiac Catheterization Laboratory. *Pediatr. Cardiol.* **2014**, *35*, 870–878. [CrossRef] [PubMed]
40. Kawasaki, T.; Fujii, K.; Akahane, K. Estimation of Organ and Effective Doses for Neonate and Infant Diagnostic Cardiac Catheterizations. *Am. J. Roentgenol.* **2015**, *205*, 599–603. [CrossRef]
41. Verghese, G.R.; McElhinney, D.B.; Strauss, K.J.; Bergersen, L. Characterization of radiation exposure and effect of a radiation monitoring policy in a large volume pediatric cardiac catheterization lab. *Catheter. Cardiovasc. Interv.* **2012**, *79*, 294–301. [CrossRef] [PubMed]
42. Keiller, D.A.; Martin, C.J. Radiation dose to the heart in paediatric interventional cardiology. *J. Radiol. Prot.* **2015**, *35*, 257–264. [CrossRef]
43. Manica, J.L.; Duarte, V.O.; Ribeiro, M.; Hartley, A.; Petraco, R.; Pedra, C.; Rossi, R. Standardizing Radiation Exposure during Cardiac Catheterization in Children with Congenital Heart Disease: Data from a Multicenter Brazilian Registry. *Arq. Bras. Cardiol.* **2020**, *115*, 1154–1161. [PubMed]
44. Kottou, S.; Kollaros, N.; Plemmenos, C.; Mastorakou, I.; Apostolopoulou, S.C.; Tsapaki, V. Towards the definition of Institutional diagnostic reference levels in paediatric interventional cardiology procedures in Greece. *Phys. Med.* **2018**, *46*, 52–58. [CrossRef] [PubMed]
45. Harbron, R.; Pearce, M.S.; Salotti, J.A.; McHugh, K.; McLaren, C.; Abernethy, L.; Reed, S.; O'Sullivan, J.; Chapple, C.-L. Radiation doses from fluoroscopically guided cardiac catheterization procedures in children and young adults in the United Kingdom: A multicentre study. *Br. J. Radiol.* **2015**, *88*, 20140852. [CrossRef]
46. Martinez, L.C.; Vano, E.; Gutierrez, F.; Rodriguez, C.; Gilarranz, R.; Manzanas, M.J. Patient doses from fluoroscopically guided cardiac procedures in pediatrics. *Phys. Med. Biol.* **2007**, *52*, 474. [CrossRef]
47. Paul, J.-F.; Rohnean, A.; Elfassy, E.; Sigal-Cinqualbre, A. Radiation dose for thoracic and coronary step-and-shoot CT using a 128-slice dual-source machine in infants and small children with congenital heart disease. *Pediatr. Radiol.* **2011**, *41*, 244–249. [CrossRef]
48. Walsh, M.A.; Noga, M.; Rutledge, J. Cumulative radiation exposure in pediatric patients with congenital heart disease. *Pediatr. Cardiol.* **2015**, *36*, 289–294. [CrossRef] [PubMed]
49. Watson, T.G.; Mah, E.; Schoepf, U.J.; King, L.; Huda, W.; Hlavacek, A.M. Effective Radiation Dose in Computed Tomographic Angiography of the Chest and Diagnostic Cardiac Catheterization in Pediatric Patients. *Pediatr. Cardiol.* **2013**, *34*, 518–524. [CrossRef] [PubMed]
50. Yakoumakis, E.; Kostopoulou, H.; Makri, T.; Dimitriadis, A.; Georgiou, E.; Tsalafoutas, I. Estimation of radiation dose and risk to children undergoing cardiac catheterization for the treatment of a congenital heart disease using Monte Carlo simulations. *Pediatr. Radiol.* **2013**, *43*, 339. [CrossRef] [PubMed]
51. Kobayashi, D.; Meadows, J.; Forbes, T.J.; Moore, P.; Javois, A.J.; Pedra, C.A.; Du, W.; Gruenstein, D.H.; Wax, D.F.; Hill, J.A.; et al. Standardizing radiation dose reporting in the pediatric cardiac catheterization laboratory—A multicenter study by the CCISC [Congenital Cardiovascular Interventional Study Consortium]. *Catheter. Cardiovasc. Interv.* **2014**, *84*, 785–793. [CrossRef]

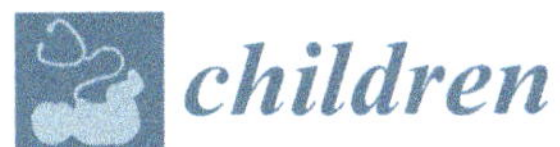

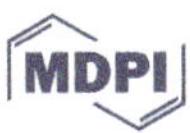

Review

Patient-Specific 3D-Printed Models in Pediatric Congenital Heart Disease

Zhonghua Sun [1,2]

1   Discipline of Medical Radiation Science, Curtin Medical School, Curtin University, Perth, WA 6845, Australia; z.sun@curtin.edu.au; Tel.: +61-8-92667509
2   Curtin Health Innovation Research Institute (CHIRI), Curtin University, Perth, WA 6845, Australia

Abstract: Three-dimensional (3D) printing technology has become increasingly used in the medical field, with reports demonstrating its superior advantages in both educational and clinical value when compared with standard image visualizations or current diagnostic approaches. Patient-specific or personalized 3D printed models serve as a valuable tool in cardiovascular disease because of the difficulty associated with comprehending cardiovascular anatomy and pathology on 2D flat screens. Additionally, the added value of using 3D-printed models is especially apparent in congenital heart disease (CHD), due to its wide spectrum of anomalies and its complexity. This review provides an overview of 3D-printed models in pediatric CHD, with a focus on educational value for medical students or graduates, clinical applications such as pre-operative planning and simulation of congenital heart surgical procedures, and communication between physicians and patients/parents of patients and between colleagues in the diagnosis and treatment of CHD. Limitations and perspectives on future research directions for the application of 3D printing technology into pediatric cardiology practice are highlighted.

Keywords: three-dimensional printing; congenital heart disease; children; model; personalized medicine; application

Citation: Sun, Z. Patient-Specific 3D-Printed Models in Pediatric Congenital Heart Disease. *Children* **2023**, *10*, 319. https://doi.org/10.3390/children10020319

Academic Editor: Bibhuti B. Das

Received: 27 December 2022
Revised: 25 January 2023
Accepted: 6 February 2023
Published: 7 February 2023

1. Introduction

Three-dimensional (3D) printing technology is being increasingly used in the medical field, with studies documenting its application in a range of areas, from its original application in maxillofacial and orthopedic surgery to cardiovascular disease [1–12]. Extensive research has proved the usefulness and established the clinical value of 3D-printed models in maxillofacial surgery and orthopedics. Meanwhile, the investigation of 3D-printed models for use in cardiovascular disease is an emerging but rapidly growing area with research that has confirmed its great potential in this domain. High-quality 3D-printed models derived from cardiac images such as computed tomography (CT), magnetic resonance imaging (MRI) and echocardiography are highly accurate in replicating normal cardiac anatomy and pathology, thus serving as a valuable and complementary tool to current image visualizations in the diagnostic assessment of cardiovascular disease [13–35].

Of various cardiovascular abnormalities, congenital heart disease (CHD) represents a very challenging area due to the complexity of the congenital anomalies, the broad spectrum of conditions and the high variability between individuals. In the pediatric sub-specialization, a basic understanding of common CHD is necessary and plays an important role in clinical decision making and patient management. However, the standard visualization techniques, including cardiac CT, MRI and echocardiography, are limited in their ability to convert 2D images into a 3D object on a flat screen and so do not allow full comprehension of complex intracardiac anatomy and defects [19,36]. To overcome these limitations, 3D-printed physical models demonstrate superior advantages and strengths over the current image visualizations by providing realistic 3D representations of the spatial relationships between these cardiac structures and abnormal changes that are difficult to acquire on traditional 2D and 3D image reconstructions. In addition to its enhancement in understanding complex anatomy, 3D-printed heart models serve as a valuable tool to guide surgical planning, to train junior or inexperienced pediatric residents, and to educate healthcare professionals or parents of patients [13–26,28–35]. This review aims to provide a summary of the current applications of 3D-printed models in pediatric CHD, and highlights limitations and future research directions about 3D printing in pediatric cardiology practice. The reason we focus on pediatric CHD is due to the increased use of 3D printing technology in CHD, in particular in the field of pediatric CHD where the rarity of pathology and the smaller size of the patients present challenges for clinicians in the diagnosis and management of CHD conditions. Three-dimensional-printed heart models with the unique advantage of an improved demonstration of complex cardiac defects at high fidelity could overcome these challenges. It is expected that this comprehensive review of the current literature on 3D printing in pediatric CHD will provide readers with a useful resource about the clinical value and applications of 3D-printed models in pediatric CHD.

2. Generation of 3D-Printed Heart Models

The steps from processing the original 2D digital imaging and communications in medicine (DICOM) images to 3D volume data, and from there to the segmentation of the image is well explained in the literature, and usually involves semi-automatic along with manual editing processes. Figure 1 shows a flow chart representing the creation of a 3D-printed heart model from an example of cardiac CT images. In general, to ensure the quality of the 3D-printed model, high resolution imaging data comprises an essential component in the production of an accurate 3D-printed model. Cardiac CT is the most commonly used modality in 3D printing due to its high spatial resolution, although cardiac MRI and echocardiography are also used in some studies when printing CHD models [37].

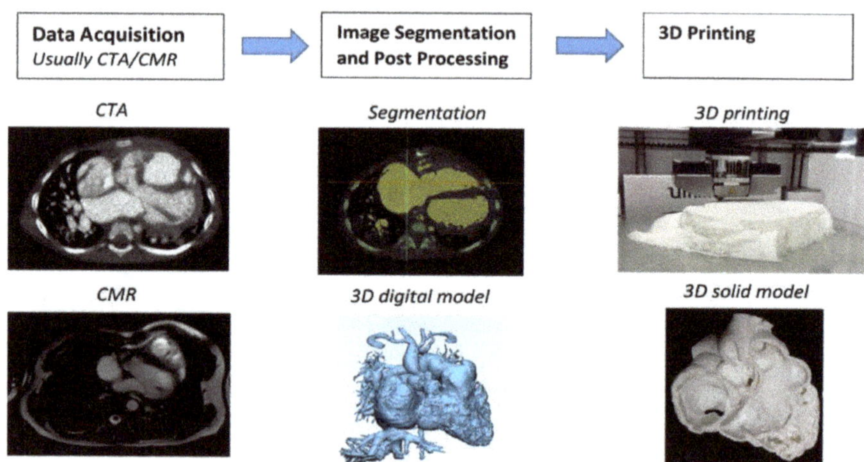

Figure 1. Steps to generate 3D printed heart models. CTA-computed tomography angiography, CMR-cardiac magnetic resonance. Reprinted with permission under the open access from Sun et al. [7].

Mimics is the most commonly used commercial software tool in image post-processing of 3D datasets for 3D printing, while 3D Slicer is an open-source tool commonly used for segmentation of volumetric data for 3D printing. Usually, hollow heart models are generated to show both outside and inside views of cardiac anatomy and pathology as shown in Figure 2, while blood pool models can also be printed to accurately demonstrate the spatial relationships between cardiac structures [38] as shown in Figure 3.

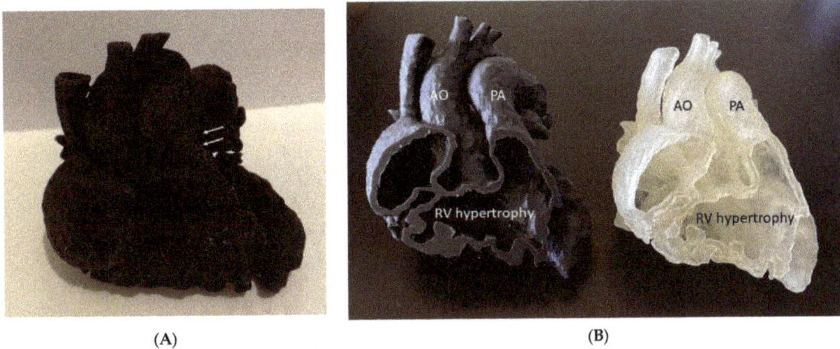

Figure 2. Three-dimensional-printed heart model of a case with Tetralogy of Fallot (ToF). (**A**): The model was printed in one piece. (**B**): The model was printed in two halves (with the same material, Agilus30, but different colors) showing the internal cardiac chambers and vascular abnormalities. Arrows indicate the pulmonary artery stenosis. AO—aorta (overriding aorta); PA—pulmonary artery; RV—right ventricle.

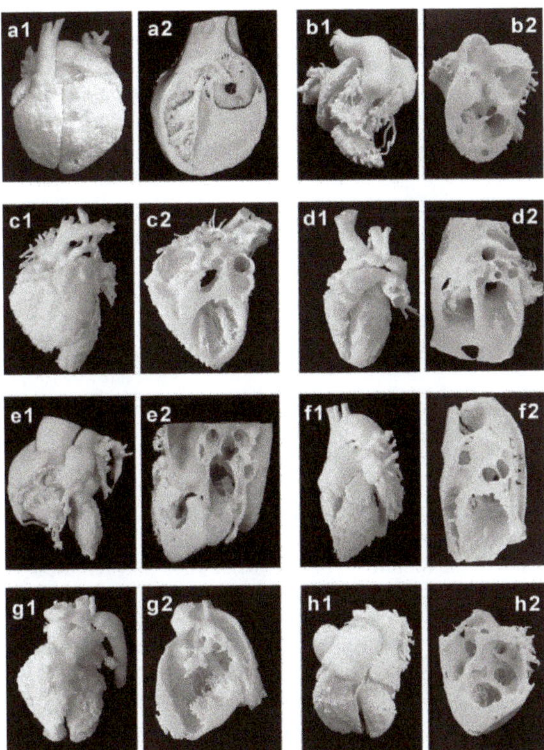

Figure 3. Three-dimensional printing of the blood pool and myocardium (showing inside views of cardiac structures at different angles) models for eight typical CHD cases (**a–h**). (**a1–h1**) are blood pool models, while (**a2–h2**) are myocardium models showing internal cardiac structures. Case 1: congenital corrected transposition of the great arteries. Case 2: double outlet right ventricle. Case 3: Williams syndrome. Case 4: coronary artery fistula. Case 5: Tetralogy of Fallot. Case 6: patent ductus arteriosus. Case 7: coarctation of the aorta. Case 8: ventricular septal defect. Reprinted with permission under the open access from Liang et al. [38].

3. Accuracy of 3D-Printed Heart Models Derived from Imaging Modalities

Three-dimensional-printed models must accurately replicate anatomical details with high accuracy so that the models can be reliably used for different purposes. Current research has shown a very small difference between 3D-printed models and original source imaging data, whether they are acquired with CT, echocardiography, MRI or rotational angiography. Table 1 summarizes the findings of dimensional measurements between a 3D-printed model and the original source images based on the current literature [39–45]. It is noted that the mean difference in dimensional measurements between 3D-printed models and original images is less than 0.5 mm indicating the high accuracy of the 3D models, with excellent correlations between different observers and measurement approaches.

Table 1. Accuracy of 3D-printed heart model in comparison with original source images according to the current literature. Modified from Lee et al. [39].

Studies	No. of 3D-Printed Models	Comparisons	Mean Difference (mm)	Analysis Method
Lee et al. [39]	3	3D model vs. original CT 3D model vs. CT of 3D model 3D model vs. STL files Original CT images vs. STL files	0.21 ± 0.37 mm −0.11 ± 0.47 mm 0.1 ± 0.28/ 0.17 ± 0.48 mm 0.12 ± 0.23/ 0.12 ± 0.25 mm	Pearson's correlation/ Bland–Altman plot
Valverde et al. [40]	40 (20 selected for accuracy comparison)	3D model vs. both CT and MRI 3D model vs. original CT 3D model vs. original MRI	0.27 ± 0.73 mm −0.16 ± 0.85 mm −0.30 ± 0.67 mm	Bland–Altman plot
Olejník et al. [41]	8	CT images vs. STL 3D model vs. in vivo	0.19 ± 0.38 mm 0.13 ± 0.26 mm	Bland–Altman plot
Olivieri et al. [42]	9	3D model vs. echo	0.4 ± 0.9 mm	Pearson's correlation/ Bland–Altman plot
Lau et al. [43]	1	3D model vs. CT	0.23 mm	Pearson's correlation
Mowers et al. [44]	5	2D echo vs. digital 3D 2D echo vs. 3D model	0 mm 0.3 mm	Pearson's correlation/ Bland–Altman plot
Parimi et al. [45]	5	3D model vs. rotational angiography	No significant difference between 3D models and biplane angiography measurements ($p = 0.14$)	Pearson's correlation/ Bland–Altman plot

DICOM—digital imaging and communications in medicine, CT—computed tomography, MRI—magnetic resonance imaging, STL—standard tessellation language.

4. Three-Dimensional-Printing Materials for Printing Patient-Specific Models

While commonly used 3D printers including fused deposition modelling (FDM), stereolithography (SLA), polyjet and selective laser sintering (SLS) are the most well known printers in the literature. Printing materials play an important role in determining the final printed models that are most appropriate to serve the purpose of different applications. The models can be printed with rigid materials (such as polylactic acid, rigid resin and rigid photopolymer (VeroClear)) as shown in many early studies [37], however, for printing heart or vascular models, soft and elastic materials with tissue properties similar to normal heart or vascular tissues are more important for the production of realistic heart models. Elastic materials include thermoplastic polyurethane (TPU), Tango materials such as TangoPlus, TangoGray, and Agilus A30 and Visiject CE-NT, and show great promise in printing CHD models. This is especially important when using 3D-printed models to simulate cardiac surgery or interventional cardiac procedures, as operators need to acquire similar tactile experience when performing simulation procedures on realistic 3D printed models [37]. Figure 4 is an example of a 3D-printed aorta model using Visijet CE-NT A30 material, a material which is soft and elastic and has the same tissue properties as cardiovascular tissues [46].

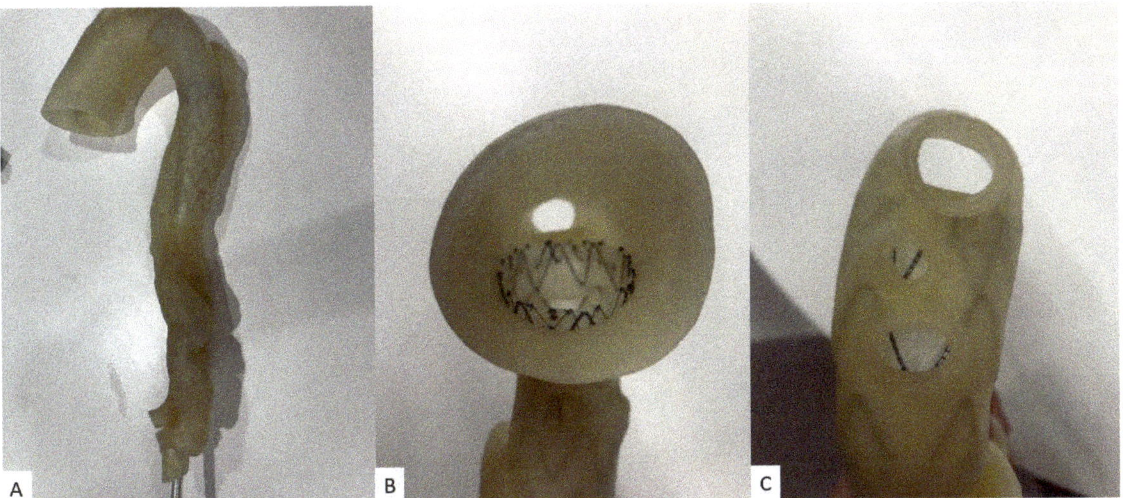

Figure 4. Three-dimensional-printed type B aortic dissection model for simulation of endovascular aortic repair of type B aortic dissection. The printing material was Visijet CE-NT A30. An aortic stent graft was placed into the true lumen of the 3D-printed model (**A**) with axial (**B**) and caudal views (**C**) showing the proximal aortic arch and vessels. Reprinted with permission under the open access from Wu et al. [46].

The cost of the printing materials is a key factor that could hinder the widespread use of 3D printing in clinical practice. It has been reported that the use of low-cost printed models is feasible and accurate for the determination of CHD cases [19,47,48]. A recent study has further confirmed the accuracy and clinical value of using low-cost 3D printed CHD models [49]. Lau et al. selected a CHD case of double outlet right ventricle (DORV) with models printed using low-cost TPU 95A (AUD $50) and high-cost TangoPlus (AUD $300), respectively. Both materials are flexible, although the TPU material is not as flexible as TangoPlus. Contrast-enhanced CT scans were performed on these 3D-printed models and measurements were conducted at 10 different anatomical locations to compare the model's accuracy to that of the original CT images (Figure 5). Their results show a strong correlation between measurements from both 3D-printed models and original CT images. Further, these two models were ranked with the same scores by clinicians, wherein both the authors of the study and then the clinicians perceiving the same clinical value or efficacy. Gomez-Ciritza et al. reported the same findings based on their seven-year experience of using low-cost 3D-printed heart models [21]. The authors produced 138 models based on cardiac CT or MRI images in patients with CHD with the mean cost of each model being 85 euro. These 3D-printed heart models were used in different applications from surgical planning of CHD and interventional procedures to education and communication with patients, colleagues and relatives.

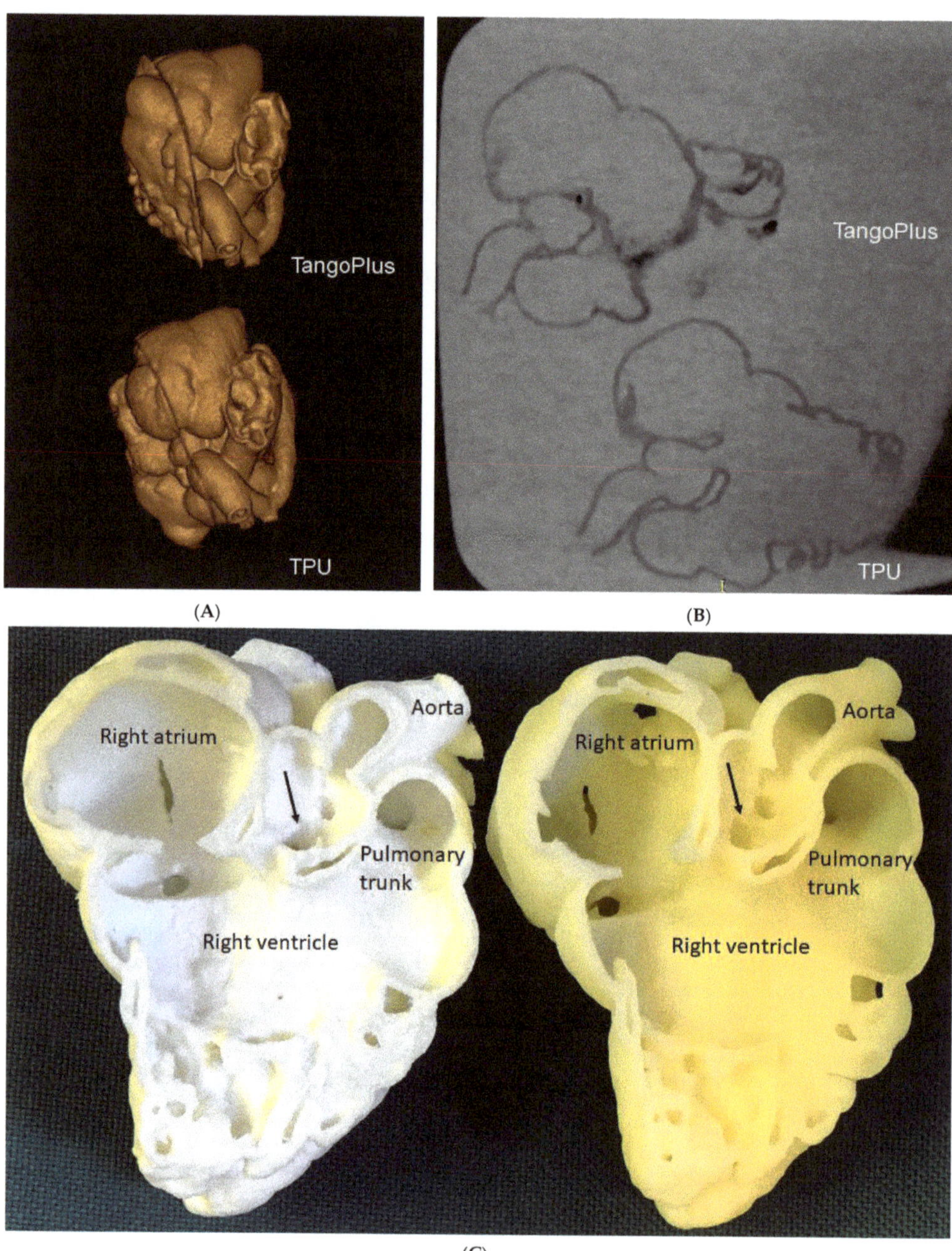

Figure 5. Three-dimensional-printed CHD models with the use of different materials for comparison of model accuracy. (**A**): Three-dimensional CT volume rendering of the 3D-printed models showing similar anatomical details. (**B**): Two-dimensional axial CT views of the 3D printed models. (**C**): Inside view of cardiac chambers and aortic structures on both models. The white model is printed with TPU, while the yellow model is printed with TangoPlus. Arrows refer to the subaortic ventricular septal defect.

The specific purpose of the 3D-printed CHD models determines the selection of appropriate printing materials. For example, if 3D-printed models are used for the educational purpose of learning cardiac anatomy and pathology, rigid or relatively soft and low-cost materials are acceptable. If the 3D-printed models are primarily used for pre-surgical planning or simulation of complex cardiac procedures, soft and elastic materials (or high-cost materials) with tissue properties similar to normal cardiovascular tissues are necessary to allow users to gain learning experience on the 3D models prior to operating on patients.

5. Educational and Clinical Value of 3D-Printed Heart Models in CHD

Three-dimensional-printed models are useful in medical and clinical education as the 3D-printed personalized models demonstrate superior advantages over current image visualization tools for the enhancement of students and medical graduates' understanding of the complex 3D cardiac anatomy and pathology. Of the current applications of 3D printing in cardiovascular disease, 3D-printed CHD models represent the most common application in medical education according to the current literature [37,50–53]. Studies have provided strong evidence in support of the use of 3D-printed models in CHD education, both for medical students, medical graduates (pediatric residents) and healthcare professionals.

Table 2 summarizes representative studies reporting the educational and clinical value of 3D-printed models in pediatric CHD. These studies have shown that 3D-printed heart models significantly enhance medical students, pediatric residents, clinicians and pediatric cardiac nurses' knowledge in learning normal cardiac anatomy and CHD (Figure 6) [25,26,28–31,33–35,38,54,55]. Three-dimensional-printed CHD models were rated highly in terms of their accuracy and satisfaction scores by the study or experimental groups when compared with the control groups, and this is particularly obvious when assessing the complex CHD in comparison with simple CHD [34]. In their recent report, Lau and Sun did not show significant improvements in knowledge retention among second and third year medical students when 3D-printed CHD models were compared with the current teaching methods using DICOM images and digital 3D heart models, although slightly higher scores were achieved in the 3D printing group (Figure 7) [25].

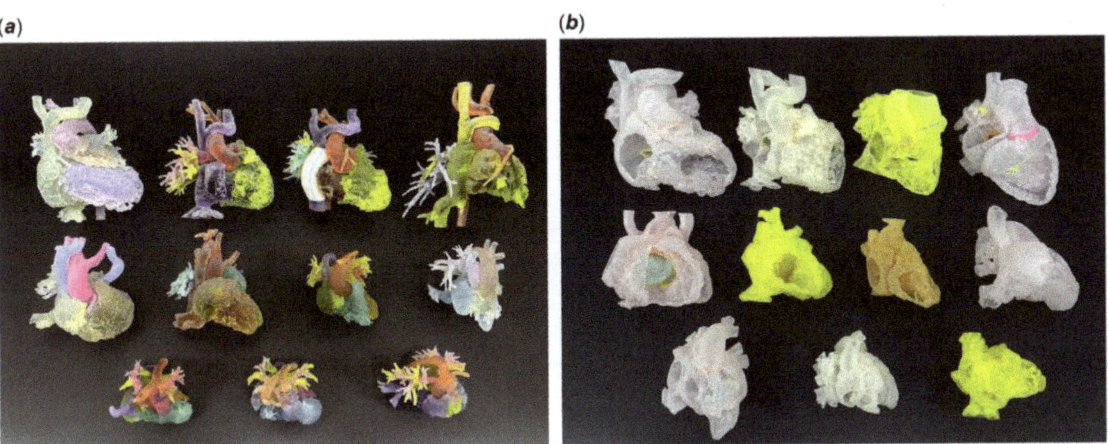

Figure 6. Three-dimensional-printed models of different kinds of complex CHD. (**a**) Blood pool models, (**b**) hollow models. Reprinted with permission from Lee C and Lee J [55].

Table 2. Application of 3D-printed models in medical and clinical education. Modified from Sun and Wee [37].

Author	Study Design	Sample Size and Participants	Original Data Source	Application in CHD	Key Findings
Lau & Sun [25]	Cohort study	53 medical students	CT	ASD, VSD, ToF and DORV.	Slightly higher scores were achieved in the 3D-printed model group than those in the control group (7.79 $\pm$ 2.63 vs. 7.04 $\pm$ 2.64, $p > 0.05$), while 3D-printed models did not improve knowledge acquisition.
Karsenty et al. [26]	RCT	347 medical students	CT	CHD including ASD, VSD, CoA and ToF.	Use of 3D printing improved objective knowledge when compared to the control group ($p < 0.0001$).
Smerling et al. [28]	Cross-sectional study	45 medical students	CT	Three-dimensional-printed heart models including pulmonic stenosis (PS), ASD, ToF, d-TGA, CoA and HLHS.	Three-dimensional-printed models significantly enhanced students' knowledge for all of these cardiac pathologies ($p < 0.001$).
Su et al. [29]	RCT	63 medical students	CT	Three-dimensional-printed VSD models: perimembranous, subarterial and muscular VSD.	Three-dimensional-printed models significantly improved VSD learning when compared to the control group ($p < 0.05$).
Lau et al. [30]	Cross-sectional study	29 participants (radiologists, sonographers and radiographers)	CT	ASD, VSD, ToF and DORV.	Both 3D-printed models and VR were useful in education and pre-operative planning when compared to conventional visualisations.
Jones & Seckeler [31]	RCT	36 pediatric medical students	CT & MRI	Three-dimensional-printed models of vascular rings and pulmonary artery slings.	Three-dimensional-printed models significantly enhanced participants' knowledge in learning anatomy and pathology ($p < 0.01$).
Loke et al. [19]	RCT	35 pediatric residents	CT, MRI and 3D echocardiography	Three-dimensional-printed models: A normal infant heart, an adult repaired ToF and an infant unrepaired ToF.	Higher satisfaction scores were achieved with 3D-printed models ($p = 0.03$).
Valverde et al. [33]	Non-RCT	127 participants	Echocardiography and CMR.	Value of 3D-printed models on medical education in criss-cross hearts.	Three-dimensional-printed models significantly increased knowledge in learning criss-cross heart anatomy ($p < 0.001$).
White et al. [34]	RCT	60 pediatric and emergency medicine residents	NA	Three-dimensional-printed models of four cases including VSD and ToF.	The 3D printing group scored significantly higher than the control group ($p = 0.037$) on ToF postlecture test, while the control group scored higher on the VSD postlecture test ($p = 0.012$).
Tan et al. [35]	RCT	132 nursing students	NA	Three-dimensional-printed model of a ASD case in teaching clinical nursing in congenital heart surgery.	Use of Three-dimensional-printed models significantly improved clinical nurses in learning congenital heart surgery.
Biglino et al. [54]	Cross-sectional study	100 cardiac nurses	NA	Nine 3D-printed models: a heathy heart, and other types of CHD.	Three-dimensional-printed models serve as useful tools in training adult and pediatric cardiac nurses for learning and understanding CHD.

Table 2. *Cont.*

Author	Study Design	Sample Size and Participants	Original Data Source	Application in CHD	Key Findings
Liang et al. [38]	Cross-sectional study	Expert group (n = 40 with 20 cardiac surgeons and 20 sonographers) and student group (40 postgraduate medical students)	CT	Eight types of CHD: PDA, CoA, VSD ccTGA, DORV, WA, CAF and ToF.	3D-printed models significantly improved the CHD diagnosis in both the expert and student groups ($p = 0.000–0.001$). Three-dimensional printing was found to be more important in the diagnosis of more complex CHD than simple CHD ($p = 0.000$).
Lee C and Lee J [55]	Cross-sectional study	74 participants including 41 residents, 14 physicians, 10 nurses and 9 perfusionists.	CT	Eleven complex CHD cases included ToF, AVSD, DORV, single ventricle with DILV/BCPA.	Subjective improvements were found in all learning categories post-seminar scores when compared with pre-seminar scores: understanding anatomy (8.4 ± 1.1 vs. 4.8 ± 2.1), 3D structure (8.9 ± 1.0 vs. 4.6 ± 2.2), pathophysiology (8.5 ± 1.0 vs. 4.8 ± 2.2), and surgery (8.8 ± 0.9 vs. 4.9 ± 2.3), with all $p < 0.001$ respectively.

ASD—atrial septal defect; AVSD—atrioventricular septal defect; BCPA—bidirectional cavopulmonary anastomosis; CAF—coronary artery fistula; CHD—congenital heart disease; CoA—coarctation of aorta; CT—computed tomography; CMR—cardiac magnetic resonance; ccTGA—corrected transposition of the great arteries; DILV—double inlet left ventricle; d-TGA—d-transposition of the great arteries; DORV—double outlet right ventricle; HLHS—hypoplastic left heart syndrome; MRI—magnetic resonance imaging; NA—not available; PDA—patent ductus arteriosus; RCT—randomized controlled trial; ToF—Tetralogy of Fallot; VR—virtual reality; VSD—ventricular septal defect; WS—William syndrome.

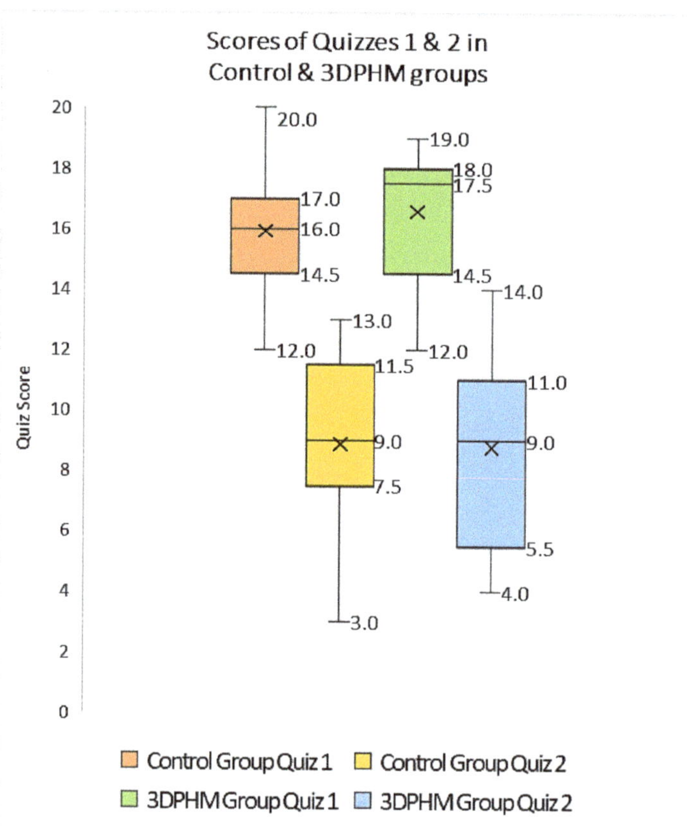

Figure 7. Boxplot showing the scores (out of 20) of quizzes one and two in 3D printing and control groups for 3DPHM-3D printed heart model. Reprinted with permission under the open access from Lau and Sun [25].

Another innovative tool in CHD education is the use of either virtual reality (VR), augmented reality (AR) or mixed reality (MR) as an alternative to 3D-printed models in education and pre-surgical planning of CHD. A user is immersed in a virtual environment during VR visualization, while AR is different from VR with virtual objects overlaying on the real world. MR extends the ability of VR and AR by allowing the user to interact with combined virtual and real objects (such as 3D-printed physical models) [56–60]. Figure 8 shows the workflow of these visualization technologies including 3D printing, VR and AR.

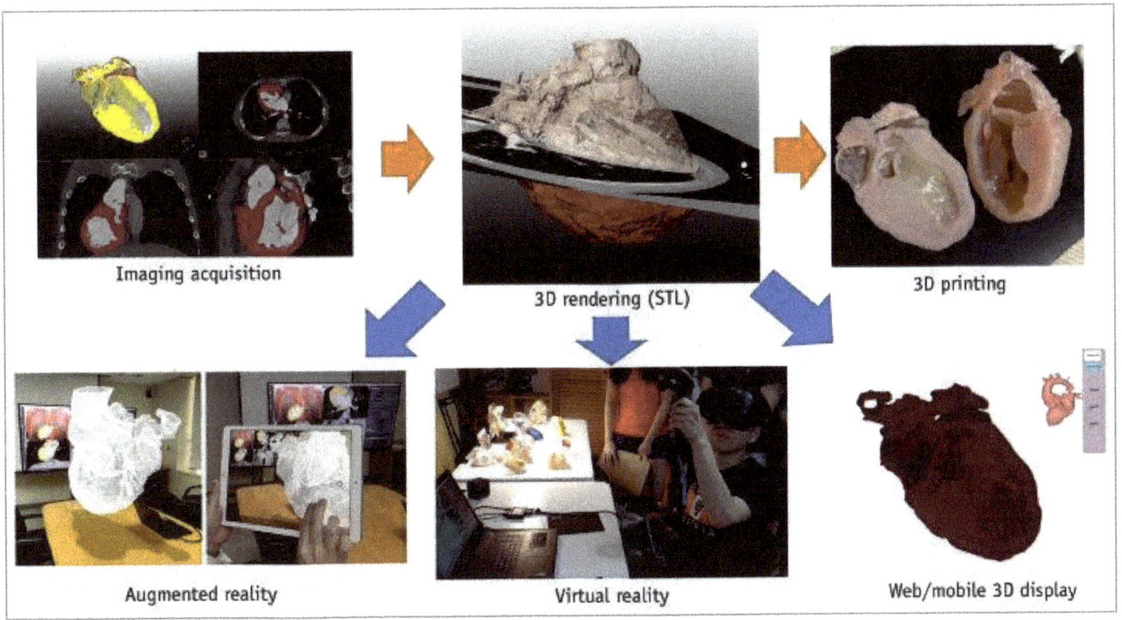

Figure 8. Workflow of advanced visualization technology. Segmented 3D volume data can be used for 3D printing, virtual reality, augmented reality and interactive or mobile 3D displays. Reprinted with permission under the open access from Goo et al. [60].

VR, AR and MR can be used for education, planning and simulation of CHD surgical procedures. In their recent review, Barteit et al. analyzed 27 studies with applications of AR and MR mainly in surgery planning (48%) and anatomy learning (15%) [61]. Lau et al. also reported the similar value of VR as opposed to 3D printing for CHD medical education through the assessment of four selected CHD cases by 29 participants [30]. VR was ranked as the most useful tool in these two areas when compared with 3D-printed models, though no significant differences were found between these two modalities. More than 70% of participants indicated that VR and 3D-printed models offered additional benefits over conventional image visualizations. In their randomized controlled trial (RCT), Patel et al., compared VR with desktop 2D views of CHD cases, with 24 and 27 participants allocated to each group, respectively [58]. Participants' impressions of CHD education with the aid of VR was 29% higher than the desktop group ($p = 0.01$). This study shows that VR may increase learner's engagement in understanding CHD.

Factors that could limit the use of 3D printing technology on a daily basis include image post-processing and segmentation time, as well as printing cost issues, hence, VR could be a potential alternative to 3D printing in medical education for CHD, and this has been confirmed by Raimondil and colleagues [62]. Investigators compared 3D printing, 3D PDF and VR in three cases of CHD and asked a senior pediatric cardiac surgeon to assess the performance of these three modalities in visualizing anatomical structures. The median post-processing time to generate VR models was only 5 min which is significantly shorter than the 8 h for 3D models (3D printing and 3D PDF) (Figure 9). Their study shows the feasibility of generating VR views directly from the raw imaging data without undergoing any preliminary segmentation process. This could be a promising technique for routine clinical application where 3D printing facilities are not available.

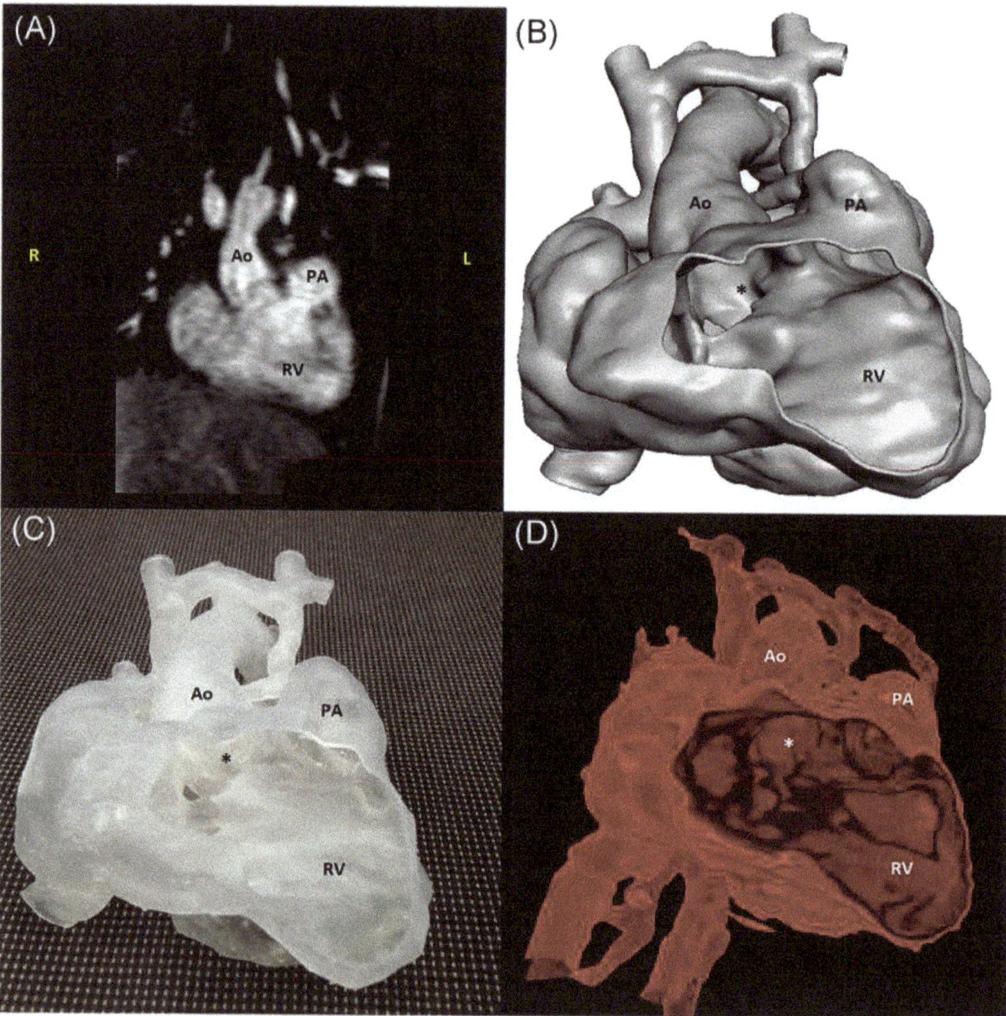

Figure 9. Images of a case with DORV with hyperplasia of the left ventricle and subaortic VSD: CMR scan (**A**), 3D PDF reconstruction (**B**), 3D-printed model (**C**), a screenshot of the DIVA software (**D**). * refers to ventricular septal defect. Ao—aorta; CMR—cardiac magnetic resonance; DORV—double outlet right ventricle; PA—pulmonary artery; RV—right ventricle; VSD—ventricular septal defect. DIVA refers to the user-friendly software for VR visualization. Reprinted with permission from Raimondil et al. [62].

6. 3D-Printed Models in CHD: Clinical Applications

Clinical value of 3D-printed models in CHD has been confirmed by a number of studies which are most commonly based on single center experiences or some case reports [21,23,39,63–83]. The clinical applications comprise three main areas, including pre-surgical planning of congenital heart surgery, simulation or training of congenital heart surgery procedures, and enhancing physician–patient or between colleagues' communication through use of personalized 3D-printed heart models.

6.1. Pre-Surgical Planning of CHD Surgery

Table 3 summarizes the current literature regarding the use of 3D-printed models in the surgical treatment of pediatric patients with CHD. These studies showed that the use of 3D-printed heart CHD models assisted pre-surgical planning, with up to 50% of surgical decisions changed by 3D-printed models according to a multi-center study [40]. Similarly, a number of studies reporting their single center experience with inclusion of either small or large number of cases also confirmed the usefulness of 3D-printed heart models in guiding surgical procedures in the management of pediatric CHD [21,23,63–67]. Two studies by Gomez-Ciriza and Ryan et al. presented their seven- and three-year experiences with more than 100 3D heart models printed in their clinical practices [21,65]. Gomez-Ciriza and colleagues reported similar findings to Valverde et al. [40], in which about 48% of surgical planning was modified with aid of 3D-printed heart models (Figure 10) [21]. In contrast, based on a three-year experience, Ryan et al. did not show significant differences between 3D-printed models (79 models of different CHD types) and standard of care in surgical planning of CHD [65].

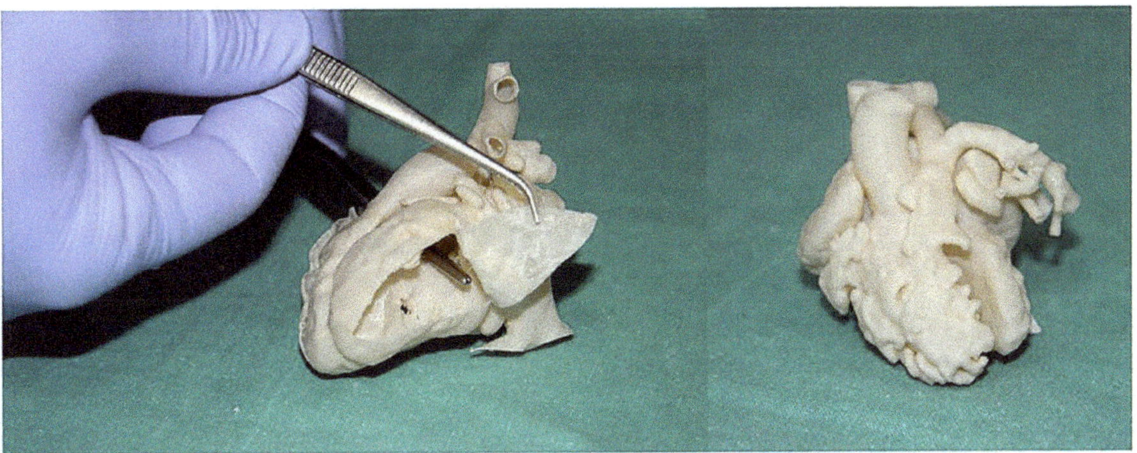

Figure 10. Surgical and interventional planning on 3D-printed heart models. DORV case, internal vision from the left ventricle (left). DORV (another case), external view (right). DORV-double outlet right ventricle. Reprinted with permission under the open access from Gomez-Ciriza et al. [21].

Table 3. Clinical value of 3D-printed CHD models in the surgical planning of CHD surgery. Modified from Sun and Wee [37].

Author	Study Design	Sample Size and Participants	Original Data Source	Application in CHD	Key Findings
Valverde et al. [40]	Prospective multicenter study	Forty patients with complex CHD.	CT and MRI	Three-dimensional-printed models of 19 DORV and 21 other types of CHD.	The surgical decision was changed in 47.5% cases with aid of 3D-printed models.
Chen et al. [63]	Cross-sectional study	Five patients with (PA with VSD or MAPCA	Echocardiography and CT	Three-dimensional-printed models and VR/MR in surgical outcomes.	Three-dimensional-printed models assisted surgeons to pre-operatively analyse surgery plans, while VR facilitated understanding of intracardiac structures.
Gomez-Ciriza et al. [21]	Cross-sectional study	Forty-three participants	CT and MRI	One hundred thirty-eight low-cost 3D-printed models were developed for surgical planning and interventional simulations.	Use of 3D-printed models has a positive impact on CHD surgery with initial surgical plan modified in 47.5% of the cases after reviewing the models.
Guo et al. [64]	Cross-sectional study	Surgeon, patients and nonmedical professionals	CT	Seven HOCM models were printed for surgical management and pre-operative conversation.	Three-dimensional-printed models were useful for surgical planning and pre-operative communication.
Kiraly et al. [23]	Cross-sectional study	Single center team learning experience of 3D-printed models in pediatric surgeries	CT	Fifteen models of pediatric patients with CHD and their impact on complex CHD surgeries.	Three-dimensional-printed models significantly contributed to improved surgical plans with intracardiac repair modified in 13 out of 15 cases.
Ryan et al. [65]	Cross-sectional study	Single center experience of 3D-printed models in CHD	CT and MRI	One hundred sixty-four models were printed for various purposes.	Three-dimensional-printed models contributed to a mean reduction in overall time when compared with standard of care, although the reductions did not reach significant differences.
Zhao et al. [66]	Cross-sectional study	Twenty-five patients with DORV	CT	Use of 3D-printed models in pre-operative repair of complex DORV.	Three-dimensional-printed models significantly reduced operating time and improved postoperative outcomes ($p < 0.05$).
Ghosh et al. [67]	Cross-sectional study	Single center three-year experience with 112 3D-printed CHD models for pre-operative planning.	MRI and CT	Use of 3D-printed models in pre-procedural planning of CHD.	Demand for the use of 3D-printed models in clinical practice has tripled over a three-year period. Incorporation of 3D printing technology into pre-procedural care of pediatric CHD surgeries is feasible.

ASD—atrial septal defect; CHD—congenital heart disease; CT—computed tomography; DORV—double outlet right ventricle; HOCM—hypertrophic obstructive cardiomyopathy; MRI—magnetic resonance imaging; NA—not available; PA—pulmonary atresia; MAPCA—major aortopulmonary collateral arteries; Soc—standard of care; VR—virtual reality; VSD—ventricular septal defect.

6.2. Hands-on Surgical Training for Congenital Heart Surgery Procedures and Medical Education

Congenital heart surgery is a technically challenging field of in pediatrics because of the wide variation of CHD, the rarity of each pathology and the smaller size of the patients. These technical challenges place strong demands for the development of appropriate training programs for surgical trainees to acquire technical skills comparable to experienced surgeons. Three-dimensional-printed heart models with high fidelity for replicating complex anatomy serve as a valuable simulation-based training program for surgical trainees to develop their technical skills prior to performing operations on patients. The hands-on surgical training (HOST) course enables participants to perform surgical procedures on 3D-printed models [68–70,84]. In their recent review, Hussein et al. analyzed five studies, with three of these using 3D-printed models for the simulation of congenital heart surgery [68,84–86]. These studies supported the idea of using 3D-printed models to prepare surgeons for the simulation of various congenital heart surgery procedures with efficacy.

Table 4 is a summary of studies documenting single center experience of how 3D-printed heart models have been used as a HOST course for congenital heart surgery and medical education [68,85–90]. In addition to successfully simulating congenital heart surgery procedures and achieving high satisfaction scores from the participants who acquired the technical skills, 3D-printed models are also useful for simulating interventional cardiac procedures (Figures 11 and 12) [21,88]. The education of medical students and clinicians is another area that has proved the potential value of incorporating 3D-printed models into medical curricula and clinical practice, through HOST courses [84,88,89]. Hon et al. have reported the value of HOST courses for preparing preclinical medical students to work as surgical assistants, as well as consultant cardiac surgeons when performing congenital heart surgery simulations on 3D-printed models [89]. Their results show that early exposure and incorporation of HOST simulation into medical curricula could stimulate the interest of medical students in pursuing highly specialized fields such as congenital heart surgery (Figure 13). Similar findings have been reported by Olivieri et al., who recruited 70 participants for training sessions involving the performance of congenital heart simulation procedures [90]. Three-dimensional-printed models were assessed to be more useful than standard hands-off (8.4 out of 10) training instruments, and served as reliable simulation training tools for congenital cardiac intensive care clinics and enhanced interdisciplinary team communication.

Table 4. Clinical applications of 3D-printed models for HOST in congenital heart surgery procedures. Modified from Sun and Wee [37].

Author	Study Design	Sample Size and Participants	Original Data Source	Application in CHD	Image Processing Software	3D Printer	3D Printing Material	Key Findings
Yoo et al. [68]	Cross-sectional study	Fifty participants (surgeons and surgical trainees) participated in the survey.	CT and MRI	HOST using 3D-printed CHD models.	Mimics (Materalise, Belgium) Average cost per model: $60	Objet Connex 260 printer.	TangoPlus FullCure resin and VeroWhite	HOST serves as a valuable surgical simulation platform for practicing congenital heart surgery on 3D-printed models.
Hussein et al. [85]	Cross-sectional study	Seven trainees completed 12 sessions through HOST program for congenital heart surgery.	NA	Twelve 3D-printed heart models were incorporated into year long currciulum.	NA	Polyjet (Stratasys J750, Eden Prairie, MN, USA).	Agilus30	Ninety-one percent of procedural times were improved by a mean of 25% ($p < 0.001$). Eighty-four percent of trainees' mean time improved between the two attempts with an improvement of 23% ($p = 0.002$).
Scanlan et al. [86]	Cross-sectional study	Four physicians and four pediatric cardiac surgery fellows assessed suitability of 3D-printed models for simulation of tricuspid valve annuloplasty and atrioventricular canal repair procedures.	Echocardiograpy	Three valve models (MV, TV and CAV) were printed with different materials for simulation of congenital heart valve procedures.	3D Slicer Directly printed model: $7.90 Molded: $45	Object 500 Connex (Stratasys, Eden Prairie, MN, USA)	Valve models printed in TangoPlus FLX 930, while valve mold printed in VeroGray RDG850 or VeroBlue GDG840	Surgeon assessment showed that the molded valve models were more realistic for cutting and suturing than directly printed models ($p < 0.01$). Complete atrioventricular canal repair was highly rated by surgeons using the molded valves compared with the directly printed valves ($p < 0.01$).
Hoashi et al. [88]	Cross-sectional study	Twenty models of CHD were created for surgical simulation with all operations performed by a young consultant surgeon.	NA	Understanding the relationship between intraventricular communications and great vessels and utility of 3D models for simulations of intracardiac procedures.	NA $2000–3000 per model	Stereolithography (SOUP2, 600GS, Japan)	Super flexible polyurethan resins	The median cardiopulmonary bypass time and cross-clamp time was 345 (110–570) min and 114 (35–293) min, respectively. No mortality was observed during the median follow-up of 1.3 (0.1–2.5) years.
Brunner et al. [87]	Cross-sectional study	Nineteen medical students and doctors participated in the hands-on training program.	CT	Hands-on training on simulation of interventional cardiology procedures on common CHD models.	Mimics (Materalise, Belgium)	Agilista 3200W Polyjet 3D printer	Silicone rubber	Practicing on 3D-printed models significantly reduced the mean fluoroscopy time and increased confidence in interventions on real patients.

Table 4. *Cont.*

Author	Study Design	Sample Size and Participants	Original Data Source	Application in CHD	Image Processing Software	3D Printer	3D Printing Material	Key Findings
Hon et al. [89]	Cross-sectional study	Fifteen preclinical medical students participated in the HOST course.	NA	Medical students rehearsed their knot-typing and simple suturing skills on 3D printed models.	NA	NA	Agilus30 (Stratasys, Eden Prairie, MN, USA)	All students were highly satisfied with 3D-printed models helping their understanding of CHD (4.80 ± 0.41) and learning complex anatomy (4.87 ± 0.35), with training sessions improving their assisting skills (4.93 ± 0.26).
Olivieri et al. [90]	Cross-sectional study	Seventy participants enrolled in the study including 22 physicians, 38 critical care nurses and 10 ancillary providers.	CT or MRI	Ten CHD cases were selected for cardiac surgery simulation.	Mimics (Materalise, Belgium)	Objet500 Connext (Stratays, Eden, Prairie, MN, USA)	Rigid plastic materials.	Three-dimensional-printed models were scored more useful (8.4 out of 10) than standard hands-off with 90% of participants scoring 8 out of 10 or higher.

CHD—congenital heart disease; CT—computed tomography; CAV—common atrioventricular valve; DORV—double outlet right ventricle; HLHS—hypoplastic left heart syndrome; MRI—magnetic resonance imaging; MV—mitral valve; NA—not available; TV—tricuspid valve.

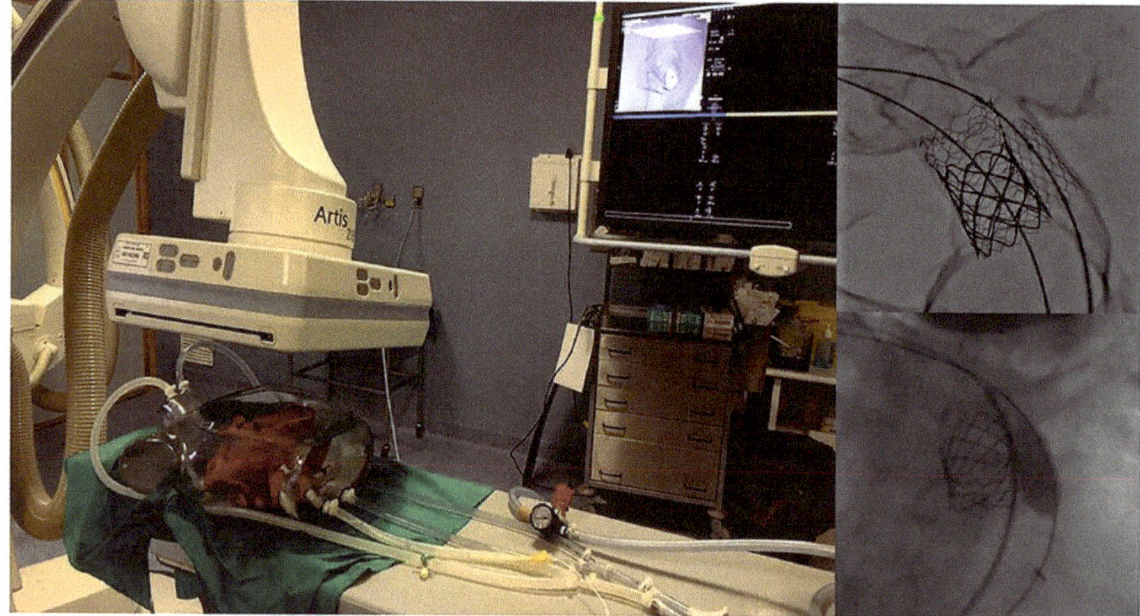

Figure 11. Catheterization applications. Left image shows the fluid inlets and outlets to superior and inferior vena cava and aortic arch/branches, respectively. Interventional planning with 3D-printed model (up right) and real intervention in the patient (down right). Reprinted with permission under the open access from Gomez-Ciriza et al. [21].

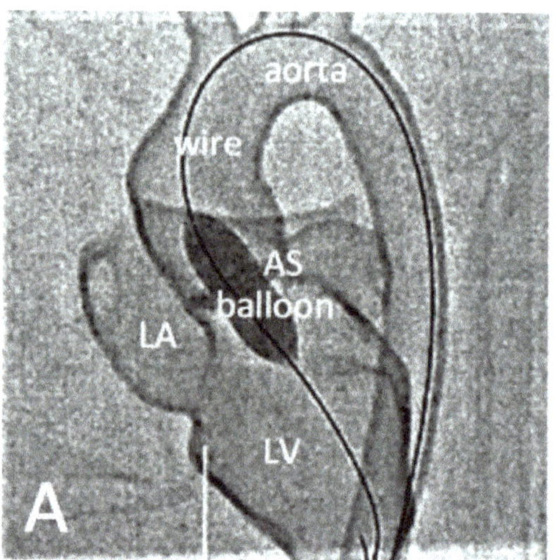

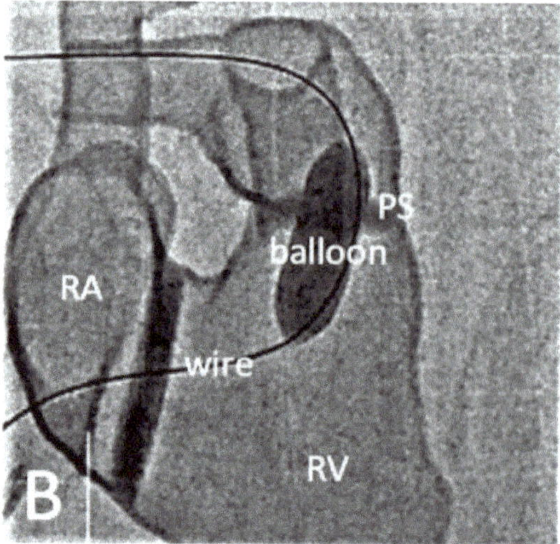

Figure 12. Fluoroscopic visualization of balloon dilatation of valvular stenosis with use of a 3D-printed heart model. (**A**) Balloon dilatation for treatment of a valvular aortic stenosis (AS). (**B**) Balloon dilatation for treatment of a valvular pulmonary stenosis (PS). Reprinted with permission under the open access from Brunner et al. [88].

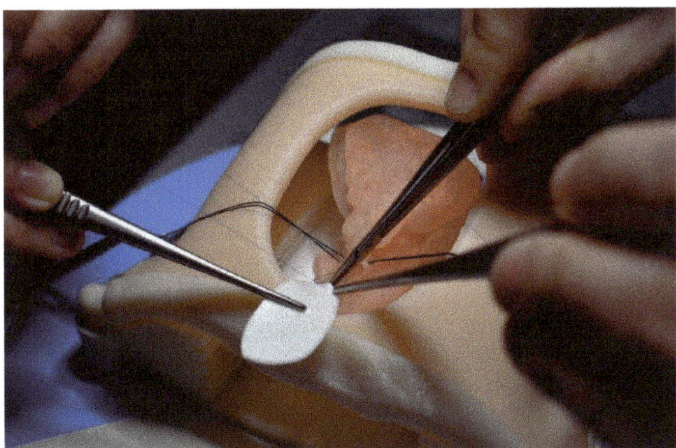

Figure 13. Example of simulation of Tetralogy of Fallot repair on a 3D-printed heart model. Reprinted with permission under the open access from Hon et al. [89].

6.3. Improving Physician–Patient Communication/Facilitating Communication with Colleagues

Physician–patient communication plays an important role in the clinical setting with patients' compliance and satisfaction with physicians having an impact on clinical outcomes [91]. Visual aids are commonly used in clinical practice for physicians to explain information to patients regarding the disease condition and treatment options [92]. However, conventional approaches of using 2D diagrams make it difficult for patients to imagine a 3D structure, and this is particularly challenging in CHD as patient and family tend to not possess adequate knowledge and understanding of complex heart anatomy or congenital defects. Three-dimensional-printed models have overcome this limitation by presenting a physically touchable model to the patient with improved understanding of both anatomy and pathology, thus enhancing communication between a physician and their patient and between a physician and their colleagues.

A number of studies have reported the value of using 3D-printed models in improving physician–patient communication. In their recent review, Traynor et al. analyzed 19 studies about the use of 3D printing technology in patient communication [93]. Of these studies, seven documented findings on cardiology and cardiovascular surgery [43,50,64,94–97], of which four studies were conducted by the same research group [94–97]. Results of these studies confirm that 3D-printed models helped communication with patients/parents and with colleagues (Figure 14), with a significant improvement in knowledge or understanding of the CHD condition, and overall satisfaction. This was confirmed by a recent study comparing 3D-printed heart models with MR in CHD [98]. The 3D-printed heart models were ranked as the best modality by 90% of participants (30 out of 34 physicians surveyed) and the most preferred communication tool with patients when compared with original DICOM and MR ($p < 0.01$).

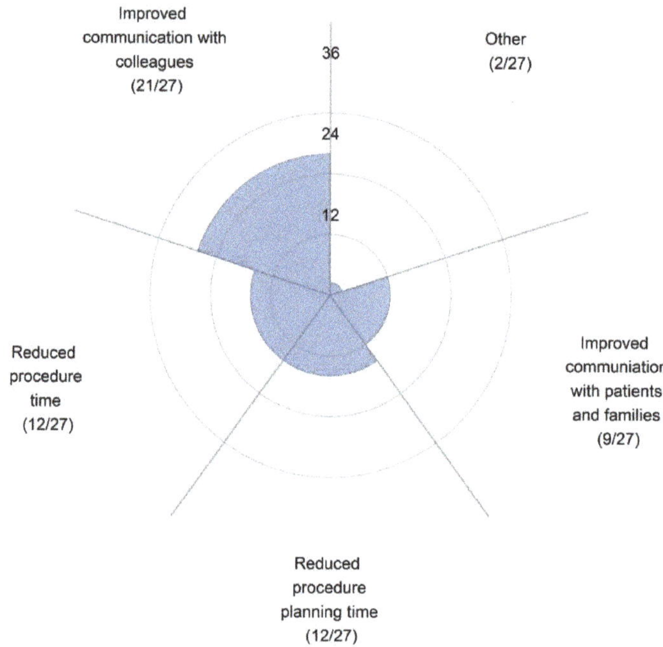

Figure 14. Survey responses show that 3D-printed models were most useful in improving communication with colleagues. Reprinted with permission under the open access from Illmann et al. [50].

Deng and colleagues conducted a RCT to study the clinical value of 3D-printed heart models in surgical consent for CHD repair [99]. Guardians of 40 patients with elective perimembranous ventricular septal defect (VSD) repair were invited to participate in the study with 20 allocated to the control and study groups, respectively. The control group received information about VSD condition and surgical indications as well as potential complications with the aid of the current approach using 2D charts, while the study group received the same information but using a 3D-printed model of the heart with VSD to assist explanation of these details. Results show significant improvements in their understanding of the VSD anatomy and the surgical procedures and potential complications ($p = 0.02$ for all of them) in the study group when compared with the control group, although there was no significant difference in overall ratings of the consent process ($p = 0.09$). This study represents the first RCT that quantifies the benefits of 3D-printed models in surgical consent, although further research with inclusion of other types of CHD conditions is needed.

7. Limitations, Challenges and Future Directions

In recent years, we have observed significant progress in the use of 3D printing technology in cardiovascular disease, with studies reporting its educational and clinical value in CHD (either educational approaches, or diagnostic methods based on 2D/3D image visualizations and standard training programs). The current evidence has proved that 3D-printed models are highly reliable and accurate in replicating cardiac anatomy and pathology (Table 1). Three-dimensional-printed models can be used as a beneficial tool in treating both adults and children with CHD [50,100]. However, the widespread application of 3D printing technology in pediatric cardiology practice is still hindered to a large extent by some limitations and barriers which need to be considered.

First, access to 3D printing facilities is limited, according to a recent international survey [50]. Illmann et al. surveyed 71 pediatric cardiologists from five continents seeking their opinions on the use of 3D-printed heart models in treating CHD patients and their access to 3D printing technology in their clinical practices. They noticed significant differences in access to 3D printing technology depending on the geographic location of the respondent, with pediatric cardiologists from the USA having more than five-times more access to 3D printing technology than their Canadian colleagues (p = 0.004). Financial barriers and preference for standard imaging modalities contribute as main reasons for limited access to 3D printing technology.

The cost of printing materials is another factor that limits its application in many practices. While low-cost 3D-printed models are acceptable for most of the educational and clinical applications [21,49], high-cost 3D-printed models are necessary for the HOST course because of the necessity to print heart models with very soft and flexible materials which enable the participants to develop tactile experience while simulating congenital heart surgery procedures. Agilus30 from Stratasys is currently the preferred material for 3D-printed heart models suitable for CHD surgery simulations (Table 4), but high cost is the main obstacle. Hussein et al. pointed out that 3D-printed model costs per trainee per year up can be as much as US$7500 when adopting the HOST program into congenital heart surgery curriculum [85]. Therefore, further cost reductions are necessary before the use of 3D-printed heart models as a training/simulation tool becomes a reality on a large scale in the near future.

Second, despite significant improvements in 3D printing technology over the last decades, the turnaround time could take several hours or even longer, including steps from initial image post-processing to printing and cleaning of the physical models. This could delay the patient treatment, especially when 3D-printed models are used for pre-surgical planning purposes. When 3D printing facilities are not accessible due to financial barriers, selection of VR or MR could be an alternative to 3D printing technology as these 3D innovative tools provide the same, or improved, advantages in terms of 3D visualization for the more efficient comprehension of CHD as opposed to 3D-printed models [30,61,98]. In their recent study, Lau et al. compared 3D-printed heart models with MR and original DICOM images in two selected pediatric CHD scenarios (ASD and VSD) with the clinical value of these modalities assessed by 34 cardiac specialists and physicians [98]. Their results show that MR was scored as the best modality in most of the clinical applications. This study further proves the potential value of using MR in pediatric cardiology practice when dealing with patients with CHD. Currently, it costs around AUD $600 and AUD $5500 to purchase an Oculus Quest 2 and Microsoft HoloLens for VR and MR demonstrations, respectively. Given the costs associated with 3D printers (including equipment setup, lab space to host the printers and technical support, etc.), printing materials and post-processing steps involved, VR and MR could be a cost-effective alternative to 3D printing technology in medical applications. Future studies are needed to compare the costs of VR/MR (multiple consoles are required for different users) and 3D-printed models (3D models can be handled by multiple students/users at the same time) in these applications.

Third, the majority of the current studies is based on case series or relatively small sample sizes (Tables 2–4), while robust studies such as RCT or multi-center studies are lacking. This could be due to several reasons, including the fact that 3D printing in pediatric cardiology is an emerging area with more evidence needed to prove its educational and clinical value in pediatric CHD before it is widely accepted. As highlighted previously, limited access to 3D printing facilities or financial barriers could explain the fact that most of the studies are case reports or case series. Further, follow-up studies are scarce, hence future studies need to focus on investigations of patient outcomes (mid- to long-term), on the way that 3D-printed models contribute to patient management and on whether it is a cost-effective approach when compared with the current or standard methods in pediatric cardiology practice.

Recent developments in 3D printing technology have made it possible to print biocompatible materials, cells and cardiovascular constructs into 3D tissues so that it now plays an important role in the treatment of pediatric congenital heart defects [101–104]. Three-dimensional bioprinting offers the potential to develop 3D cardiovascular tissue/organ structures with optimized microenvironments that include cellular morphologies and structures, with research evidence showing the capability of printing complex cardiovascular tissue constructs such as vascular grafts, myocardium and heart valves (Figure 15) [105–107]. With the use of 3D bioprinting technology, it is feasible to print a full-size model of the human heart [108,109]. Although these 3D-printed heart chambers had chamber-like contractile function and physiological features, they did not contain all of the main cardiac structures, such as endothelial cells and fibroblasts. Thus, it is still not clinically feasible to directly translate 3D-printed cardiovascular tissues to patient therapy. Further technological advancements in 3D bioprinting could overcome these limitations and challenges and there is no doubt that 3D bioprinting represents an exciting future in treating congenital heart disease and other anomalies.

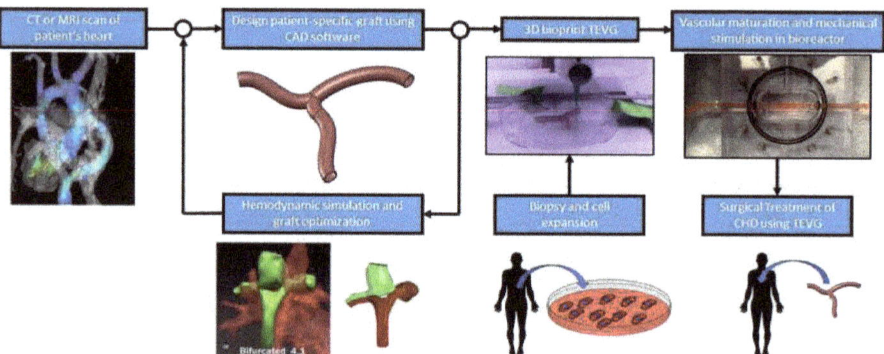

Figure 15. Proposed workflow of patient-specific TEVG fabrication. CAD-computer aided design, TEVG—tissue engineered vascular grafts. Reprinted with permission from Lee et al. [107].

In summary, 3D printing technology as an exciting and rapidly evolving field has revolutionized our current practice in the diagnosis and management of pediatric patients with CHD. Use of 3D-printed models has augmented the traditional visualization tools when diagnosing and assessing CHD conditions. Research from the current literature has shown that patient-specific 3D printed models serve as a valuable educational tool in learning anatomy and congenital heart defects. Three-dimensional-printed models are of great value in assisting surgical planning and simulation of congenital heart surgery procedures, thus greatly improving surgical care and patient management. Through the use of a hands-on surgical training program, 3D-printed personalized models significantly enhance surgical trainees' skills and confidence in performing complex cardiac operations. This has a significant clinical impact since successful simulation of congenital heart surgical procedures will result in high operation success rates with lower risks or complications when performing on patients, and thus improving patient outcomes. Three-dimensional-printed models can be used as a more effective tool than the images or diagrams that are currently used during physicians' communication with patients or with colleagues when dealing with pediatric CHD. To achieve the goal of implementing 3D printing technology into pediatric cardiology practice, a close collaboration between stakeholders and researchers is essential. This ensures that their knowledge and skills in the development of 3D-printed models are fully utilized and maximized to assist the delivery of personalized medicine, thus contributing to an optimized diagnostic strategy and clinical decision-making in pediatric patients with CHD.

Funding: This research received no external funding.

Institutional Review Board Statement: Not applicable.

Informed Consent Statement: Not applicable.

Data Availability Statement: Not applicable.

Conflicts of Interest: The author declares no conflict of interest.

References

1. Giannopoulos, A.A.; Steigner, M.L.; George, E.; Barile, M.; Hunsaker, A.R.; Rybicki, F.J.; Mitsouras, D. Cardiothoracic applications of 3-dimensional printing. *J. Thorac. Imaging.* **2016**, *31*, 253–272. [CrossRef]
2. Witowski, J.; Wake, N.; Grochowska, A.; Sun, Z.; Budzyński, A.; Major, P.; Popiela, T.J.; Pędziwiatr, M. Investigating accuracy of 3D printed liver models with computed tomography. *Quant. Imaging Med. Surg.* **2019**, *9*, 43–52. [CrossRef] [PubMed]
3. Witowski, J.S.; Pędziwiatr, M.; Major, P.; Budzyński, A. Cost-effective, personalized, 3D-printed liver model for preoper-ative planning before laparoscopic liver hemihepatectomy for colorectal cancer metastases. *Int. J. Comput. Assist. Radiol. Surg.* **2017**, *12*, 2047–2054. [CrossRef]
4. Costello, J.P.; Olivieri, L.; Krieger, A.; Thabit, O.; Marshall, M.B.; Yoo, S.-J.; Kim, P.C.; Jonas, R.A.; Nath, D.S. Utilizing Three-Dimensional Printing Technology to Assess the Feasibility of High-Fidelity Synthetic Ventricular Septal Defect Models for Simulation in Medical Education. *World J. Pediatr. Congenit. Heart Surg.* **2014**, *5*, 421–426. [CrossRef] [PubMed]
5. Costello, J.P.; Olivieri, L.J.; Su, L.; Krieger, A.; Alfares, F.; Thabit, O.; Marshall, M.B.; Yoo, S.-J.; Kim, P.C.; Jonas, R.A.; et al. Incorporating Three-dimensional Printing into a Simulation-based Congenital Heart Disease and Critical Care Training Curriculum for Resident Physicians. *Congenit. Heart Dis.* **2014**, *10*, 185–190. [CrossRef] [PubMed]
6. Javan, R.; Zeman, M.N. A Prototype Educational Model for Hepatobiliary Interventions: Unveiling the Role of Graphic Designers in Medical 3D Printing. *J. Digit. Imaging* **2017**, *31*, 133–143. [CrossRef] [PubMed]
7. Sun, Z.; Lau, I.; Wong, Y.H.; Yeong, C.H. Personalized Three-Dimensional Printed Models in Congenital Heart Disease. *J. Clin. Med.* **2019**, *8*, 522. [CrossRef] [PubMed]
8. Bagaria, V.; Bhansali, R.; Pawar, P. 3D printing-creating a blueprint for the future of orthopedics: Current concept review and the road ahead! *J. Clin. Ortho. Trauma.* **2018**, *9*, 207. [CrossRef]
9. Skelley, N.W.; Hagerty, M.P.; Stannard, J.T.; Feltz, K.P.; Ma, R. Sterility of 3D-Printed Orthopedic Implants Using Fused Deposition Modeling. *Orthopedics* **2020**, *43*, 46–51. [CrossRef]
10. Anwar, S.; Singh, G.K.; Miller, J.; Sharma, M.; Manning, P.; Billadello, J.J.; Eghtesady, P.; Woodard, P.K. 3D Printing is a Transformative Technology in Congenital Heart Disease. *JACC Basic Transl. Sci.* **2018**, *3*, 294–312. [CrossRef]
11. Gallo, M.; D'Onofrio, A.; Tarantini, G.; Nocerino, E.; Remondino, F.; Gerosa, G. 3D-printing model for complex aortic transcatheter valve treatment. *Int. J. Cardiol.* **2016**, *210*, 139–140. [CrossRef] [PubMed]
12. Ripley, B.; Kelil, T.; Cheezum, M.K.; Gonçalves, A.; Di Carli, M.F.; Rybicki, F.J.; Steigner, M.; Mitsouras, D.; Blankstein, R. 3D printing based on cardiac CT assists anatomic visualization prior to transcatheter aortic valve replacement. *J. Cardiovasc. Comput. Tomogr.* **2015**, *10*, 28–36. [CrossRef] [PubMed]
13. Lau, I.; Sun, Z. Three-dimensional printing in congenital heart disease: A systematic review. *J. Med. Radiat. Sci.* **2018**, *65*, 226–236. [CrossRef]
14. Bhatla, P.; Tretter, J.T.; Chikkabyrappa, S.; Chakravarti, S.; Mosca, R.S. Surgical planning for a complex double-outlet right ventricle using 3D printing. *Echocardiography* **2017**, *34*, 802–804. [CrossRef] [PubMed]
15. Biglino, G.; Milano, E.G.; Capelli, C.; Wray, J.; Shearn, A.I.; Caputo, M.; Bucciarelli-Ducci, C.; Taylor, A.M.; Schievano, S. Three-dimensional printing in congenital heart disease: Considerations on training and clinical implementation from a teaching session. *Int. J. Artif. Organs* **2019**, *42*, 595–599. [CrossRef]
16. Lau, I.W.W.; Sun, Z. Dimensional Accuracy and Clinical Value of 3D Printed Models in Congenital Heart Disease: A Systematic Review and Meta-Analysis. *J. Clin. Med.* **2019**, *8*, 1483. [CrossRef]
17. Anwar, S.; Rockefeller, T.; Raptis, D.A.; Woodard, P.K.; Eghtesady, P. 3D Printing Provides a Precise Approach in the Treatment of Tetralogy of Fallot, Pulmonary Atresia with Major Aortopulmonary Collateral Arteries. *Curr. Treat. Options Cardiovasc. Med.* **2018**, *20*, 5. [CrossRef]
18. Gosnell, J.; Pietila, T.; Samuel, B.P.; Kurup, H.K.N.; Haw, M.P.; Vettukattil, J.J. Integration of Computed Tomography and Three-Dimensional Echocardiography for Hybrid Three-Dimensional Printing in Congenital Heart Disease. *J. Digit. Imaging* **2016**, *29*, 665–669. [CrossRef]
19. Loke, Y.-H.; Harahsheh, A.S.; Krieger, A.; Olivieri, L.J. Usage of 3D models of tetralogy of Fallot for medical education: Impact on learning congenital heart disease. *BMC Med. Educ.* **2017**, *17*, 54–61. [CrossRef]
20. Sun, Z. Clinical Applications of Patient-Specific 3D Printed Models in Cardiovascular Disease: Current Status and Future Directions. *Biomolecules* **2020**, *10*, 1577. [CrossRef]
21. Gómez-Ciriza, G.; Gómez-Cía, T.; Rivas-González, J.A.; Forte, M.N.V.; Valverde, I. Affordable Three-Dimensional Printed Heart Models. *Front. Cardiovasc. Med.* **2021**, *8*, 642011. [CrossRef] [PubMed]
22. Moore, R.A.; Riggs, K.W.; Kourtidou, S.; Schneider, K.; Szugye, N.; Troja, W.; D'Souza, G.; Rattan, M.; Bryant, R., 3rd; Taylor, M.D.; et al. Three-dimensional printing and virtual surgery for congenital heart procedural planning. Birth. *Defects. Res.* **2018**, *110*, 1082–1090. [CrossRef] [PubMed]

23. Kiraly, L.; Shah, N.C.; Abdullah, O.; Al-Ketan, O.; Rowshan, R. Three-Dimensional Virtual and Printed Prototypes in Complex Congenital and Pediatric Cardiac Surgery—A Multidisciplinary Team-Learning Experience. *Biomolecules* **2021**, *11*, 1703. [CrossRef] [PubMed]

24. Garas, M.; Vacccarezza, M.; Newland, G.; McVay-Doonbusch, K.; Hasani, J. 3D-printed speciamens as a valuable tool in anatomy education: A pilot study. *Ann. Anat.* **2018**, *219*, 57–64. [CrossRef]

25. Lau, I.; Sun, Z. The role of 3D printed heart models in immediate and long-term knowledge retention in medical education. *Rev. Cardiovasc. Med.* **2022**, *23*, 022. [CrossRef] [PubMed]

26. Karsenty, C.; Guitarte, A.; Dulac, Y.; Briot, J.; Hascoet, S.; Vincent, R.; Delepaul, B.; Vignaud, P.; Djeddai, C.; Hadeed, K.; et al. The usefulness of 3D printed heart models for medical student education in congenital heart disease. *BMC. Med. Edc.* **2021**, *21*, 480. [CrossRef] [PubMed]

27. Lim, K.H.A.; Loo, Z.Y.; Goldie, S.J.; Adams, J.W.; McMenamin, P.G. Use of 3D printed models in medical education: A randomized control trial comparing 3D prints versus cadaveric materials for learning external cardiac anatomy. *Anat. Sci. Educ.* **2015**, *9*, 213–221. [CrossRef] [PubMed]

28. Smerling, J.; Marboe, C.C.; Lefkowitch, J.H.; Pavlicova, M.; Bacha, E.; Einstein, A.J.; Naka, Y.; Glickstein, J.; Farooqi, K.M. Utility of 3D Printed Cardiac Models for Medical Student Education in Congenital Heart Disease: Across a Spectrum of Disease Severity. *Pediatr. Cardiol.* **2019**, *40*, 1258–1265. [CrossRef] [PubMed]

29. Su, W.; Xiao, Y.; He, S.; Huang, P.; Deng, X. Three-dimensional printing models in congenital heart disease education for medical students: A controlled comparative study. *BMC Med. Educ.* **2018**, *18*, 178. [CrossRef]

30. Lau, I.; Gupta, A.; Sun, Z. Clinical Value of Virtual Reality versus 3D Printing in Congenital Heart Disease. *Biomolecules* **2021**, *11*, 884. [CrossRef] [PubMed]

31. Jones, T.W.; Secker, M.D. Use of 3D models of vascular rings and slings to improve resident education. *Congenit. Heart. Dis.* **2017**, *12*, 578–582. [CrossRef] [PubMed]

32. Krishnasamy, S.; Mokhtar, R.A.R.; Singh, R.; Sivallingam, S.; Abdul Aziz, Y.F.; Mathaneswaran, V. 3D rapid prototyping heart model validation for teaching and learning-A pilot project in a teaching institution. *Braz. J. Cardiothorac. Surg.* **2021**, *36*, 707–716.

33. Valverde, I.; Gomez, G.; Byrne, N.; Anwar, S.; Cerpa, S.M.A.; Talavera, M.M.; Pushparajah, K.; Forte, V.M.N. Criss-cross heart three-dimensional printed models in medical education: A multicentre study on their value as a supporting tool to conventional imaging. *Anat. Sci. Educ.* **2022**, *15*, 719–730. [CrossRef] [PubMed]

34. White, S.C.; Sedler, J.; Jones, T.W.; Seckeler, M. Utility of three-dimensional models in resident education on simple and complex intracardiac congenital heart defects. *Congenit. Heart Dis.* **2018**, *13*, 1045–1049. [CrossRef] [PubMed]

35. Tan, H.; Huang, E.; Deng, X.; Ouyang, S. Application of 3D printing technology combined with PBL teaching model in teaching clinical nursing in congenital heart surgery: A case-control study. *Medicine* **2021**, *100*, 20. [CrossRef] [PubMed]

36. Cantinotti, M.; Valverde, I.; Kutty, S. Three-dimensional printed models in congenital heart disease. *Int. J. Cardiovasc. Imaging* **2017**, *33*, 137–144. [CrossRef]

37. Sun, Z.; Wee, C. 3D Printed Models in Cardiovascular Disease: An Exciting Future to Deliver Personalized Medicine. *Micromachines* **2022**, *13*, 1575. [CrossRef]

38. Liang, J.; Zhao, X.; Pan, G.; Zhang, G.; Zhao, D.; Xu, J.; Li, D.; Lu, B. Comparison of blood pool and myocardial 3D printing in the diagnosis of types of congenital heart disease. *Sci. Rep.* **2022**, *12*, 7136. [CrossRef]

39. Lee, S.; Squelch, A.; Sun, Z. Quantitative Assessment of 3D Printed Model Accuracy in Delineating Congenital Heart Disease. *Biomolecules* **2021**, *11*, 270. [CrossRef]

40. Valverde, I.; Gomez-Ciriza, G.; Hussain, T.; Suarez-Mejias, C.; Velasco-Forte, M.N.; Byrne, N.; Ordoñez, A.; Gonzalez-Calle, A.; Anderson, D.; Hazekamp, M.G.; et al. Three-dimensional printed models for surgical planning of complex congenital heart defects: An international multicentre study. *Eur. J. Cardio-Thoracic Surg.* **2017**, *52*, 1139–1148. [CrossRef]

41. Olejník, P.; Nosal, M.; Havran, T.; Furdova, A.; Cizmar, M.; Slabej, M.; Thurzo, A.; Vitovic, P.; Klvac, M.; Acel, T. Utilisation of three-dimensional printed heart models for operative planning of complex congenital heart defects. *Kardiol. Pol.* **2017**, *75*, 495–501. [CrossRef]

42. Olivieri, L.J.; Krieger, A.; Loke, Y.-H.; Nath, D.S.; Kim, P.C.; Sable, C.A. Three-Dimensional Printing of Intracardiac Defects from Three-Dimensional Echocardiographic Images: Feasibility and Relative Accuracy. *J. Am. Soc. Echocardiogr.* **2015**, *28*, 392–397. [CrossRef]

43. Lau, I.W.W.; Liu, D.; Xu, L.; Fan, Z.; Sun, Z. Clinical value of patient-specific three-dimensional printing of congenital heart disease: Quantitative and qualitative assessments. *PLoS ONE* **2018**, *13*, e0194333. [CrossRef]

44. Mowers, K.L.; Fullerton, J.B.; Hicks, D.; Singh, G.K.; Johnson, M.C.; Anwar, S. 3D echocardiography provides highly accurate 3D printed models in congenital heart disease. *Pediatr. Cardiol.* **2021**, *42*, 131–141. [CrossRef] [PubMed]

45. Parimi, M.; Buelter, J.; Thanugundla, V.; Condoor, S.; Parkar, N.; Danon, S.; King, W. Feasibility and Validity of Printing 3D Heart Models from Rotational Angiography. *Pediatr. Cardiol.* **2018**, *39*, 653–658. [CrossRef]

46. Wu, C.A.; Squelch, A.; Jansen, S.; Sun, Z. Optimization of computed tomography angiography protocols for follow-up type B aortic dissection patients by using 3D printed model. *Appl. Sci.* **2021**, *11*, 6844. [CrossRef]

47. Valverde, I.; Gomez, G.; Gonzalez, A.; Suárez-Mejías, C.; Adsuar, A.; Coserria, J.F.; Uribe, S.; Gomez-Cia, T.; Hosseinpour, A.R. Three-dimensional patient-specific cardiac model for surgical planning in Nikaidoh procedure. *Cardiol. Young* **2014**, *25*, 698–704. [CrossRef] [PubMed]

48. Garekar, S.; Bharati, A.; Chokhandre, M.; Mali, S.; Trivedi, B.; Changela, V.P.; Solanki, N.; Gaikwad, S.; Agarwal, V. Clinical Application and Multidisciplinary Assessment of Three Dimensional Printing in Double Outlet Right Ventricle with Remote Ventricular Septal Defect. *World J. Pediatr. Congenit. Heart Surg.* **2016**, *7*, 344–350. [CrossRef]

49. Lau, I.; Wong, Y.H.; Yeong, C.H.; Aziz, Y.F.A.; Sari, N.A.; Hashim, S.A.; Sun, Z. Quantitative and qualitative comparison of low- and high-cost 3D-printed heart models. *Quant. Imaging Med. Surg.* **2019**, *9*, 107–114. [CrossRef]

50. Illmann, C.F.; Hosking, M.; Harris, K.C. Utility and Access to 3-Dimensional Printing in the Context of Congenital Heart Disease: An International Physician Survey Study. *CJC Open* **2020**, *2*, 207–213. [CrossRef] [PubMed]

51. Meyer-Szary, J.; Luis, M.S.; Mikulski, S.; Patel, A.; Schulz, F.; Tretiakow, D.; Fercho, J.; Jaguszewska, K.; Frankiewicz, M.; Pawłowska, E.; et al. The Role of 3D Printing in Planning Complex Medical Procedures and Training of Medical Professionals—Cross-Sectional Multispecialty Review. *Int. J. Environ. Res. Public Health* **2022**, *19*, 3331. [CrossRef] [PubMed]

52. Yamasaki, T.; Toba, S.; Sanders, S.P.; Carreon, C.K. Perfusion-distension fixation of heart specimens: A key step in immortalizing heart specimens for wax infiltration and generating 3D imaging data sets for reconstruction and printed 3D models. *Cardiovasc. Pathol.* **2022**, *58*, 107404. [CrossRef] [PubMed]

53. Talanki, V.R.; Peng, Q.; Shamir, S.B.; Baete, S.H.; Duong, T.Q.; Wake, N. Three-dimensional printed anatomic models derived from magnetic resonance imaging data: Current state and image acquisition recommendations for appropriate clinical scenarios. *J. Magn. Reson. Imaging.* **2022**, *55*, 060–1081. [CrossRef] [PubMed]

54. Biglino, G.; Capelli, C.; Koniordou, D.; Robertshaw, D.; Leaver, L.-K.; Schievano, S.; Taylor, A.M.; Wray, J. Use of 3D models of congenital heart disease as an education tool for cardiac nurses. *Congenit. Heart Dis.* **2016**, *12*, 113–118. [CrossRef]

55. Lee, C.; Lee, J.Y. Utility of three-dimensional printed heart models for education on complex congenital heart diseases. *Cardiol. Young* **2020**, *30*, 1637–1642. [CrossRef]

56. Sutherland, J.; Belec, J.; Sheikh, A.; Chepelev, L.; Althobaity, W.; Chow, B.J.W.; Mitsouras, D.; Christensen, A.; Rybicki, F.J.; La Russa, D.J. Applying Modern Virtual and Augmented Reality Technologies to Medical Images and Models. *J. Digit. Imaging* **2019**, *32*, 38–53. [CrossRef]

57. Dhar, P.; Rocks, T.; Samarasinghe, R.M.; Stephenson, G.; Smith, C. Augmented reality in medical education: Students' experience and learning outcomes. *Med. Educ. Online* **2021**, *26*, 1953953. [CrossRef] [PubMed]

58. Patel, N.; Costa, A.; Sanders, S.P.; Ezon, D. Stereoscopic virtual reality does not improve knowledge retention of congenital heart disease. *Int. J. Cardiovasc. Imaging* **2021**, *37*, 2283–2290. [CrossRef]

59. Maresky, H.S.; Oikonomou, A.; Ali, I.; Ditkofsky, N.; Pakkal, M.; Ballyk, B. Virtual reality and cardiac anatomy: Exploring immersive three-dimensional cardiac imaging, a pilot study in undergraduate medical anatomy education. *Clin. Anat.* **2019**, *32*, 238–243. [CrossRef]

60. Goo, H.W.; Park, S.J.; Yoo, S.J. Advanced medical use of three-dimensional imaging in congenital heart disease: Augmented reality, mixed reality, virtual reality and three-dimensional printing. *Korean. J. Radiol.* **2020**, *21*, 133–145. [CrossRef]

61. Barteit, S.; Lanfermann, L.; Barnighausen, T.; Neuhann, F.; Beiersmann, C. Aug-mentted reality, mixed and virtual reality-based head-mounted devices for medical education: Systematic review. *JMIR. Serious Games* **2021**, *9*, e29080. [CrossRef]

62. Raimondi, F.; Vida, V.; Godard, C.; Bertelli, F.; Reffo, E.; Boddaert, N.; El Beheiry, M.; Masson, J.B. Fast-track virtual reality for cardiac imaging in congenital heart disease. *J. Card. Surg.* **2021**, *36*, 2598–2602. [CrossRef]

63. Cen, J.; Liufu, R.; Wen, S.; Qiu, H.; Liu, X.; Chen, X.; Yuan, H.; Huang, M.; Zhuang, J. Three-Dimensional Printing, Virtual Reality and Mixed Reality for Pulmonary Atresia: Early Surgical Outcomes Evaluation. *Heart Lung Circ.* **2020**, *30*, 296–302. [CrossRef] [PubMed]

64. Guo, H.; Wang, Y.; Dai, J.; Ren, C.; Li, J.; Lai, Y. Application of 3D printing in the surgical planning of hypertrophic obstructive cardiomyopathy and physician-patient communication: A preliminary study. *J. Thorac. Dis.* **2018**, *10*, 867–873. [CrossRef] [PubMed]

65. Ryan, J.; Plasencia, J.; Richardson, R.; Velez, D.; Nigro, J.J.; Pophal, S.; Frakes, D. 3D printing for congenital heart disease: A single site's initial three-year experience. *3D. Print. Med.* **2018**, *4*, 10. [CrossRef]

66. Zhao, L.; Zhou, S.; Fan, T.; Li, B.; Liang, W.; Dong, H. Three-dimensional printing enhances preparation for repair of double outlet right ventricular surgery. *J. Card. Surg.* **2018**, *33*, 24–27. [CrossRef]

67. Ghosh, R.M.; Jolley, M.A.; Mascio, C.E.; Chen, J.M.; Fuller, S.; Rome, J.J.; Silvestro, E.; Whitehead, K.K. Clinical 3D modeling to guide pediatric cardiothoracic sur-gery and intervention using 3D printed anatomic models, computer aided design and virtual reality. *3D. Pring. Med.* **2022**, *8*, 11. [CrossRef]

68. Yoo, S.J.; Spray, T.; Austin, E.H.; Yun, T.J.; van Arsdell, G.S. Hands-on surgical training of congenital heart surgery suing 3-dimensional print models. *J. Thorac. Cardiovasc. Surg.* **2017**, *153*, 15301–15540. [CrossRef] [PubMed]

69. Hussein, N.; Honjo, O.; Haller, C.; Coles, J.G.; Hua, Z.; Van Arsdell, G.; Yoo, S.-J. Quantitative assessment of technical performance during hands-on surgical training of the arterial switch operation using 3-dimensional printed heart models. *J. Thorac. Cardiovasc. Surg.* **2020**, *160*, 1035–1042. [CrossRef]

70. Hussein, N.; Lim, A.; Honji, O.; Haller, C.; Coles, J.G.; Van Arsdell, G.; Yoo, S.J. Development and validation of a procedure-specific assessment tool for hands-on surgical training in congenital heart surgery. *J. Thorac. Cardiovasc. Surg.* **2020**, *160*, 229–240. [CrossRef]

71. Averkin, I.I.; Grehov, E.V.; Pervunina, T.M.; Komlichenko, E.V.; Vasichkina, E.S.; Zaverza, V.M.; Nikiforov, V.G.; Latipova, M.L.; Govorov, I.E.; Kozyrev, I.A.; et al. 3D-printing in preoperative planning in neonates with complex congenital heart defects. *J. Matern. Fetal. Neonatal Med.* **2022**, *35*, 2020–2024. [CrossRef] [PubMed]

72. Betancourt, L.G.; Wong, S.H.; Singh, H.R.; Nento, D.; Agarwal, A. Utility of three-dimensional printed model in biventricular repair of complex congenital cardiac defects: Case report and review of literature. *Children* **2022**, *9*, 184. [CrossRef] [PubMed]

73. Brüning, J.; Kramer, P.; Goubergrits, L.; Schulz, A.; Murin, P.; Solowjowa, N.; Kuehne, T.; Berger, F.; Photiadis, J.; Weixler, V.H.-M. 3D modeling and printing for complex biventricular repair of double outlet right ventricle. *Front. Cardiovasc. Med.* **2022**, *9*, 1024053. [CrossRef]

74. Liang, J.; Lu, B.; Zhao, X.; Wang, J.; Zhao, D.; Zhang, G.; Zhu, B.; Ma, Q.; Pan, G.; Li, D. Feasibility analyses of virtual models and 3D printing for surgical simulation of the double-outlet right ventricle. *Med. Biol. Eng. Comput.* **2022**, *60*, 3029–3040. [CrossRef]

75. Spanaki, A.; Kabir, S.; Stephenson, N.; van Poppel, M.P.M.; Benetti, V.; Simpson, J. 3D Approaches in Complex CHD: Where Are We? Funny Printing and Beautiful Images, or a Useful Tool? *J. Cardiovasc. Dev. Dis.* **2022**, *9*, 269. [CrossRef]

76. Yoo, S.-J.; Hussein, N.; Barron, D.J. Congenital Heart Surgery Skill Training Using Simulation Models: Not an Option but a Necessity. *J. Korean Med. Sci.* **2022**, *37*, e293. [CrossRef] [PubMed]

77. Bernhard, B.; Illi, J.; Gloeckler, M.; Pilgrim, T.; Praz, F.; Windecker, S.; Haeberlin, A.; Gräni, C. Imaging-based, patient-specific three-dimensional printing to plan, train, and guide cardiovascular interventions: A systematic review and meta-analysis. *Heart. Lung. Circ.* **2022**, *31*, 1203–1218. [CrossRef] [PubMed]

78. Mattus, M.S.; Ralph, T.B.; Keller, S.M.P.; Waltz, A.L.; Bramlet, M.T. Creation of patient-specific silicone cardiac models with ap-plications in presurgical plans and hands-on training. *J. Vis. Exp.* **2022**, *10*, 180.

79. Peel, B.; Lee, W.; Hussein, N.; Yoo, S.-J. State-of-the-art silicone molded models for simulation of arterial switch operation: Innovation with parting-and-assembly strategy. *JTCVS Tech.* **2022**, *12*, 132–142. [CrossRef]

80. Qiu, H.; Wen, S.; Ji, E.; Chen, T.; Liu, X.; Li, X.; Teng, Y.; Zhang, Y.; Liufu, R.; Zhang, J.; et al. A novel 3D visualized operative procedure in the single-stage complete repair with unifocalization of pulmonary aresia with ventricular septal defect and major aortopulmonary collateral arteries. *Front. Cardiovasc. Med.* **2022**, *9*, 836200. [CrossRef]

81. Magagna, P.; Caprioglio, F.; Gallo, M.; Salvador, L. 3D printing to manage postinfarct ventricular septal defect. *J. Card. Surg.* **2021**, *37*, 449–450. [CrossRef] [PubMed]

82. Wei, L.; Sun, G.; Wu, Q.; Zhang, W.; Tang, M.; Zhao, T.; Hu, S. Case Report: Three-Dimensional Printing–Assisted Surgical Treatment of Complex Body Vein Ectopic Drainage. *Front. Cardiovasc. Med.* **2022**, *9*, 782601. [CrossRef]

83. Longinotti, L.; Castaldi, B.; Bertelli, F.; Vida, V.L.; Padalino, M.A. Three-dimensional Printing for Hybrid Closure of Complex Muscular Ventricular Septal Defects. *Ann. Thorac. Surg.* **2021**, *113*, e129–e132. [CrossRef]

84. Hussein, N.; Honjo, O.; Haller, C.; Hickey, E.; Coles, J.G.; Williams, W.G.; Yoo, S.-J. Hands-On Surgical Simulation in Congenital Heart Surgery: Literature Review and Future Perspective. *Semin. Thorac. Cardiovasc. Surg.* **2020**, *32*, 98–105. [CrossRef]

85. Hussein, N.; Honjo, O.; Barron, D.J.; Haller, C.; Coles, J.G.; Yoo, S.-J. The Incorporation of Hands-On Surgical Training in a Congenital Heart Surgery Training Curriculum. *Ann. Thorac. Surg.* **2020**, *112*, 1672–1680. [CrossRef]

86. Scanlan, A.B.; Nguyen, A.V.; Ilina, A.; Lasso, A.; Cripe, L.; Jegatheeswaran, A.; Sil-vestro, E.; McGowan, F.X.; Mascio, C.E.; Fuller, S.; et al. Comparison of 3D echocardiography-derived 3D printed valve models to molded models for simulated repair of pediatric atrioventricular valve. *Pediatr. Cardiol.* **2018**, *39*, 538–547. [CrossRef]

87. Brunner, B.S.; Thierij, A.; Jakob, A.; Tengler, A.; Grab, M.; Thierfelder, N.; Leuner, C.J.; Haas, N.A.; Hopfner, C. 3D-printed heart models for hands-on training in pediatric cardiology-the future of modern learning and teaching? *GMS. J. Med. Educ.* **2022**, *39*, Doc23.

88. Hoashi, T.; Ichikawa, H.; Nakata, T.; Shimada, M.; Ozawa, H.; Higashida, A.; Kurosaki, K.; Kanzaki, S.; Shiraishi, I. Utility of a super-flexible three-dimensional printed heart model in congenital heart surgery†. *Interact. Cardiovasc. Thorac. Surg.* **2018**, *27*, 749–755. [CrossRef] [PubMed]

89. Hon, N.W.L.; Hussein, N.; Honjo, O.; Yoo, S.-J. Evaluating the Impact of Medical Student Inclusion Into Hands-On Surgical Simulation in Congenital Heart Surgery. *J. Surg. Educ.* **2020**, *78*, 207–213. [CrossRef]

90. Olivieri, L.J.; Su, L.; Hynes, C.F.; Krieger, A.; Alfares, F.A.; Ramakrishnan, K.; Zurakowski, D.; Marshall, M.B.; Kim, P.C.W.; Jonas, R.A.; et al. "Just-In-Time" Simulation Training Using 3-D Printed Cardiac Models After Congenital Cardiac Surgery. *World J. Pediatr. Congenit. Heart Surg.* **2016**, *7*, 164–168. [CrossRef] [PubMed]

91. Stewart, M.A. Effective physician-patient communication and health outcomes: A review. *Can. Med. Assoc. J.* **1995**, *152*, 1423–1433.

92. Pratt, M.; Searles, G.E. Using Visual Aids to Enhance Physician-Patient Discussions and Increase Health Literacy. *J. Cutan. Med. Surg.* **2017**, *21*, 497–501. [CrossRef] [PubMed]

93. Traynor, G.; Shearn, A.I.U.; Milano, E.G.; Ordonez, M.V.; Forte, M.N.V.; Caputo, M.; Schievano, S.; Mustard, H.; Wray, J.; Biglino, G. The use of 3D-printed models in patient communication: A scoping review. *J. 3D Print. Med.* **2022**, *6*, 13–23. [CrossRef]

94. Biglino, G.; Koniordou, D.; Gasparini, M.; Capelli, C.; Leaver, L.K.; Khambadkone, S.; Schievano, S.; Taylor, A.M.; Wray, J. Piloting the use of patient-specific cardiac models as a novel tool to facilitate communication during clinical consultations. *Pediatr. Cardiol.* **2017**, *38*, 813–818. [CrossRef] [PubMed]

95. Biglino, G.; Capelli, C.; Wray, J.; Schievano, S.; Leaver, L.-K.; Khambadkone, S.; Giardini, A.; Derrick, G.; Jones, A.; Taylor, A.M. 3D-manufactured patient-specific models of congenital heart defects for communication in clinical practice: Feasibility and acceptability. *BMJ Open* **2015**, *5*, e007165. [CrossRef] [PubMed]

96. Biglino, G.; Moharem-Elgamal, S.; Lee, M.; Tulloh, R.; Caputo, M. The Perception of a Three-Dimensional-Printed Heart Model from the Perspective of Different Stakeholders: A Complex Case of Truncus Arteriosus. *Front. Pediatr.* **2017**, *5*, 209. [CrossRef]

97. Biglino, G.; Capelli, C.; Leaver, L.K.; Schievano, S.; Taylor, A.M.; Wray, J. Involving patient, family and medical staff in the evaluation of 3D printing models of congenital heart disease. *Common. Med.* **2015**, *12*, 157–169. [CrossRef] [PubMed]

98. Lau, I.; Gupta, A.; Ihdayhid, A.; Sun, Z. Clinical Applications of Mixed Reality and 3D Printing in Congenital Heart Disease. *Biomolecules* **2022**, *12*, 1548. [CrossRef] [PubMed]

99. Deng, X.; He, S.; Huang, P.; Luo, J.; Yang, G.; Zhou, B.; Xiao, Y. A three-dimensional printed model in preoperative consent for ventricular septa defect repair. *J. Cardiothorac. Surg.* **2021**, *16*, 229. [CrossRef] [PubMed]

100. Chessa, M.; Van De Bruaene, A.; Farooqi, K.; Valverde, I.; Jung, C.; Votta, E.; Sturla, F.; Paul Diller, G.; Brida, M.; Sun, Z.; et al. Three-dimensional printing, holograms, computational modelling, and artificial intelligence for adult congenital heart disease care: An exciting future. *Eur. Heart. J.* **2022**, *43*, 2672–2684.

101. Alonzo, M.; AnilKumar, S.; Roman, B.; Tasnim, N.; Joddar, B. 3D Bioprinting of cardiac tissue and cardiac stem cell therapy. *Transl. Res.* **2019**, *211*, 64–83. [CrossRef]

102. Zhang, J.; Wehrle, E.; Rubert, M.; Muller, R. 3D bioprinting of human tissues: Biofabrication, bioinks and bioreactors. *Int. J. Mol. Sci.* **2021**, *22*, 3971. [CrossRef]

103. Wang, Z.; Lee, S.J.; Cheng, H.-J.; Yoo, J.J.; Atala, A. 3D bioprinted functional and contractile cardiac tissue constructs. *Acta Biomater.* **2018**, *70*, 48–56. [CrossRef] [PubMed]

104. Kato, B.; Wisser, G.; Agrawal, D.K.; Wood, T.; Thankam, F.G. 3D bioprinting of cardiac tissue: Current challenges and perspectives. *J. Mater. Sci. Mater. Med.* **2021**, *32*, 54. [CrossRef] [PubMed]

105. Jiang, S.; Feng, W.; Chang, C.; Li, G. Modeling human heart development and congenital defects using organoids: How close are we? *J. Cardiovasc. Dev. Dis.* **2022**, *9*, 125. [CrossRef] [PubMed]

106. Lee, A.; Hudson, A.R.; Shiwarski, D.J.; Tashman, J.W.; Hinton, T.J.; Yerneni, S.; Bliley, J.M.; Campbell, P.G.; Feinberg, A.W. 3D bioprinting of collagen to rebuild components of the human heart. *Science* **2019**, *365*, 482–487. [CrossRef] [PubMed]

107. Lee, W.; Hong, Y.; Dai, G. 3D bioprinting of vascular conduits for pediatric congenital heart repairs. *Transl. Res.* **2019**, *211*, 35–45. [CrossRef]

108. Bliley, J.; Tashman, J.; Stang, M.; Coffin, B.; Shiwarski, D.; Lee, A.; Hinton, T.; Feinberg, A. FRESH 3D bioprinting a con-tractile heart tube using human stem cell-derived cardiomyocytes. *Biofabrication* **2022**, *14*, 024106. [CrossRef]

109. Mirdamadi, E.; Tashman, J.W.; Shiwarski, D.J.; Palchesko, R.N.; Feinberg, A.W. FRESH 3D Bioprinting a Full-Size Model of the Human Heart. *ACS Biomater. Sci. Eng.* **2020**, *6*, 6453–6459. [CrossRef]

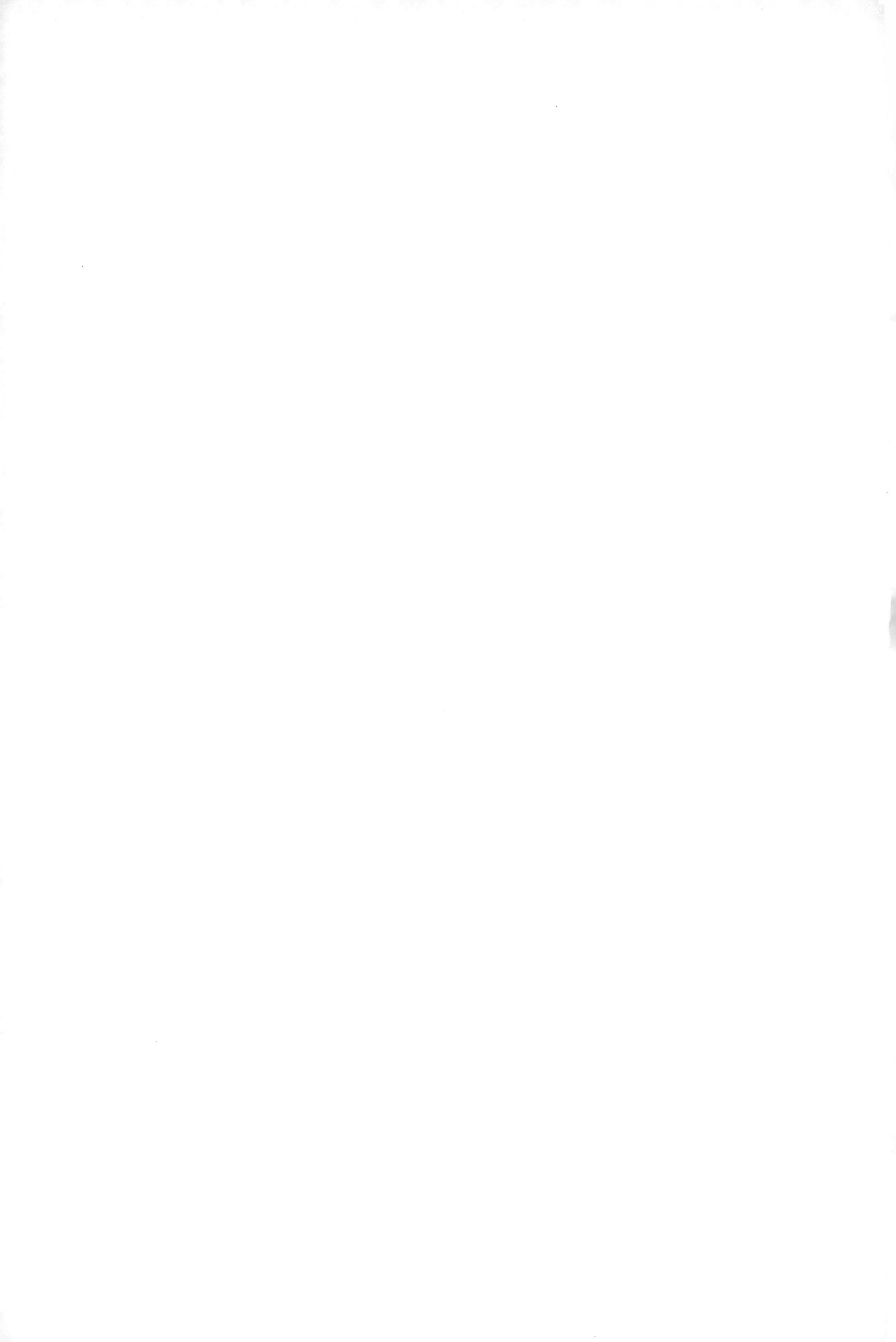

MDPI

St. Alban-Anlage 66

4052 Basel

Switzerland

Tel. +41 61 683 77 34

Fax +41 61 302 89 18

www.mdpi.com

Children Editorial Office

E-mail: children@mdpi.com

www.mdpi.com/journal/children

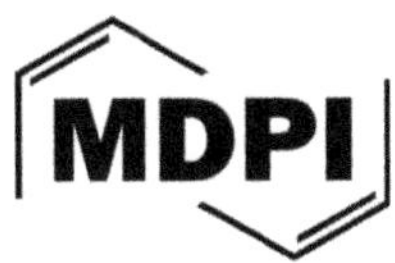